124770

Health Promotion
Management and Self-Care

D1408801

MP

Morton Publishing Company
295 West Hampden, Suite 104
Englewood, Colorado 80110

© 1982 by Morton Publishing Company

Printed in the United States of America

ISBN: 0-89582-069-2

Acknowledgments

This text was written with the cooperation of members of the Department of Health Sciences, Brigham Young University, Provo, Utah. The Publisher wishes to express appreciation to the following individuals for their contributions: Molly Brog, M.S., Robert Burgener, Ph.D., Maxilyn Capell, M.A., Paul Coon, M.S., Kathryn Frandsen, Brent Q. Hafen, Ph.D. (editor), Steve Heiner, Ed.D., Willard Hirschi, M.A., Richard Hurley, Ph.D., Sherald James, M.S., Keith Karren, Ph.D., Laura Lewis, M.H.Ed., Hal Meyer, M.S., Ray Petersen, M.H.Ed., Ronald Rhodes, Ph.D. (editor), McKay Rollins, Ph.D., Richard Salazar, Ph.D., and Alton Thygerson, Ed.D. (editor).

Photo Credits

Black-and-white photos courtesy of:

Stock Boston
  Susie Fitzhugh
  Michael Hayman
  Arthur Grace
  Jean-Claude Lejeune
  Elizabeth Hamlin
  Peter Simon
  Owen Franken

  Sam Sweezy
  Frederik D. Bodin
  Peter Vandermark
  Anna Kaufman Moon
  David Powers
  Frank Siteman

World Health Organization
Ulrike Welsch
Steve Heiner
The Food and Drug Administration
March of Dimes Birth Defects Foundation
United Press International Inc.
The *Denver Post*
Ron Moscati, Buffalo *Courier Express*
H. Armstrong Roberts
Wide World Photos

Color Photos courtesy of:

Drug Enforcement Administration, U.S. Department of Justice, Washington, D.C.
Mary Dooros
Sterling K. Clarren, M.D., Assistant Professor, University of Washington
© Lennart Nilsson, *Behold Man*
Dr. Joseph Mancuso, Spenco Medical Center, Waco, Texas
Paul Wexler, M.D., Rose Medical Center, Denver, Colorado
N. Branson Call, M.D., Ophthalmic Plastic and Reconstructive Surgeon, Salt Lake City, Utah
Eugene L. Robertson, M.D., Plastic and Reconstructive Surgeon, Provo, Utah
U.S. Public Health Service, Communicable Disease Center

Illustrations by Susan Strawn

Contents

Part I: Introduction

    Chapter 1: Facts That Figure   1

Part II: Behavioral Aspects of Health   23

    Chapter 2: Finding Yourself: A Lifetime of Health   25
    Chapter 3: Coping and Adjusting: Dealings with Feelings   55
    Chapter 4: Sexuality: His and Hers   113
    Chapter 5: Substance Abuse: The Crutches That Cripple   141
    Chapter 6: Life Crises: The Beginning to the End   193

Part III: Health Maintenance   243

    Chapter 7: Nutrition: Basic Life Support   245
    Chapter 8: Overweight and Obesity: Girth Control   285
    Chapter 9: Fitness: Keep Moving   325
    Chapter 10: Reproduction and Childbirth: New Beginnings   357

Part IV: Reducing Risks

    Chapter 11: Cardiovascular Disease: Have a Heart   415
    Chapter 12: Cancer: Beating the Odds   443
    Chapter 13: Chronic Diseases: Everybody Gets Something   471
    Chapter 14: Infectious Disease: Don't Get Bugged   495
    Chapter 15: Environmental Hazards: Cleaning Up Your Act   527

Part V: Self-Care   545

    Chapter 16: Consumer Health: Have It Your Way   547
    Chapter 17: Self-Care: To Each His Own   569
    Chapter 18: Emergency Care: Ready or Not   607

Appendix: Methods of Birth Control   629
Index   649

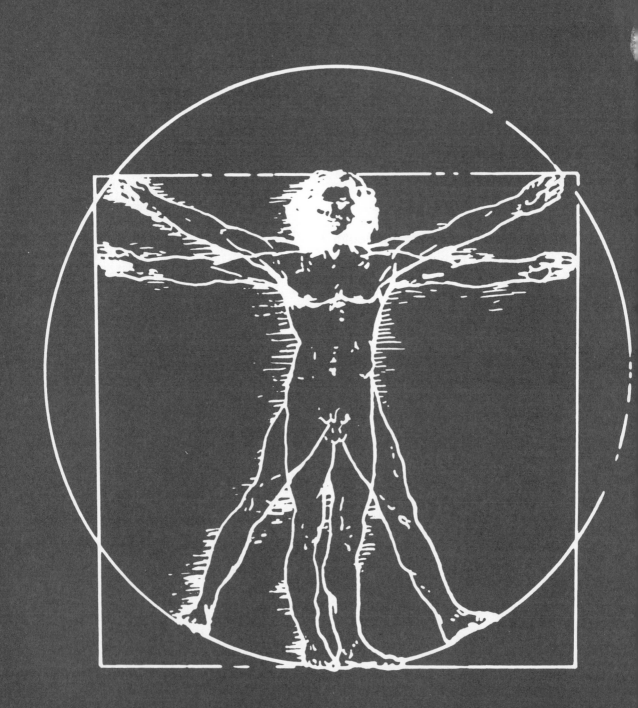

Part I

Introduction

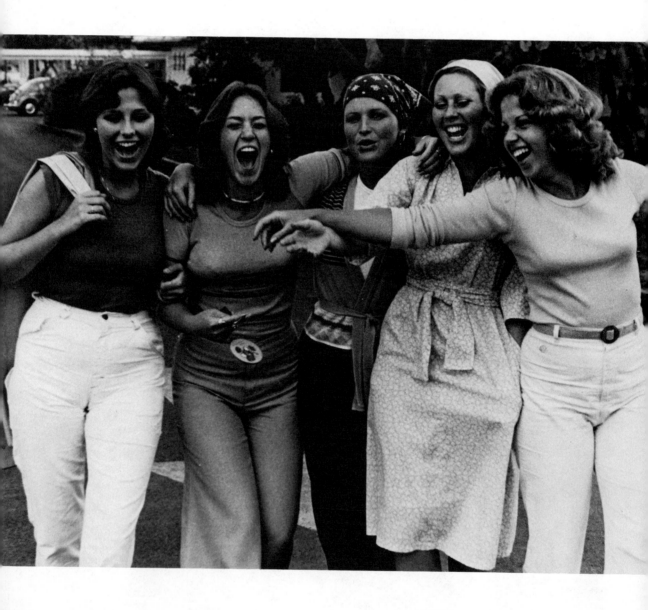

1
Introduction: Facts That Figure

How long will you live, and how effective will your life be?

The answer depends on *you* — on how much you eat, on where you live, on whether you sleep with a window open, on whether you eat fresh fruits and vegetables (an apple a day?), on whether you wear a seat belt, on whether your grandfather had a stroke, on how many times you exercise each week, and how much you earn during your lifetime, on how many cigarettes you smoke or don't smoke every day. All of those factors — and many more — determine not only how long you will live, but what *kind* of a life you will live.

And what is important is that *you* have control over most of those factors. Of course, none of us can control whether our grandmother suffered a heart attack at the age of sixty or whether our father died from cancer of the colon. But each of us does control many other factors that decide how soon we will die and how healthy we will be until then.

Not too many years ago, medicine was a mystery. Nobody thought about sickness (or wellness, for that matter) until they came down with a rumbling stomach, a stabbing earache, a throbbing head. Today, we know more about our bodies. We also know more about how to choose a doctor; we can discuss intelligently the results of lab tests and the therapeutic value of various kinds of treatments. We can participate in our own health care because we know more about disease and what causes it. We know how drugs act on our bodies and what benefits and side effects we can expect from them.

Most important, we know how to *prevent* disease. We have discovered what causes disease; we know what risk factors are involved. And we know how to reduce our risk of developing disease — even serious diseases like cancer, heart disease, and emphysema — and how to increase our chances of living a long, healthy, happy life. If you do not know as much as you should about these subjects, this book will help you learn.

THE STATE OF THE UNION

The health of American people has never been better.[1] Our ability to treat and prevent disease has grown tremendously through our understanding of what causes disease. A report released by the Surgeon General's Office at the beginning of this decade indicated that increased medical care and greater health expenditures have brought about a greater state of health — but that disease prevention and the promotion of health are even more significant factors.

Still, we *can* do better. In a period of two decades, the amount of money that we as a nation spent on health care increased more than 700 percent, yet the increase has not yielded the striking improvements for which we might have hoped. Why? Because most of the money has been aimed at treatment and rehabilitation rather than *prevention.*[2]

Some strides in prevention have been gained, but we still lag behind other industrial nations concerning our health status. Twelve other countries do better in preventing deaths from cancer; twenty-six others have a lower death rate from circulatory disease. Eleven others do a better job of keeping babies alive during the first year of life. Fourteen others have a higher level of life expectancy for men, and six others have a higher level for women.[3]

We *can* improve — we can begin to approach our potential — if we realign our priorities, if we make a solid commitment to living better health habits, and if we identify and assess risks on an individual basis to prevent the initial occurrence of disease.

THE TOP TEN KILLERS

The ten most frequent causes of death in the United States today can to a great extent be prevented — or at least held in check — if you know the risk factors for each and if you take appropriate measures to reduce your risk.

Heart Disease

Heart disease — including heart attack, rheumatic fever, hypertension, stroke, arteriosclerosis, congestive heart failure, and congenital heart defects — claims more than one million lives each year in the United States alone. More than twenty-eight million more are injured by heart disease each year but do not die. Heart disease is the leading cause of death in this country today.

Cancer

A single name for more than one hundred separate diseases, cancer is the number two killer in America, claiming almost one-half million victims each year. Lung cancer is the most often fatal; colon or rectum cancer is second in the number of victims claimed, followed by stomach cancer, lymph gland cancer, leukemia, kidney or bladder cancer, breast cancer, uterine cancer, prostate cancer, mouth cancer, and skin cancer.

Stroke

During a stroke, blood circulation in the brain is disturbed as a result of: (1) a blood clot that breaks off from an artery and travels elsewhere in the body to become lodged; (2) an artery that bulges and bursts; (3) a

LEADING CAUSES OF DEATH IN THE UNITED STATES,
Number of Deaths (in thousands)

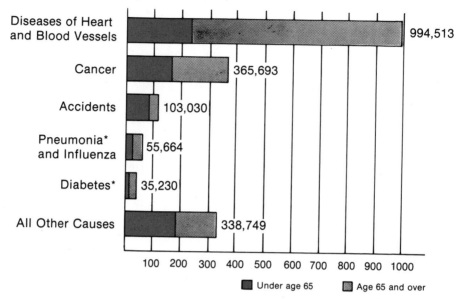

Diseases of Heart and Blood Vessels — 994,513
Cancer — 365,693
Accidents — 103,030
Pneumonia* and Influenza — 55,664
Diabetes* — 35,230
All Other Causes — 338,749

100 200 300 400 500 600 700 800 900 1000

■ Under age 65   ▨ Age 65 and over

*Deaths from certain causes of mortality in early infancy, cirrhosis of the liver, suicide, and homicide exceed those from pneumonia and influenza, and diabetes for persons under age 65.

Figure 1-1. Source: National Center for Health Statistics, U.S. Public Health Service, DHEW.

blood clot that forms within an artery and blocks blood flow; or (4) a weak artery that leaks blood, leading to hemorrhage.

Strokes cause more than 200,000 deaths in the United States each year. A leading cause of stroke is high blood pressure, which affects more than twenty-one million Americans.

Accidents

Accidents of all kinds kill about 100,000 people every year in the United States and injure more than 10.5 million; 380,000 a year are not killed but are left physically disabled for life. The tragedy of accidental death is that youths are adversely affected the most. They are cut down in their prime and have no opportunity to contribute their potential.

Accidents are the leading cause of death for persons between the ages of one and thirty-eight years.

Influenza and Pneumonia

Influenza and pneumonia together claim almost 60,000 lives each year in the United States. The flu viruses affect about 50 million Americans every year. They can be fatal to those with lung or heart disease or to pregnant women or elderly persons.

Diabetes Mellitus

Every year, four million Americans are affected by diabetes; diabetes alone kills more than 37,000 people each year in the United States, and its complications (such as heart disease) claim over 300,000 victims. Diabetes can be controlled by insulin, by careful control of the diet, by intake of regular meals, and by careful monitoring of strenuous exercise.

Cirrhosis of the Liver

More than 33,000 Americans each year die as a result of cirrhosis of the liver, a disease that can result from fat accumulations in the liver, viral infections, tissue destruction as a result of too much alcohol, or destruction as a result of syphilis.

Arteriosclerosis

Arteriosclerosis (hardening and thickening of the arteries) causes 30,000 deaths a year in the United States; it is also an underlying cause of heart attacks and strokes, which claim an additional 900,000 lives each year in the United States alone. Cell debris, calcium, and fat deposits combine to build up and thicken the walls of the arteries, eventually thickening and clogging the arteries and disrupting the blood flow.

Diseases of Infancy

Birth defects claim about 50,000 lives each year, mainly from congenital anomalies, malformations, low birth weight, respiratory distress

LIFE EXPECTANCY
BY SEX AND RACE

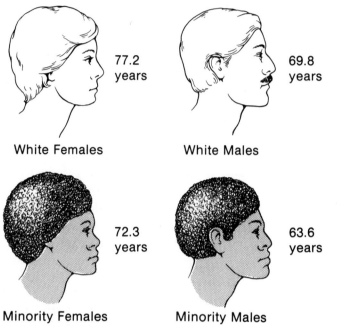

White Females — 77.2 years

White Males — 69.8 years

Minority Females — 72.3 years

Minority Males — 63.6 years

Figure 1-2. Although blacks and other minorities still have a shorter life expectancy than whites, much progress has been made.

syndrome, and hyaline membrane disease. After the first month of life, Sudden Infant Death Syndrome (SIDS) is the number one killer of infants (the syndrome usually strikes between the ages of two and four months).

While you cannot control diseases that you had as an infant, you can to a large extent control the risk you run of giving birth to a baby with such a disease.

Suicide

More than 25,000 people in the United States die each year from suicide.

Those are the top ten killers — grim, constantly threatening, ever present. The good news? You can control your risk of developing most of them. This book will help you learn how.

6

CONTRIBUTORS TO HEALTH

A number of factors combine to contribute to good health:[4]

1. **Health.** Your general health and fitness level — influenced by your weight, your diet, how much you drink and smoke, and your blood pressure — is one of the greatest contributors to longevity and to disease prevention.

2. **Exercise.** Start off slowly, but start. You will prolong your life by increasing the capacity of your heart and by strengthening your lungs and their power to circulate oxygenated blood throughout your body.

3. **Emotional Outlook.** Your relationship with your husband or wife, your relationship with your parents, your relationship with your roommates, your ability to mix with other people, how satisfied you are with the way you live, whether your life-style is pleasant, and how well people get along with you are important to good health and longevity. A positive and optimistic outlook on life coupled with a contentment with your place in life and a general satisfaction with your personal worth will make you healthier and more resistant to chronic disease.

4. **Where You Live.** It makes a difference where you live. Those who live in rural and small urban areas are less prone to suffer from stress that leads to heart disease and high blood pressure. Because of a myriad of factors, the state in which you live can have an effect on how long you live. Those who live in Hawaii and Utah have the longest life spans; Minnesota, North Dakota, and Wisconsin are "healthy" places to live, too. Residents of Washington, D.C. have the lowest life expectancy, followed by residents of South Carolina, Mississippi, and Louisiana.

5. **Life-style.** The unique pattern of your daily life — the food that you eat, the way you get to school or work, the people with whom you live, the drugs that you take, the hobbies that you enjoy, the sports in which you participate — all affect your health.

6. **Health Habits.** Your health habits — whether you have a physical

exam when needed, whether you have a Pap smear regularly, whether you examine your breasts monthly, whether you eat three meals a day — determine what kind of health you have. Good health and longevity are linked to seven basic health habits: eating three meals a day, eating breakfast every day, exercising moderately two or three times a week, getting enough sleep, not smoking, not drinking alcohol, and keeping your weight near its ideal level.

7. **Individual Attitude.** The way you look at life can play a major part in what your health is like. Laughing, believing in a religious faith, loving others, and your attitudes toward yourself are important determinants of good health and well-being.

8. **Nutrition.** Eating the right foods — stocking your body with the essential proteins, minerals, and vitamins — leads to good health. A machine that is not properly fueled and well oiled cannot be expected to perform at its peak. Nutrition is the basic building block that contributes to your body's well-being.

9. **Education.** People who are well educated are healthier because they have a basic understanding of the rules of sanitation, immunization, nutrition, and other health maintenance practices.

10. **Employment.** Your employment determines how healthy you are because it can introduce environmental hazards that you would probably never enounter otherwise. You may be forced to work with asbestos, for instance, or you may spend fourteen hours a day breathing in fine particles of coal dust. Or you may sit in a soft chair behind a desk where your only exercise may be pushing a pencil.

11. **Environment.** Your environment in general — social, economic, and physical — influences your health. The water you drink and the air you breathe need to be clean; you need to enjoy your friends and family members; you need to have financial resources to meet your nutritional needs.

12. **Psychological Makeup and Intelligence.** You will be healthy if you can, most of the time, avoid getting depressed, avoid being bored, and avoid being under too much stress. Those who have a high regard for their own health and physical well-being, who use their mental abilities, who challenge themselves intellectually, and who

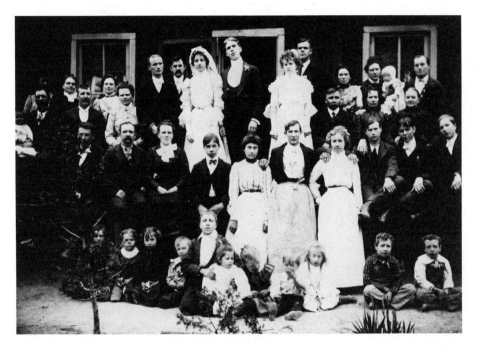

Families influence health.

are psychiatrically sound are usually more healthy.

13. **Ability to Adjust.** How well can you adjust to meet changing circumstances in your own life determines to a large extent your level of health.

14. **Others.** Other factors that lead to good health include good driving, wearing seat belts, having a balanced family development, being able to manage stress, and being able to manage the risk factors that lead to disease development.

DISEASE RISK FACTORS

Heredity

Of course, you cannot control your heredity, but you can be alert to conditions that may develop due to heredity, and you can take steps to prevent or lessen the severity of the condition. Certain diseases and dispositions toward diseases seem to be inherited — they include heart disease, stroke, cancer, phlebitis, embolisms, pneumonia, tuberculosis, aneurysms, Parkinson's disease, Chiari's syndrome, suicide, and some diseases of the liver. Some forms of anemia, such as sickle-cell anemia, are also hereditary.

But just because you inherit the tendency toward a condition does not mean that you are helpless. You have the responsibility of finding out what hereditary factors are at work on you, and then you can use the information to help pinpoint potential problem areas and devise measures that will reduce risks.

Obesity

Overweight is a serious health problem, both physically and emotionally. In fact, obesity is a major contributing factor to most serious diseases. It is indirectly responsible for eight of the ten leading causes of death — all but accidents and suicide. In some cases, it may even be an indirect cause of an accident or suicide.

High Blood Pressure

When the pumping effort of the heart is increased due to high blood pressure, the heart enlarges and damage occurs to the arteries. When the arteries in the brain are damaged, stroke results; when the damaged arteries are in the eyes, loss of vision can result; damaged arteries in the kidneys lead to loss of function and kidney failure.

One of the most common causes of high blood pressure is overweight. A particular cause is using too much table salt. Both of these are factors that you can control.

Smoking

The facts are in. Among men who have lung cancer, those who smoke have an 88 percent higher mortality rate than those who do not smoke; women smokers have a 28 percent higher mortality rate from lung cancer than women who do not smoke. The incidence of lung cancer among women has doubled in the last ten years; 80 percent of all lung cancer is directly attributable to smoking. Smoking causes other diseases, too — and it makes many more diseases worse.

Age

Depending on your age, you run a higher risk for developing certain conditions. Arthritis, for example, strikes people of all ages, but it is much more common after middle age due to wear and tear on joints. One in four heart attack deaths occur before the age of sixty-five; three-fourths of them afflict those older than sixty-five. Children and young adults are more prone to accidents and suicide.

Race

Members of certain racial groups run higher risks in some areas. Blacks, for example, are twice as likely as members of any other racial group to develop high blood pressure. Blacks, too, are the only racial group susceptible to sickle-cell anemia.

Stress

Stress has long been recognized as a leading contributor to heart disease, but only recently have medical researchers linked stress to a number of diseases — including cancer and the common cold.

Alcohol

Alcohol is now considered to be our nation's number one drug problem; alcoholism has become a crippling disease that affects more than 12 million Americans. Ingestion of alcohol — sometimes in only moderate amounts — leads to pneumonia, cirrhosis of the liver, birth defects, and a breakdown of the body's ability to resist disease. Alcohol is also frequently implicated in motor vehicle accidents, homicide, and suicide.

High Serum Cholesterol Levels

Cholesterol — one of the two principal blood fats — is generally high in people who eat excessive animal fats (especially liver, pork, lamb, and dark fowl) and dairy products (cheese and eggs). If your blood cholesterol content is high, you run a much greater risk of developing stroke, heart disease, or vascular disease.

Diabetes

If you have diabetes, you run the risk of developing a number of other conditions, including heart disease and tuberculosis.

Other general risk factors that lead to development of disease include chronic fatigue, frequent infection, lack of exercise, and electro-cardiogram abnormalities.

ASSESSING RISK

The benefit of learning risk factors as they relate to diseases and disease conditions is that you can define your *own* risk factors — you can find out what habits and life-styles in *your* background make you susceptible to certain diseases. And then you can do something about it!

Some diseases may involve a single significant risk. Most diseases, however, involve many contributing factors resulting from many risks. Heart disease is related to people who are at risk because they are under too much stress, they smoke, they drink alcohol, they are overweight, they eat too many animal fats, they do not exercise enough, or they have uncontrolled high blood pressure. In assessing risks, you are one step

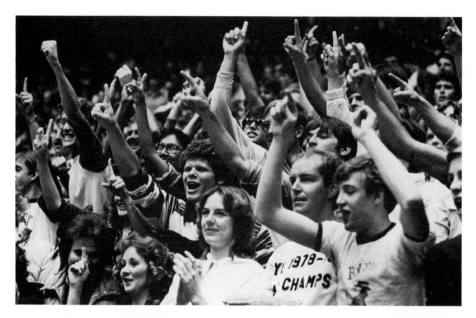

Happiness and health are learning to live with yourself and others.

further toward identifying and preventing the development of the associated disease. You can — and should — use your risk factors to your advantage in creating a higher level of wellness.

LIMITATIONS OF RISK ANALYSIS

Every person is born with a hereditary endowment that affects his maximum longevity. No one can predict exactly what his potential genetic life span will be, but we do know that acquired risk factors (including accidents) can shorten that life span.

In assessing your own risk factors, keep in mind the fact that you probably cannot add many years to your own hereditary potential. But you *can* eliminate the factors that may subtract years from the maximum potential that is available to you.[5]

EMPHASIS ON PREVENTION

A report issued from the Surgeon General's Office pinpoints prevention as the single most important factor that will lead to better health for Americans. If we identify our priorities and keep a sharp focus on what we can do to reduce our own risks, the goal of prevention is attainable and possible.

Role of the Individual

The edict released form the Surgeon General's Office stated:

. . . the health of this Nation's citizens can be significantly improved through actions individuals can take themselves, and through actions decision makers in the public and private sectors can take to promote a safe and healthier environment for all Americans at home, at work, and at play. For the individual often only modest life-style changes are needed to substantially reduce risk for several diseases. And many of the personal decisions required to reduce risk for one disease can reduce it for others. Within the practical grasp of most Americans are simple measures to enhance the prospects of good health. . . .[6]

What the good news boils down to is this: *you* can control how healthy you are. The most tragic health situation in this country today is that too many people neglect their own health, surrendering to someone else (a doctor, a nurse, a folk healer) the complete responsibility. Of course, there are many times when you must see a doctor. It would be stupid to treat yourself for what might be a serious health problem — that, too, constitutes neglect. The ideal situation is an intelligent partnership with your doctor — knowing when you need help, accepting and following directions, and taking what measures you can to stay healthy.

You are responsible for being in tune with your body, for knowing when medical help is needed, for making an appointment with a doctor, for following instructions. *You* are the one who is responsible for following through with treatment, for taking your prescription as directed, for exercising.

14

LIFE-STYLE AND HEALTH

In a recent research report it was found that good health practices rather than health status were responsible for the fact that certain people live longer.

The seven health habits that made the difference were:

1. never smoking cigarettes
2. regular physical activity
3. moderate to no use of alcohol
4. 7-8 hours of sleep regularly
5. maintaining proper weight
6. eating breakfast
7. not eating between meals

The research results show that at every age level from 20 to 70, those persons who followed all seven of the health habits listed above had significantly longer life spans than those who followed only six.

Men who were 60 years of age or older and had followed all seven health practices had better health status than men of 30 who followed none to three of them.

The study also showed that men at age 45 who practiced none to three of the good health habits could expect to live to about 66.5 years old. Those at 45 who followed four or five of the good health practices could anticipate living to be 73 years old; and those who followed six or seven could expect to live to 75 years old.

Lester Breslow and James E. Enstrom, "Persistence of Health Habits and Their Relationship to Mortality," *Preventive Medicine*, 9:469-483 (1980).

The Concept of Wellness

There is still more: *you are responsible for keeping yourself well. You* have the ability to identify what you are doing now that will shorten your life span; *you* have the ability to change what you can and the intelligence to adapt to situations that you cannot change. *You* are in control of your body, and of all the things that affect it.

This book is about staying well. Specifically, it's about *you* staying well. Every chapter has information that will help you cope with changes that take place in your body, that will teach you how to care for yourself and prevent disease, and that will help you identify your own personal risks.

At the end of each chapter, a self-evaluation will specifically pinpoint your areas of risk. Once you determine your weaknesses and risks from the self-evaluation, return to the chapter and take special note of the information that will help you prevent disease.

You can start by taking the self-evaluation that follows. It will start you on the way to becoming — and staying — healthy and responsible.

Notes

1. Julius B. Richmond, *Healthy People: The Surgeon General's Report on Health Promotion and Disease Prevention, 1979* (U.S. Department of Health, Education, and Welfare, Public Health Service, Office of the Assistant Secretary of Health and Surgeon General), DHEW Publication Number (PHS) 79-55071, pp. v, 3.
2. Ibid., p. 6.
3. Ibid.
4. Departmental Task Force on Prevention, *Disease Prevention and Health Promotion: Federal Programs and Prospects* (U.S. Department of Health, Education, and Welfare, Public Health Service, Office of the Assistant Secretary of Health, September 1978), DHEW Publication Number (PHS) 79-55071B, p. 7; Ralph Grawunder, "How Long Will You Live Predictor," *Personal Health Appraisal,* pp. 185-191; and Palmore, Erdmore, and Jeffers, *Prediction of Life Span* (Lexington, Massachusetts: D.C. Heath and Company, 1971).
5. Irving S. Wright, "Can Your Family History Tell You Anything About Your Chances for a Long Life?" *Executive Health* 14, (No. 5), February 1978.
6. Richmond, p. 10.

Self-Evaluation

All of us want good health. But many of us do not know how to be as healthy as possible. Health experts now describe *life-style* as one of the most important factors affecting health. In fact, it is estimated that as many as seven of the top ten leading causes of death could be reduced through common-sense changes in life-style. That's what this brief test, developed by the Public Health Service, is all about. Its purpose is simply to tell you how well you are doing to stay healthy. The behaviors covered in the test are recommended for most Americans. Some of them may not apply to persons with certain chronic diseases or handicaps, or to pregnant women. Such persons may require special instructions from their physicians.

	Almost Always	Some-times	Almost Never
Cigarette Smoking			
If you never smoke, enter a score of 10 for this section and go to the next section on *Alcohol and Drugs*.			
1. I avoid smoking cigarettes.	2	1	0
2. I smoke only low tar and nicotine cigarettes *or* I smoke a pipe or cigars.	2	1	0
Smoking Score:			
Alcohol and Drugs			
1. I avoid drinking alcoholic beverages *or* I drink no more than 1 or 2 drinks a day.	4	1	0
2. I avoid using alcohol or other drugs (especially illegal drugs) as a way of handling stressful situations or the problems in my life.	2	1	0
3. I am careful not to drink alcohol when taking certain medicines (for example, medicine for sleeping, pain, colds, and allergies), or when pregnant.	2	1	0
4. I read and follow the label directions when using prescribed and over-the-counter drugs.	2	1	0
Alcohol and Drugs Score:			

	Almost Always	Some-times	Almost Never

Eating Habits

1. I eat a variety of foods each day, such as fruits and vegetables, whole grain breads and cereals, lean meats, dairy products, dry peas and beans, and nuts and seeds.

	Almost Always	Some-times	Almost Never
1.	4	1	0
2.	2	1	0
3.	2	1	0
4.	2	1	0

2. I limit the amount of fat, saturated fat, and cholesterol I eat (including fat on meats, eggs, butter, cream, shortenings, and organ meats such as liver).

3. I limit the amount of salt I eat by cooking with only small amounts, not adding salt at the table, and avoiding salty snacks.

4. I avoid eating too much sugar (especially frequent snacks of sticky candy or soft drinks).

Eating Habits Score:

Exercise/Fitness

1. I maintain a desired weight, avoiding overweight and underweight.

2. I do vigorous exercises for 15-30 minutes at least 3 times a week (examples include running, swimming, brisk walking).

3. I do exercises that enhance my muscle tone for 15-30 minutes at least 3 times a week (examples include yoga and calisthenics).

4. I use part of my leisure time participating in individual, family, or team activities that increase my level of fitness (such as gardening, bowling, golf, and baseball).

	Almost Always	Some-times	Almost Never
1.	3	1	0
2.	3	1	0
3.	2	1	0
4.	2	1	0

Exercise/Fitness Score:

	Almost Always	Sometimes	Almost Never
Stress Control			
1. I have a job or do other work that I enjoy.	2	1	0
2. I find it easy to relax and express my feelings freely.	2	1	0
3. I recognize early, and prepare for, events or situations likely to be stressful for me.	2	1	0
4. I have close friends, relatives, or others whom I can talk to about personal matters and call on for help when needed.	2	1	0
5. I participate in group activities (such as church and community organizations) or hobbies that I enjoy.	2	1	0
Stress Control Score:			
Safety			
1. I wear a seat belt while riding a car.	2	1	0
2. I avoid driving while under the influence of alcohol and other drugs.	2	1	0
3. I obey traffic rules and the speed limit when driving.	2	1	0
4. I am careful when using potentially harmful products or substances (such as household cleaners, poisons, and electrical devices).	2	1	0
5. I avoid smoking in bed.	2	1	0
Safety Score:			

What Your Scores Mean

Scores of 9 and 10

Excellent! Your answers show that you are aware of the importance of this area to your health. More important, you are putting your knowledge to work for you by practicing good health habits. As long as you continue to do so, this area should not pose a serious health risk. It is likely that you are setting an example for your family and friends to follow. Since you got a very high test score on this part of the test, you may want to consider other areas where your scores indicate room for improvement.

Scores of 6 to 8

Your health practices in this area are good, but there is room for improvement. Look again at the items you answered with a "Sometimes" or "Almost Never." What changes can you make to improve your score? Even a small change can often help you achieve better health.

Scores of 3 to 5

Your health risks are showing! Would you like more information about the risks you are facing and about why it is important for you to change these behaviors. Perhaps you need help in deciding how to successfully make the changes you desire. In either case, help is available.

Scores of 0 to 2

Obviously, you were concerned enough about your health to take the test, but your answers show that you may be taking serious and unnecessary risks with your health. Perhaps you are not aware of the risks and what to do about them. You can easily get the information and help you need to improve, if you wish. The next step is up to you.

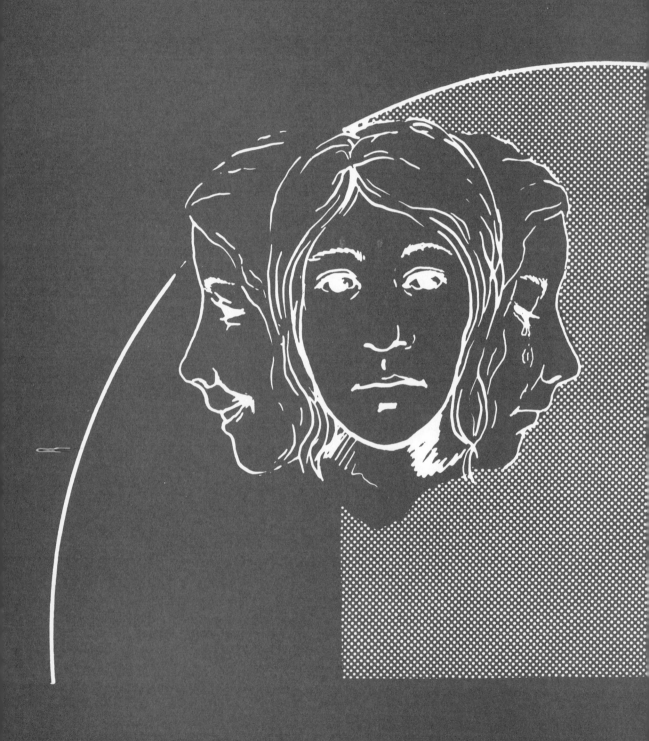

Part II
Behavioral Aspects of Health

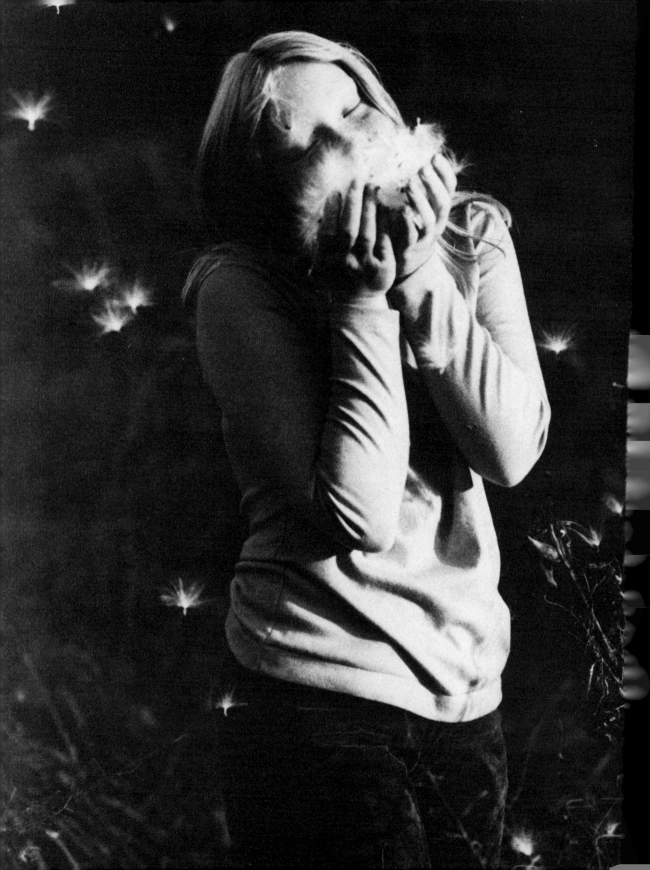

2
Finding Yourself: A Lifetime of Health

He was a poor all-around student. He had never made a healthy adjustment to school, and his teachers had always considered him to be a problem. Even his parents had regarded him as "different" — he had started talking much later than normal, and his father had always been ashamed of his son's lack of athletic ability. The boy could not seem to make and keep friends. He had odd mannerisms; he made up his own religion and often chanted hymns to himself. Finally, when he was a senior in high school, his physician issued a certificate excusing him from school for six months because of a nervous breakdown.

The boy?

Albert Einstein.[1]

The home environment was troubled. The father was alcoholic but extremely fond of his rather homely daughter; the little girl lived in a fantasy world for years, imagining herself to be the mistress of her father's household. Her mother rejected her — after all, she was so unattractive — and the girl started to develop problems. When she was five, she swallowed a penny to attract attention. As an older child, she began to lie and to steal sweets.

After the death of both her parents, she went to live with her grandmother, who was granted legal custody. The grandmother — a widow — had poorly managed her own four young children still at home. A son, drinking to the point of alcoholism, left home without telling anyone where he was going; a daughter, emotionally distraught over a love affair, remained locked in her room for years.

The grandmother vowed to be more strict with the young girl than she had been with her own children. She put her in braces to improve her posture, dressed her oddly, and refused to let her have playmates. To maintain complete control over the child, her grandmother refused to enroll her in school.

The little girl?

She grew up to become one of our most respected citizens, Eleanor Roosevelt.

When the baby was born with an extremely large head (usually a sign of brain fever), his mother refused to listen to friends and relatives who claimed that he was probably abnormal. Three of his siblings had died before his birth, presumably of similar conditions. At the age of six, he was sent to school; his teacher diagnosed him as being mentally ill. His mother, outraged by the teacher's diagnosis, withdrew the boy from school and vowed to teach him herself.

The boy?

Thomas Edison.

The point of these three examples is simple: endowed with a will to survive and succeed, we can rise above any adversity, any ill situation. The key? Self-esteem, a recognition of our own worth as individuals. It is appropriate to begin a study of health with an examination of self-esteem, because all health and well-being begins here.

FINDING YOURSELF

Each person is an individual in the purest sense — each has a unique set of genetic determinants that make him different from every other person who lives or who has ever lived. No mind, no body, and no spirit is the same as any other; no happiness, no hate, and no love experienced by one man is exactly like that experienced by another.

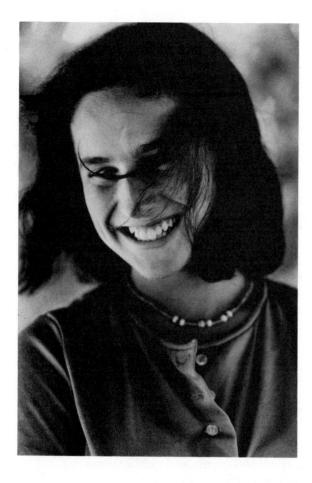

Finding yourself depends greatly on the quality of your feelings about yourself.

But as individual — and as different — as we are, we all struggle with the same basic questions: Who am I? Where did I come from? Where am I going? Is there a life after this one? (A great British humanitarian remarked as he slipped from mortality, "What a great adventure this will be!") Am I the architect of my own destiny? How can I make my life count?

The questions are as old as life itself, but our complex society has changed some of the answers — and has changed many of the ways in which we seek answers. Never before in the history of this planet have our opportunities been so great or our dangers so harrowing.

In seeking to find ourselves, we realize that every individual has certain basic needs. Each of us needs food, shelter, water, air, and security to stay alive. But we have other needs that make living more than just staying alive — we need beauty, justice, goodness, wholeness, and order in our lives as much as we need food and water. As you study health, you will learn to satisfy the basic needs that enable you to live a healthy life. Once those basic needs have been satisfied, you will find the determination and motivation to satisfy the needs that enable you to grow and develop self-esteem.

WHAT IS SELF-ESTEEM?

One of the most critical aspects of good mental health is the ability to like and respect yourself — the development of self-esteem. No value judgment is more important to man than the judgment that he passes on himself — not a conscious, verbalized judgment, but a feeling that you experience constantly as a reflection of your attitudes, perceptions, beliefs, ideas, and feelings about yourself. Self-esteem is the epitome of qualities that you attribute to yourself.

Self-concept takes us one step further, giving us a total view of ourselves in four dimensions:

1. **Body image,** our physical and sexual self.
2. **Social self,** our ethical, racial, religious, and cultural makeup.
3. **Cognitive self,** our thinking and knowing self.
4. **Self-esteeem,** our evaluation of the self.

Where does self-concept come from? No one is born with it; it is learned as our experiences and environment forge the ways in which we view ourselves. As we interact with and receive feedback from others, we learn to view ourselves in either a positive or negative way.

Early associations with parents, siblings, peers, teachers, and other sigificant people help formulate self-concept. While self-concept is for-mulated early in life (with parents serving as the most important determinants), it can change throughout life as a result of ever-changing influences and relationships. Despite change, early shaping by parents

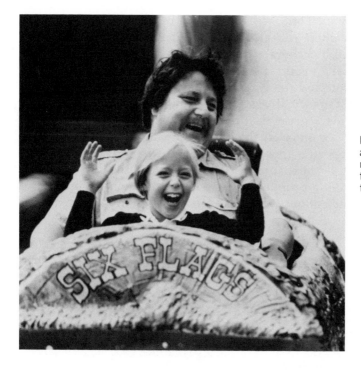

Parents who feel good about their children raise children who feel good about themselves.

carries its influence until death. Parents — the primary role models, primary feedback agents, and primary evaluators of behavior — have a profound effect on self-concept that lasts for a lifetime.

A good self-concept brings high self-esteem: the knowledge that you are a competent individual who is able to think, judge, and know. (It does not mean, however, that you believe yourself to be infallible.) A person with good self-esteem realizes that he is as worthy and as important as every other human being, and because he recognizes the truth of that concept, gone is his compulsion to prove his worth to others.

It should be noted that proving yourself *to* others is not the same as receiving proof *from* others. The feedback that you receive from generous acts of selfless service will usually engender appreciative comments that make you feel good about yourself. When such behavior-response relationships have been well established, you tend to feel good about yourself every time you give of yourself even if the positive feedback does not always occur. You see yourself as being important to others because of what you mean to them in much the same way as you see

29

those important to you. Thus, self-esteem is a result of those potentials (what you are) as well as those behaviors (what you can do) that are expressly appreciated by others — first parents, then peers.

What happens when you realize a glaring discrepancy between your perception of yourself and the way you think you ought to be? Everyone has felt this discrepancy at least once — and what happens to you at that moment depends a great deal on your basic sense of self-worth. If your sense of self-worth is usually high, you will probably retain faith in yourself and bridge (or appreciably narrow) the gap. On the other hand, if your sense of self-worth is low, you will probably become a victim of a self-fulfilling prophecy: you believe the negative inferences that others have made about you, and eventually you make them come true.

"Our self-esteem is an emotion — not an intellectual inventory of our favorable characteristics, but how warm, friendly, and appreciative we actually feel toward ourselves. It is the degree that we consciously or unconsciously accept and like ourselves, despite our mistakes and human frailties. It is not egotism. It is a man's feelings about himself as a person, a feeling that has profound effects on emotions, values, desires, and goals. Our basic need and urge is to 'feel good' about ourselves, mentally, physically, and emotionally."

— L. S. Barksdale
Essays on Self-Esteem
(Idyllwild, California:
The Barksdale Foundation),
p. 41

If everyone is equally valuable, why do some begin to believe the negative feedback that they receive? Simple — it's human nature. Told something about yourself often enough, it's easy to start believing it. A counselor at a community college held several sessions with a student who was having problems adjusting to a vocational training course. During the consultations, the counselor administered several tests, among them an I.Q. test.

During the next session, the student remarked, "I know I can't do very well. My abilities are limited — there's a certain level I can't go beyond."

"Why do you feel that way about yourself?" the counselor probed.

The student explained that his eighth-grade teacher had told him that his I.Q. was eighty-five and that he would never do very well in school. The counselor was shocked — the student's test had revealed a completely normal I.Q.

Sometimes the crippling is done with good intentions — a parent who was psychologically crippled as a child and who did not realize that it goes on to cripple his or her child in the same way — and the terrible crippling continues through generations. As a general rule, any behavior that causes a child to feel incapable, inadequate, unloved, unable, or less than worthy can be considered crippling. A child's self-esteem can become hopelessly crippled if his basic needs are constantly abused, if he is excluded from his parents' emotional lives, and if he is disciplined without warmth and respect. If a child is to develop self-confidence and self-respect, his parents must respect him and have confidence in him.

Early in life, a low self-esteem can be programmed into a child through any of the following sources:

- Low esteem on the part of the parents
- Belittling by parents, teachers, and peers
- Lack of appreciation expressed by parents, teachers, and peers
- Parents who compare their children and their characteristics and talents

CHILDREN LEARN WHAT THEY LIVE

If a child lives with criticism, He learns to condemn.
If a child lives with hostility, He learns to fight.
If a child lives with ridicule, He learns to be shy.
If a child lives with shame, He learns to feel guilty.
If a child lives with tolerance, He learns to be patient.
If a child lives with encouragement, He learns confidence.
If a child lives with praise, He learns to appreciate.
If a child lives with fairness, He learns justice.
If a child lives with security, He learns to have faith.
If a child lives with approval, He learns to like himself.
If a child lives with acceptance and friendship, He learns to find love in the world.

— Dorothy Law Nolte

A CHILD'S SELF IMAGE

In earlier China, mothers would tightly bind their young daughters' feet and keep them bound for years, causing terrible deformity. It was done with good intent, because tiny feet and a mincing walk were considered attractive in a Chinese girl. In time, the crippled daughter would grow up, marry, and have daughters of her own. Then the irony: the crippled mother would get out the bandages and cripple her daughters just as she was crippled. Through generation after generation, like echoes in á canyon, the crippling continued. An old Russian proverb states the problem succinctly: "The little girl who is beaten will beat her doll-baby." We do unto others as we have been done unto.

So it happens that many small children are crippled by parents who were themselves crippled psychologically as children.

As a general rule, we can say that any behavior of significant people that causes a young child to think ill of himself, to feel inadequate, incapable, unworthy, unwanted, unloved, or unable, is crippling to the self. Where respect and warmth are missing, where the child's questions go unanswered, where his offers to help are rejected, where his discipline is based on failure and punishment, where he is excluded from his parents' emotional life, and where his basic rights are abused, there his self is undermined. It is vital for parents to remember the simple rule that they must have respect for and confidence in their children before their children can have self-respect or self-confidence.

— William W. Purkey

- Parents who are overly demanding
- Adverse family, economic, social, cultural, and ethnic conditions
- A sense of guilt over affluence
- Repeated defeats and failures
- Lack of purpose in life
- Dependence on others for a sense of worth
- Never accepting challenges; doing only what comes easiest
- An unflattering physical appearance
- Lack of motivation to be independent
- Parents that push children to fill needs that they themselves never achieved
- Rivalry with an exceptionally talented brother or sister
- Parents who are overpossessive, overpermissive, or tyrannical
- Parents who place a high value on material possessions

- Procrastination
- Parents who rear the child with a system of reward and punishment

Stanley Coopersmith, a professor of psychology at the University of California/Davis, studied 1,748 normal middle-class boys and their families for six years; his studies began when the boys were preadolescent and concluded when they reached young adulthood.

The results?

Coopersmith found that parents have the power to endow a child with high self-esteem. A child tends to see himself as his parents see him — or as he *thinks* his parents see him.[2] The homes of the self-confident, successful young men had three things in common:

1. There was love in the family. There was plenty of hugging and kissing, but there was more: there was genuine concern and respect for the children. A child feels that he is a person of great worth when he discovers that he is an object of intense interest and pride.
2. There was a high degree of democracy within the family. Each child was encouraged to present his own ideas for discussion — and no matter how bizarre they were, those ideas were greeted with enthusiasm and respect.
3. The parents were less permissive than the parents of children with low self-esteem; a child whose parents are too permissive can become alarmed and insecure. Many such children believe that their parents do not establish or enforce rules because the parents do not care what happens to the child.

SYMPTOMS OF LOW SELF-ESTEEM

An individual who is suffering from low self-esteem probably manifests several of the following symptoms:[3]

1. **Bullying or bragging.** An individual who has a soft interior and who feels highly susceptible often resorts to bullying, a way of creating a tough, protective exterior. Such individuals are often simply crying out for attention of *any* kind — and most people pay attention to a bully.
2. **Fearfulness and timidity.** A little bit of shyness is normal; we all feel a little uncertain when we encounter the unknown. A fearfulness

that interferes with normal living, however, can be regarded as the by-product of a crippling self-esteem.

3. **Inability to make decisions.** An individual with poor self-esteem is afraid of making a wrong choice and of getting rebuked for it — so he does not make any choices at all. High self-esteem is accompanied by the realization that everyone makes mistakes and that mistakes are nothing to fear.

4. **No desire to express opinions.** Similarly, a person suffering from low self-esteem believes that his opinions have no worth. As a result, he becomes withdrawn, passive, and seemingly uninterested in what is going on around him. He takes the safest course: by not venturing an opinion, he does not get scorned or ridiculed by others. A person who has a good sense of self-esteem speaks up for his opinions and eagerly accepts the chance to defend them.

5. **Expectation of failure.** No one can force another person to succeed, but many who suffer from low self-esteem continue to set impossibly high goals for themselves. Each time such a person fails to reach a goal (even though the the goal was unrealistic), his low sense of worth is reinforced. He comes to expect failure — and he proves himself right.

6. **Can make no sense out of life.** An individual with low self-esteem views his future with alarm and insecurity — he is in a terrible mess, and things are bound to get worse. He cannot make decisions, set goals, or aim for anything specific. He lacks a set of values that could guide him in some direction.

"It is everyone's fundamental right to feel that he is as good as another person and that we are all children of God, born with rights to happiness and to the feelings that we are human beings of dignity. Your greatness comes from your recognition of the best in yourself, from the human dignity that you give yourself, from the sense of self-respect that is your present to yourself every day of the year — not just on Christmas."

— Maxwell Maltz
The Magic Power of Self-Image Psychology
(Englewood Cliffs, New Jersey:
Prentice-Hall, Inc.), pp. 199-204.

Eleanor Roosevelt, who rose above massive odds as a child, once quipped, "No one can make you feel inferior without your consent." You are often your own worst enemy — but you have the power to change all that.

If you think that your self-esteem could use a boost, try some of the following:

1. Identify your needs and strive to fulfill them. You have probably never sat down and actually listed out your needs — but do it now. You will be surprised at how many there are. You will be equally surprised at how easily you can fulfill them. Once you realize that you have taken control of meeting your own needs, you will gain a sense of self-value as you become an important person in your life.

2. List your goals. Write each one down in as much detail as you can. Then look at them with an objective eye. Is each one realistic? Can you, with your best talents and abilities, hope to achieve each one? If you have set unrealistic or impossible goals for yourself, eliminate or revise them. Nothing can be more defeating than failing to achieve what you set out to do.

3. Figure out who you are in relation to others. You need to establish your own sense of worth and identity. You need to do things because you want to — not because others want you to. You are as good as the next person, and you have just as much right to pursue your own course and fill your own needs.

4. Dwell on your successes — not your failures. Use your memory and your imagination to relive your past. Consider your failures in a new light: what can you learn from them? How can you avoid making the same mistake? Then forget about them. Dwell instead on your successes, those personal triumphs, those moments of progress and courage. Look forward to your future in light of the successes that you have had in the past.

5. While you can use the past to bolster your self-image, do not be chained to the past. You can do nothing to change it. Instead, concentrate on the present and the future.

6. Avoid self-pity like the plague that it is — it is the most destructive emotion of all. Come to a new understanding that you are really

distinct from what you do. No matter how many mistakes you have made, no matter how messed up things have been, you are worthwhile, and you do not have to fail.

7. Act as you want to be. Sounds oversimplified, but it works. If you act confident and self-assured, you will be.

8. Become a little child again. React to life with absorption, curiosity, and concentration. Begin to see things through a child's eyes, and allow yourself to experience new wonder at all around you.

9. Break out of the rut by trying something new. Take a class in a new field, try a new food, meet a new person. Try not to always stick with the safe and secure; develop a healthy curiosity in the unknown.

10. Be honest and direct in your dealings with others. It is a temptation to put on pretenses and play games with people who are close to you — but doing so compromises your integrity and sincerity.

11. Trust your own feelings. Do not worry about what others tell you to feel, and do not worry if your feelings are different than the popular ones. Your feelings are valid, and they are worthy; pay attention, and learn their value. Be prepared to be unpopular if your views do not coincide with the current tide — and remember that the world's greatest people were often the dissenters.

12. Take on responsibility — it enables you to take control of your life and bolsters self-esteem.

13. Make commitments. When you decide what you want to do, work hard to achieve it.

SELF-ACTUALIZING INDIVIDUALS

In his study of the human personality, Abraham Maslow developed a core of personality traits that make up the *self-actualizing individual:* a person who lives in a way that enables him to move beyond his basic needs and to fulfill his "growth" needs — those needs that allow for development of high self-esteem. In developing his list of personality traits, Maslow examined the lives of people whom he believed to be self-actualizers — among them Walt Whitman, Abraham Lincoln, Jane Addams, Albert Einstein, Eleanor Roosevelt, Albert Schweitzer, Thomas Jefferson, Ludwig van Beethoven, and Helen Keller.

THE IGNORANT BUMBLE-BEE

"The bumble-bee cannot fly. According to the theory of aerodynamics, and as may be readily demonstrated through laboratory tests and wind tunnel experiments, the bumble-bee is unable to fly. This is because the size, weight, and shape of his body, in relation to the total wing-spread that he has, make flying impossible.

"But the bumble-bee, being ignorant of these profound truths, goes ahead and flies anyway, and manages to produce a little honey every day!"

According to Maslow, those with the highest self-esteem exhibit the following characteristics:

1. They are able to perceive reality and tolerate it and are able to accept uncertainty.
2. They accept themselves and others.
3. They are spontaneous in thought and behavior.
4. Their orientation toward life is one of problem solving instead of an orientation centered on self.
5. They have a keen, unhostile sense of humor.
6. They need privacy and detachment sometimes.
7. They are relatively independent of their environments. They do not consciously try to be unconventional, but they follow their own paths.
8. They appreciate with continued freshness and pleasure the basics of life.
9. They are at times profoundly spiritual.
10. They are able to identify with and show concern for mankind.
11. They have deep interpersonal relationships with only a few people instead of with many.
12. They are highly imaginative and creative in their approach to life.
13. They are democratic.
14. They are able to view life objectively; they keep the ends distinguished from the means.

In a nutshell, those who are self-actualizing — those who have high self-concepts — act on their environments instead of reacting. They decide what they will achieve, how they will feel toward themselves, what goals they will set. By acting instead of reacting, you can formulate goals, values, and ideals that will improve your own self-esteem.

HAPPINESS: A BY-PRODUCT OF SELF-ESTEEM

You might wonder why self-esteem is so important, why we all seem to strive for it. The answer in part lies in happiness, that balanced state of equilibrium that we all seek.

The state of normal, healthy, adults is a happy one. As children, we were spontaneously cheerful; as we grew, we learned self-defeating behaviors — behaviors that occur over and over — thoughts, feelings, and attitudes about ourselves that hinder our spiritual, social, and emotional growth.[4] It takes a long time to change those self-defeating behaviors, because they are powerful habits. But they *can* be changed, because they are learned behaviors. No one inherits self-defeating behaviors.

Concentrate on living your life minute by minute — not year by year, or decade by decade. You possess the power to control your life much more easily when you take it a little at a time.

Concentrate on the journey, not the destination. If you are in too big of a hurry to get that promotion, finish your education, meet the right marriage partner, you will miss all the fun of getting there.

Begin to think of yourself as responsible and in control of your own happiness. Perhaps you had parents who were thoughtless and cruel. Undoubtedly those parents had an effect on your childhood, but let it stop there. Avoid the temptation to dip into your past for scapegoats — quit blaming your present behavior on what happened to you ten or fifteen years ago. You can make decisions now that will help erase the past and its unhappiness *if* you accept responsibility for yourself.

Decide that you are going to appreciate yourself and others, no matter what. Happiness comes when you realize your own sense of intellect, beauty, worth, and personality.

Three of the keys to happiness — and to a high sense of self-esteem — lie in your development of a sense of values, your ability to make sound decisions, and your ability to set and reach your goals.

38

VALUE SYSTEMS

Self-worth is inherently related to the fulfillment of morals, standards, and values — to the understanding of right and wrong behavior.

No one can develop a set of values for you; you must decide what is important to you — what will allow you the highest degree of growth and attainment. You must search within yourself to decide what reflects the wrong and the right in behavior. In establishing a set of values for yourself, you might consider your own experience (real or vicarious), your religious beliefs, science and art, and the traditions and customs that surround the culture you have embraced.

As you decide which values to accept, you must also make the difficult decision about which values to reject. One clever doctor outlined a few of the values common in our society that he feels deserve a critical examination:[5]

1. **Happiness is linked to possessions.** The current line of thought seems to run like this: the more things you have, the happier you are; the way to become happier is to accumulate more things. Too often, we measure ourselves in terms of what we have instead of in terms of what we are. If we extend this view to others, they begin to feel like possessions numbered among our many other possessions. They fail to realize how unique and valuable they are, and we eventually fall into the same trap.

2. **You can measure happiness by your accomplishments.** What you achieve is important, but it is not as important as what you *are*. It is hard to separate the two, but try this: take away everything that you have ever done. Strip yourself of roles, throw away your badges, discard all your titles, take your diploma off the wall above your desk. What you are left with is the basic: it is what you are. How comfortable do you feel with that core of yours? When you have developed a high self-esteem, you will feel comfortable, happy, important, special, and worthwhile to yourself.

    You can extend this feeling to others. Once you have learned to separate what you do from what you are, you can make important distinctions with other people. You can tell a child, "I like you, but I don't like what you just did." You can tell a depressed roommate, "You failed at something, but you are not a failure."

3. **We are all alike.** Sure, we have similarities, but each of us is a unique person with individual needs and souls. We cannot be alike — nor should we be alike. We need to stop trying to make everyone be like us, and we need to stop trying to be like everyone else. Learn to respect differences — they are what make us interesting.

4. **If you are happy, you have no problems.** Too many people define mental health as the absence of problems. In reality, mental health consists of the ability to cope with problems. As humans, we are all bound to occasionally experience some hurt, some boredom, some loneliness, and some frustration — and to think that we won't is a grand delusion. Instead of believing that we must avoid problems, we need to concentrate on ways to cope with problems — ways to improve our lives by turning rough spots into stepping stones.

Your own set of values should contain truth and morality, but it should also include the behaviors that help you recognize your own worth and the worth of others. Once you have developed your own values system, it will serve as a guide in helping you make important decisions throughout your life.

MAKING DECISIONS

Every day our lives are filled with decisions. Some are small — what clothing to wear, what to eat for lunch, which book to read next. Others are pivotal, life-shaping decisions that may change the course of life — who to marry, what occupation to pursue, how to handle a roommate who stole a copy of next week's law exam. Sometimes the hardest decision of all is simply to make a decision instead of evading the issue at hand.

Too often we choose not to choose. We let circumstances push us along, and we become what those circumstances dictate. Too many of us have no direction — we really do not know where we are going in life, and we have not made some of the most important decisions of all: what we want to become, and how we will accomplish it.

No one can avoid making decisions. Perhaps one of the greatest opportunities and fulfillments of your life is the freedom to direct your life. Of course, there are religious, legal, social, and cultural restraints, but your options are greater now than to any collective group of people throughout history. Two hundred years ago, your entire life might have been controlled by where you were born. Before the Industrial Revolution, the lives of people were tied up in the basics: getting the wheat planted, making the soap, harvesting the corn. All of the decisions were centered around meeting the basic needs of food, water, shelter, and warmth. There simply wasn't time to worry about the growth needs — the need for justice, beauty, goodness.

All of the small decisions that you make work together to help determine your personality. Each decision that you make carries with it a consequence, and the way in which you handle those consequences also helps to determine your personality.

One of the most crucial processes that you will ever learn is making decisions — but too many of us never learn! Most of our decisions are haphazard at best, and we seem to manage our lives from one crisis to the next. Planning ahead — making important decisions — will allow you to take control of your life as much as is possible.

The decision-making process is made up of three vital steps: planning, acting, and evaluating.

Planning

First, identify the decision that you have to make. This sounds obvious, but too often we do not even realize when we have the chance

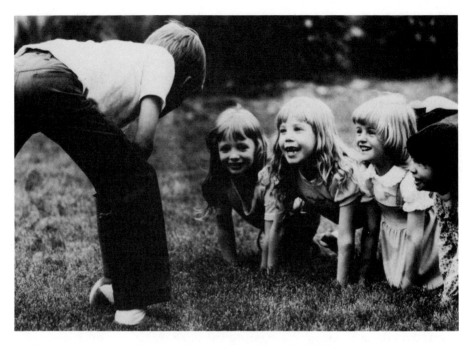

We are enhanced when we are involved.

to make a choice. If the decision is a broad one, you might consider tackling it in pieces, narrowing and isolating each facet to simplify the whole.

Once you have identified your decision, four steps are involved in planning:

1. **List the possible alternatives.** Use a pencil and paper — it will clarify your thinking. List as many alternatives as you can possibly come up with; do not worry at first about listing only the feasible ones, but list anything that pops into your mind. Then go through your list of alternatives, one by one, and try to identify the possible consequences of each one. How does each one fit into your time limit? Is each one feasible? What would be the projected results of each one? Review the list carefully, and eliminate any alternative that would not be a good one — throw out the ones with too may undesirable consequences, not enough good results, or those that simply will not work for you.

42

2. **Prioritize.** Plenty of factors go into every decision. Figure out which ones are the most important to you, then use your list of priorities to assist you in making the decision. In deciding which shirt to buy, for example, price might not be as important to you as wearability, excellent workmanship, and style. If style is your top priority, you would automatically reject any shirt that did not conform to that style; you would examine workmanship, wearability, and price as secondary considerations.

3. **Identify your resources and gather information.** If others will be affected by your situation, check with them. Gather as much information as you can about the decision that you have to make — talk to others who have recently had to make a similar decision, consult an expert in the field, or hit the books at the college library. While you might want to ask for others' opinions, you should not let them make your decision for you — simply add their opinions to your list of resources, and keep it at that.

4. **Anticipate the benefits of your decision.** Sometimes you will have no difficulty in making a decision — one solution may stand out, or you may automatically eliminate all but one alternative because they conflict with your basic values. But more often than not, you will need to decide between several alternatives. If you are in such a bind, try to imagine what will happen as a consequence of each choice. Consider what kinds of obstacles you will have to overcome in each situation. Use a pencil and paper. Write each alternative, and list possible good and bad reasons for choosing each one. If you can, rate each one according to its importance. You will probably need to continue research at this point.

Acting

To put it simply, go ahead: make your decision! An old Chinese proverb admonishes that the hardest part of any journey is the first step. Once you have committed yourself, move forward with determination. Do not spend too much time on the planning phase; do not be so engrossed with gathering information that you miss the chance to move while the time is right. One businessman wisely observed that making a wrong decision is better than making no decision at all — you can regroup and recover from a wrong decision, but you can can never recapture a lost opportunity.

> "The life of every man is a diary in which he means to write one story, and writes another; and his humblest hour is when he compares the volume as it is with what he hoped to make it."
>
> — James Barrie,
> British Playwright

Evaluating

Too many people leave this step out, yet it is the key to being able to make a better decision the next time around. To evaluate your decision, honestly and objectively analyze the results of the decision. Are you pleased with the results? Why, or why not? How could the circumstances be improved? Did you forget to consider a few alternatives that might have worked? Did you overlook an obvious (and painful!) obstacle? Did you neglect your own emotions? Was there someone else who could have helped you see things more clearly?

It is tough to face your own mistakes, but you can learn from them, grow a little in the process, and make a better decision the next time if you have the courage to examine your mistakes with the same gusto as you savor your victories.

SETTING GOALS

A goal is your expectation of accomplishment.[6] The ability to set and achieve goals is important to every aspect of health. Achieving goals can give you a sense of self-worth and can enhance your self-esteem. Setting goals gives you something for which to live, something to anticipate. Goals give direction to your decisions: you make certain decisions because you want to achieve certain goals. And your goals help to shape the set of values that you decide to adopt.

Basically, a life without goals is an empty, purposeless life. Without goals, there is nothing for which to reach, nothing to achieve. Decisions become meaningless, values are empty. Self-esteem plummets.

You may have never given much thought to your goals; you may even believe that you do not have any specific goals. You might be

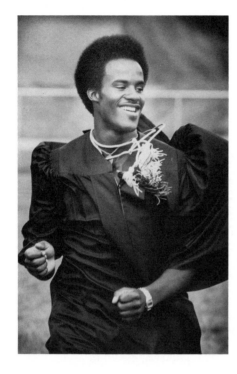

Setting and reaching realistic goals greatly enhance a feeling of self-worth.

surprised: many of the vague thoughts that you have entertained about your future are, in reality, goals to be sought and won.

There are five basic rules to consider in setting goals:[7]

1. Make your goals personal. When your goal is personal, it means a lot to you, and you are motivated to achieve it. A goal that you set for other reasons will not hold the allegiance, and you will be easily driven off course.
2. When you write down your goals, state them in positive terms rather than negative ones. "I want to be slim" instead of "I don't want to be fat" gives you a healthier, more positive outlook that will give you impetus to reach your goal.
3. Write down your goals. No one has a perfect memory, and no one can keep tens of thousands of details straight in his mind forever. When you write your goals down, they crystallize — you see them in an organized way. You are forced to concentrate on them, to keep on track.

> "A person who doubts himself is like a man who would enlist in the ranks of his enemies and bear arms against himself. He makes his failure certain by himself being the first person convinced of it."
>
> — Alexander Dumas

4. Set goals that are attainable. You might want to become president of the United States — but is that really reachable for you? Do you have the time and the money to enter the political arena? Most important, is becoming president a goal that is *compatible* with your other goals? If your other goals are to be a good mother by spending plenty of time with your children, to get a law degree, and to live in Oregon, then perhaps you should revise your presidential goal. Each goal that you make should be compatible with your other goals and should be attainable — forget those that are obviously out of the realm of possibilities.

5. At least a few of your goals should include some behavior change. Concentrate on what you want to *be* instead of what you want to *have*.

Types of Goals

No matter what kind of goal you establish, it will fall into one (or sometimes more) of the basic areas of your life: career and financial, physical, family and home, ethical and spiritual, mental and emotional, or social and cultural. You may want to categorize your goals so that you can achieve a balance in your life. Do not make ten physical goals (lose weight, learn to play racquetball, stop biting nails) while ignoring the social or career areas of your life. Strive for a balance, including goals from each area of your life.

No matter which area of your life your goal affects, there are four basic kinds of goals:[8]

1. **Short-range.** A short-range goal may be something that you aim to do by the end of the day, week, or month. Any goal that you want to achieve within a six-month period is generally considered to be

short-range. Short-range goals keep our lives interesting; they provide the spice we need from time to time. We all need short-range goals to give us a continuing sense of accomplishment — no one can wait only for something that lies twenty years down the road. We all need a pat on the back more often than that!

2. **Long-range.** While short-range goals provide us with daily or weekly direction, long-range goals — those that will take a year or more to achieve — give us direction and fiber of a pivotal nature. A long-range goal gives us basic meaning; long-range goals often affect short-range goals. If you have a long-range goal of getting a law degree, you will set up short-range goals that dictate which classes you will take during your first semester at college.

3. **Tangible.** A tangible goal involves anything that is concrete: a new house, a new car, more money, a college degree.

4. **Intangible.** Intangible goals are more difficult to make and more difficult to attain, because they deal with personality characteristics and behavior modifications that cannot be looked at. A goal to become more concerned about other people is an intangible goal; wanting to give a friend a hundred dollars is a tangible goal.

Whatever kind of goal you decide to set, keep this basic rule in mind: keep your goal simple, and set only a few goals. Setting ten goals to achieve by the end of the day will probably end in frustration and a deflated sense of self-esteem; setting three goals for the end of the day, on the other hand, can result in a sense of accomplishment and winning.

The Process

Ready to start setting goals? Follow these steps for each goal that you make:

1. Write down your goal. Be as specific as you can, including as many details as you have thought about. Be clear. This first step is important: you are crystallizing your thoughts, preparing to make a definite plan. Take the time here to make sure of your thoughts.

2. Ask yourself some important questions about the goal that you have written down. First, and probably most important: is this goal important to you? Weed out what is not really important — a process

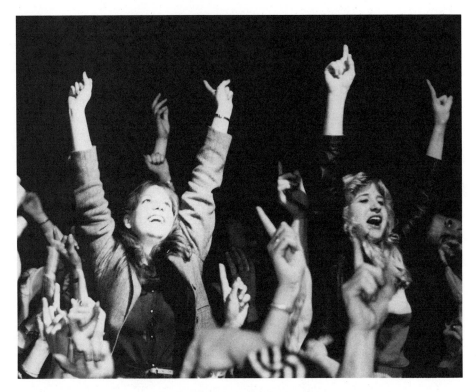

Winning is best when it is shared.

that calls for setting priorities. We are each blessed with twenty-four hours in a day, seven days a week — no more, no less. Stick to the basics, the things that have value to you. Do not clutter yourself with goals that will not matter a year from now.

Is your goal realistic? Is it specific? Is it positive? Does your goal have a time limit?

3. Rewrite your goal as a result of the questions that you asked yourself. Consider your priorities and your abilities. If the goal has a time limit, make sure that you consider it. As you rewrite, make sure that the goal is positive, realistic, and specific.

4. Decide exactly what you need to do to reach your goal. Decide what information you will need, what experience you should gain, what money you will have to spend, what skills you will have to develop, and what arrangements you will need to make to reach your goal.

> "You cannot run away from a weakness; you must sometimes fight it out or perish. And if that be so, why not now, and where you stand?"
>
> — Robert Louis Stevenson

Maybe you want to be a doctor. Write down all the actions that you will need to take: you will have to attend medical school. To go to medical school, you will need a certain amount of money. You will also need to achieve a certain grade-point average in college, and you will need to take certain courses in college to prepare yourself for medical school. You will have to cultivate some good contacts that can provide you with references. You need to gather information about medical schools and make a decision about which one you would like to attend; you need to send for applications and catalogs.

5. Plot your course of action. Decide what you will need to do, how long each will take, and when you aim to have each step completed. For example, you are saving money for medical school; you will save $2,000 each year as a result of your part-time job and $4,500 each year as a result of your summer job. By the time you enroll in medical school, you figure that you will have saved approximately $26,000. Will it be enough to finance your complete medical education?

We all have goals — at least some vague ones — yet we hurry around, living our lives amid clutter and bustle that really means little. Use your goals to give you a sense of purpose and direction. Define what you want, and then work toward it. Make sure that you do something each week toward at least one goal. These little steps will become the mortar in the brick of your life — they will have the power to give strength that will fortify you against whatever may come your way.

Notes

1. This and the two following examples are taken from studies reported in A. B. Abramovitz, *Basic Prevention: Its Nature and Value* (Madison, Wisconsin: Wisconsin State Board of Health), pp. 2-3.

2. Coopersmith's study is reported in Floyd Miller, "What Every Child Needs Most," *Reader's Digest*, January 1969.
3. Ibid.
4. Wayne W. Dyer, *Your Erroneous Zones* (New York: Avon Books, 1976), p. 133.
5. Dr. Darold A. Treffert, "Five Dangerous Ideas Our Children Have About Life," *Family Weekly*, September 19, 1976.
6. Paul Mussen and Mark R. Rosenzweig, *Psychology: An Introduction* (Lexington: D. C. Health and Company, 1973), p. 163.
7. Carolyn Monson, "Power to Attain Lies in Goal Setting," *Salt Lake Tribune*, January 4, 1981, p. W-2.
8. Ibid.

Self-Evaluation

How Happy Are You?

Have you ever wondered exactly how happy you are? Read each of the following questions below, and answer each either "yes" or "no," depending on which best describes your thoughts or behavior. If you fall somewhere in between, circle the response that comes closest to describing you.

Yes	No	1.	I live in an area of small population.
Yes	No	2.	I think that I have lots of responsibilities.
Yes	No	3.	I am able to act natural and be myself in most situations.
Yes	No	4.	I have enough money to meet my basic needs, but I am not wealthy.
Yes	No	5.	I feel that my job is ideally suited to my abilities, and I am able to excel in it.
Yes	No	6.	I enjoy doing favors for other people if it is convenient for me and if I feel it will really help them.
Yes	No	7.	I have little trouble falling asleep, and I am a pretty sound sleeper.
Yes	No	8.	I like to have my surroundings neat and clean, but I am not obsessed with cleanliness and order.
Yes	No	9.	I am rarely physically ill.
Yes	No	10.	I try to be punctual.
Yes	No	11.	I get angry with others occasionally, but I do not often hold a grudge.
Yes	No	12.	Days seem to fly by, but weeks and months seem to pass more slowly for me.
Yes	No	13.	While my situation is not the best, it is okay, and it is improving steadily.
Yes	No	14.	I do not consider myself to be incredibly good looking.
Yes	No	15.	My signature is rather bold and large.
Yes	No	16.	I consider myself to be physically fit.
Yes	No	17.	I am a hard worker.
Yes	No	18.	I sleep eight hours or less each night.

Yes   No   19.   I enjoy using my imagination to come up with unusual or different ways of approaching problems or situations in my life.

Yes   No   20.   I think that my own thoughts control my happiness, not what happens to me.

Scoring: In each instance, the "Yes" response reflects the thoughts or behaviors most often associated with happy people. The more "Yes" answers you circled, the more likely you are to be happy and satisfied with your situation in life.

What Is Your Self-Esteem?

The Barksdale Foundation, an organization dedicated to human understanding, developed the following self-esteem evaluation. To find out how you really feel about yourself, score each of the statements as follows:

0 = not at all true for me
1 = partly true or true part of the time
2 = fairly true or true about half of the time
3 = mainly true or true most of the time
4 = true all of the time

Score		Self-Esteem Statements
_____	1.	I do not feel that anyone else is better than I am.
_____	2.	I am free of shame, blame, and guilt.
_____	3.	I am a happy, carefree person.
_____	4.	I have no need to prove I am as good as or better than others.
_____	5.	I do not have a strong need for people to pay attention to me or like what I do.
_____	6.	Losing does not upset me or make me feel "less than" others.
_____	7.	I feel warm and friendly toward myself.
_____	8.	I do not feel that others are better than I am because they can do things better, have more money, or are more popular.
_____	9.	I am at ease with strangers and make friends easily.

52

_____ 10. I speak up for my own ideas, likes, and dislikes.

_____ 11. I am not hurt by others' opinions or attitudes.

_____ 12. I do not need praise to feel good about myself.

_____ 13. I feel good about others' good luck and winning.

_____ 14. I do not find fault with my family, friends, or others.

_____ 15. I do not feel that I must always please others.

_____ 16. I am open and honest and not afraid of letting people see my real self.

_____ 17. I am friendly, thoughtful, and generous toward others.

_____ 18. I do not blame others for my problems and mistakes.

_____ 19. I enjoy being alone with myself.

_____ 20. I accept compliments and gifts without feeling ashamed or "less than" others.

_____ 21. I admit my mistakes and defeats without feeling ashamed.

_____ 22. I feel no need to defend what I think, say, or do.

_____ 23. I do not need others to agree with me or tell me that I'm right.

_____ 24. I do not brag about myself, what I have done, or what my family has or does.

_____ 25. I do not feel "put down" when criticized by my friends or others.

Scoring: Add all the scores together to get the sum of all scores, or your self-esteem index. Your score reflects the following:

95 or above   Sound self esteem
75-90   You are at a disadvantage
50-75   You are at a serious disadvantage
Less than 50   You have a crippling lack of self-esteem

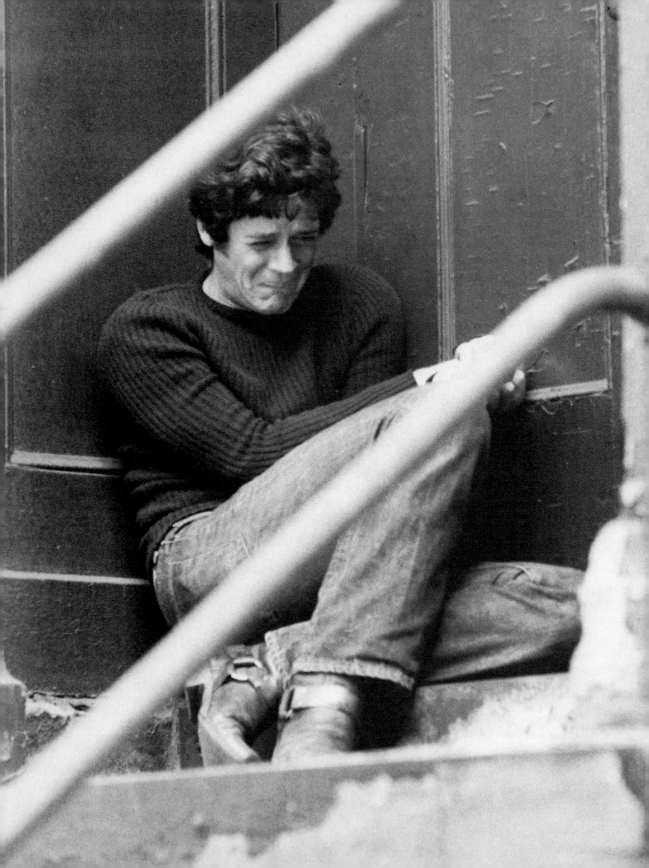

3
Coping and Adjusting: Dealings with Feelings

Life is filled with crises; no one can escape them, because they are part of being alive. As a result, each of us suffers a kind of stress that accompanies each crisis.

You have probably noticed that some people seem to sail along smoothly, with hardly a ripple upsetting their course, while others seem to be tossed furiously on the crest of thundering waves, smashed into craggy rocks along the way. We each inherit and develop abilities that enable us to deal with crisis and its ensuing stress; the difference between healthy and unhealthy people is the ability to *manage* that stress. Continued physical health seems to depend on the ability to deal with — not simply evade — stress.[1]

You can take an active part in beginning to manage the stress and the crises in your life; you can change your ability to adjust and cope. Remember, the Chinese word for "crises" is written with two symbols: one characterizing danger, and the other representing opportunity.[2]

WHAT IS CRISIS?

In psychosocial terms, a crisis is a state of temporary disequilibrium brought on by unavoidable life changes.[3] Crises are considered to be temporary, because in a healthy individual, the personality systems and defenses correct a crisis-induced imbalance within a few weeks or months. The steady, usual pattern of the individual's life is disrupted only until the body defenses have a chance to compensate.

The causes of some crises may be easy to identify, but in other cases the causes are underlying and elusive. A state of crisis may begin in anticipation before the event actually takes place — a college senior, for example, may anticipate his father's death from cancer and may enter a crisis state before his father ever dies. A crisis may also be precipitated by an event that seems mild but reminds the individual of a past crisis. One seven-year-old girl did not cry at all when her mother died, but when her kitten was killed, she experienced the grief all over again and this time was able to cry and release her feelings.

Most of the life changes that bring crisis involve relationships with other people. If a crisis is to occur, the situation must be a "no exit" one; the demand for change must be unavoidable, and the situation must be one that cannot be changed or escaped. Once such a change occurs, the individual's mental and emotional health will determine his ability to cope with the change and reduce its effects on his life.

Certain characteristics enable an individual to better cope with a crisis situation. The capacity to orient quickly to change is helpful, as is the ability to plan and make decisions in the face of change. An individual who can call on others for help and who can recognize his own need for help is better equipped to deal with crisis than is an individual who becomes paralyzed or disoriented and does not recognize the need for a helping hand.

The result of inability to cope with crisis and the change it brings is often physical and/or emotional illness.

WHAT HAPPENS DURING CRISIS? ▬▬▬▬▬▬▬

Four major phases describe what happens to an individual who faces crisis.

1. **Impact.** When the crisis first hits, the impact brings on a state of dazed shock that lasts for several hours. Because most crisis situations involve a loss — loss of a job, loss of status, loss of a loved one

56

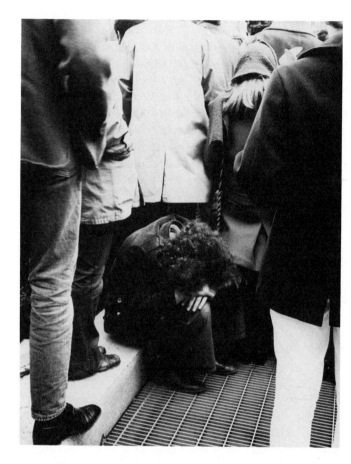

Depression is a low-down feeling.

— the impact phase consists of the individual's searching for the lost object and reminiscing about the lost object.

2. **Recoil/Turmoil.** Within several hours, the individual enters the recoil/turmoil phase, a period marked by depression, rage, anxiety, and guilt. The individual becomes detached and confused. This stage of ambiguity and uncertainty generally lasts for several days while the individual relives the past and tries to sort out the events of the crisis in his mind.

3. **Adjustment.** The adjustment phase begins as the individual begins to explore alternatives to replace his loss. A man who was fired begins making positive plans for finding a new job. A couple whose

freedom and sense of privacy was lost when their new baby was born searches for new ways of experiencing those lost senses while they enjoy their new baby. A college student who does not make the football team after a brilliant high school career begins to assess other activities in which he can excel at college. During the adjustment phase, the individual's thoughts are centered on the future, and he generally approaches the task with an attitude of hope and aggressive problem solving. He acts instead of reacting.

4. **Reconstruction.** In this final phase, the individual tests alternatives and reattaches himself over a period of several months. A woman who was laid off and who then made positive plans for finding another corporate-level position now moves forward with new determination, making appointments with prospective employers and brushing up her resume; once hired, she makes new attachments that will replace the ones at her previous job. Again, the individual's thoughts and efforts concentrate on the future, and her attitude is one of hope.

COPING WITH CRISIS

A person who is able to cope with crisis is one who is aware of the fact that he is suffering; he freely expresses his feelings of pain, frustration, or indecision. Healthy coping, however, is *not* marked by excessive or prolonged ventilation of emotion — in other words, scream loudly, but briefly! The healthy individual vents his frustrations in ways that are not destructive, and he reaches out for help and assistance. At some point along the way, he recognizes the opportunity for growth and challenge that accompanies the crisis.[4]

Here are some simple steps that you can take when confronted with a crisis. No matter how difficult they seem at first, plunge in.

1. **Decide what is causing the problem.** Look toward, not away from, your problems and feelings — you cannot begin to work out a solution until you identify a cause. This seems like a frightening step to take, but you will find that knowledge often kills fear. Once you find out more about what is causing your feelings, you can get a grip on them.

TRADITIONAL VALUES

"Religion and other moral traditions are not only useful, but scientifically valid," according to Dr. Donald T. Campbell, past president of the American Psychological Association.

At a convention in Chicago, Campbell chided his fellow psychologists for their belief in self-gratification over self-restraint, and their inclination to regard "guilt" as a "neurotic symptom."

A report in *TIME Magazine* says, "Campbell believes that there is a biological basis in favor of self-seeking, uninhibited behavior. To counter the bias, societies have evolved strong ethical and religious rules favoring the group over the individual."

Thus, "Love thy neighbor" and "Honor thy parents" serve as brakes on too much antisocial behavior. These commands were absolute and uncompromising in order to balance out the biological bias in the opposite direction.

"Psychiatrists and psychologists have assumed that the human impulses provided by biological evolution are right, and that regressive or inhibiting moral traditions are not."

Campbell said, "In the light of recent work in population genetics, this assumption may now be regarded as scientifically wrong, in my judgment."

Campbell urged the group to revise their teaching of the young so as to remove "any arrogant scientistic certainty that psychology's current beliefs are the final truth of these matters."

"All the dominant modern psychologies," he stated, "are individually hedonistic, explaining all human behavior in terms of individual pain and pleasure, individual needs and drives."

Campbell called on the professionals to "broaden our narrowly individualistic focus" and to begin studying social systems with the assumption of "an underlying wisdom in the recipes of living that tradition has supplied us. They might be better tested than the best of psychology's and psychiatry's speculations on how lives should be lived."

Try keeping a journal; as you write about your problems, you can isolate them and begin to think of how to solve your dilemma. Reviewing journals from the past allows you to relive other times of depression or tension when you mobilized your resources and pulled through. A father who had lost his son in a tragic accident pulled out an earlier journal and reread the entry that he had written after witnessing the boy's birth. The father wept afterward, but he appreciated the joy of his son's companionship for those short years more fully. This appreciation helped to start the healing process.

2. **Learn to accept what you cannot change.** Realize that the only person who you can change is yourself — you are the only person over whom you have total control. You have no control over most things and never will; you cannot right every injustice, nor can you make people over. You must come to the realization that you cannot change many situations — you can only learn to cope with them and adjust to them.

3. **Share your worries with someone else.** Verbalizing your problems and fears to someone who you love, trust, or respect helps to relieve the stress and often helps you to discover alternatives that otherwise might have escaped your eye. A good confidante will listen empathetically, and he will often ask questions that will help you to explore your feelings honestly. One young engineer said that he always talked his work problems — even the technical ones — over with his wife. "Does she understand everything you tell her about engineering?" a colleague asked him. "No, not always," answered the engineer, "but when I'm done, I do."

4. **Get enough exercise.** Exercise has all sorts of benefits: one of the greatest is that it provides a physical release for the pent-up rage and hostility that accompany a crisis. The physical changes that your body undergoes during a crisis are the same ones that it experiences in reaction to danger — and that physical and mental tension can be worked off physically. Choose any kind of exercise that will relieve your boredom, excite your senses, and provide you with fun and relaxation — jogging, tennis, swimming, handball, or walking are good ones to try. You will find that as you concentrate on your exercise, your mind will be diverted from your problems — and you will be refreshed enough later to tackle them with new vigor.

5. **Avoid self-medication.** Reaching for a bottle — whether it is filled with alcohol or pills — does not teach you to cope with a crisis. Your problems are still there when you come out of the stupor, and sometimes they have become even worse because you did not act on them immediately. Your crisis may be causing you pain, but do not add the extra pain of dependence on alcohol or drugs.

6. **Serve others.** Avoid the cesspool of self-pity; do something for someone else, and you will find yourself thinking of them instead of your crisis. Learn to love people and use things, rather than love things and use people.

7. **Avoid loneliness.** You will undoubtedly need some time alone to

LONELINESS KILLS

Anyone who has ever felt lonely — and that stacks up to include almost everyone — knows the sorrow and sense of isolation that can accompany it. But loneliness isn't just a pitiable and temporary social condition: if it's prolonged enough, loneliness can actually kill you.

The deterioration from loneliness is first emotional, then physical; studies have long shown that single, divorced, and widowed people fall prey to diseases of all kinds much more frequently than do married people. (For example, widows between the ages of twenty-five and thirty-four are five times more likely to develop coronary disease leading to death than are married women in the same age group; divorced white males are ten times more likely to develop tuberculosis than their married counterparts.)

Results of health studies like these point up the importance of strong family ties and the fostering of solid relationships between people.

The reasons for these striking differences can all be boiled down into a simple concept: loneliness kills. The implications for the medical community are vast — patients need to be touched, need to have attention from a doctor instead of simply being given a bottle of pills to cure their ills. And the implications for society as a whole cause us to reach out and look around us.

— Adapted from *Time*,
September 5, 1977, p. 45.

collect your thoughts and sort out your feelings, but the difference between aloneness and loneliness is vast. Withdrawing will not solve the crisis. Keep yourself in touch with those around you who have offered a helping hand.

8. **Try a temporary diversion.** If your well is empty — if you have tried everything and you are at the end of your rope — try a brief diversion to refresh yourself. Go see a funny movie, read a book that you have always been meaning to get around to, or go to a concert with a friend. Cut loose a little bit. You will be refreshed and will find an inner strength to tackle the problem afterward.

9. **Take active management steps.** Once you have identified your problem, create a plan of action for solving it. Try to remember the small details. Keep your options open, and be creative in solving your problems — your solution might not be the one that you originally thought of, but try it anyway.

10. **Assess your priorities.** Uncertainty runs rampant during a crisis. The result? You may find yourself running around like the proverbial chicken with its head cut off. During a time of confusion like a crisis, it is hard to decide what to do first. But take the few valuable minutes required to list on paper your priorities. Decide what is *the* most important thing that you need to do; write that down first. Order the rest of your activities the same way, listing the most important ones first. Then tackle them in that same order — and do not move on down the list to an easier task until you have completed all of the tasks before it.

11. **Have a physical checkup.** A crisis may precipitate a condition mimicking physical illness as a result of sheer stress; if the physical illness lingers, however, see your doctor. A woman who remained ill and depressed after a miscarriage finally consulted her doctor, who discovered that she had diabetes. With treatment, she was able to bounce back from the crisis of the miscarriage much more easily.

12. **Take care of yourself physically.** Your mother lies critically ill halfway across the country while you nervously pace in your dorm room. You fail an examination critical to your major course of study. Your partner breaks off a three-year relationship that you thought would be permanent. It is tempting to forget all about your normal health routines in a time of crisis — but good health and nutrition are even more important during times of stress and upset. Get plenty of sleep (consult your doctor if you simply are unable to fall asleep for more than a few nights), and eat well-balanced, nourishing meals. It is easy to raid the vending machine and try to exist on candy bars when you are not that interested in food — but remember that nutrition will give you the strength (mental and physical) to combat the situation.

STESS ━━━━━━━━━━━━━━━━━━━━━

"She gives me a pain in the neck!"

"That accident took ten years off my life!"

"Working around him makes me sick!"

"That practically scared me to death!"

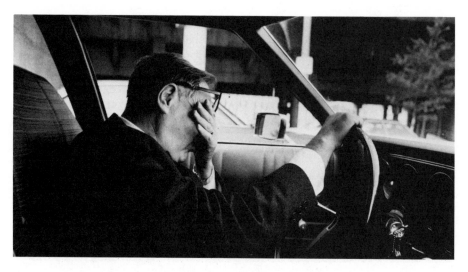

Stress is defined in a medical sense as the wear and tear caused by living.

Meaningless sayings? No. Dealing with an unpleasant person can cause neck pains. A frightening accident can age you. Facing a person who makes you feel uncomfortable or threatened can make you sick, usually with respiratory problems or the common cold. A frightening experience, one that evokes severe enough emotions, can cause death.

Stress is a natural by-product of a crisis. But it is more: stress has been defined in a medical sense as the wear and tear caused by living. The changes that come about during a crisis — and the changes that occur every day as a normal part of living — result in what we call stress as our bodies and our minds react to the changes with emotional tension.

Our very lives begin with one of the most stressful experiences that we will ever encounter: birth. While childbirth is a natural and normal process, it can hardly be pleasant for the baby. The sudden and powerful uterine contractions squeeze the infant, thrusting it into the birth canal and out of the mother's body — launching it into a world of harsh lights and deafening sound in contrast to the dark, warm comfort of the womb. From that moment of birth, stress in some form is always a part of our lives.

We are each under some kind of stress constantly. Some stress is minor: Did I remember to put a dime in the parking meter? Did I unplug the iron before I left the apartment? Other stress is severe: Will I be one of the workers laid off at the plant? Is my husband going to file for divorce if we are to unable to work things out? Will my sister die from complications of the automobile accident? Whatever its intensity, stress is present at all times. If you strive for achievement, you will undergo stress; if you have no challenges in your life, you will experience stress. Stress is, literally, the response of the body to any demand that is placed on it.[5]

Once the body is under stress, it reacts — physically as well as emotionally — to try and normalize things again. In other words, stress demands that the body adjust. That kind of wear and tear takes its toll: as many as 80 percent of all people who go to the doctor do so because of stress-related illnesses.[6] Some doctors believe that all illnesses are at least partially caused by stress.

LESSONS LEARNED FROM THE LABORATORY

From what the laboratory and the clinical study of somatic diseases has taught me concerning stress, I have developed three general principles readily applicable to everyday living. I have summarized these precepts as follows:

1. Find your own natural predilections and stress level. People differ with regard to the amount and kind of work they consider worth doing to meet the exigencies of daily life and to assure their future security and happiness. In this respect, all of us are influenced by hereditary predispositions and the expectations of our society. Only through planned self-analysis can we establish what we really want; many people suffer all their lives because they are too conservative to risk a radical change and break with traditions.
2. Altruistic egoism. The selfish hoarding of the good will, respect, esteem, support, and love of our neighbor is the most efficient way to give vent to our pent-up energy and create enjoyable, beautiful, or useful things.
3. "EARN thy neighbor's love." This motto, unlike "Love thy neighbor as thyself," is compatible with our biological structure; and although it is based on altruistic egoism, it could hardly be attacked as unethical. Who could blame a person who wants to assure homeostasis and happiness by accumulating the treasure of other people's benevolence? Yet this makes one virtually unassailable, for people would not attack and destroy those upon whom they depend.

What it comes down to is:
Fight for your highest attainable aim
But do not put up resistance in vain.
© Hans Selye, 1980 Aspen Systems Corporation

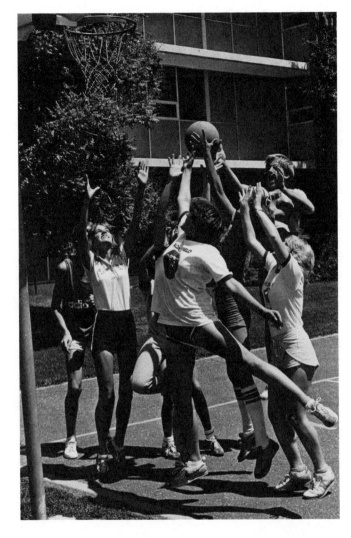

Physical activity helps
to reduce stress.

The kind of stress — and the way in which you adapt to it — determines whether or not your health and life-style will be affected. We all experience short-term stress: we experience a stressful situation, learn to adapt to it, and return to a normal (or near-normal) condition.

The trouble comes when the stress becomes long-term: there is no

THE POSITIVE POWER OF LAUGHING

Could it be possible that, amid all the wonder drugs and potions on the market, the potential for healing lies in a good burst of laughter?

Norman Cousins lay helpless in a hospital bed in 1964 suffering from an irreversible collagen disease that was causing him to literally "come unstuck." The doctors had reached a standstill when Cousins himself decided to be more than just a passive observer. He designed for himself a comprehensive therapy program that included massive doses of Vitamin C — and plenty of good laughter.

Armed with some of the funniest books he could find, he arranged to have film segments of *Candid Camera* brought to the hospital and shown in his room.

The results?

As little as ten minutes of genuine laughter killed his pain and allowed him two hours of deep, pain-free sleep. By laughing his way through, Cousins was able to win the battle and defeat the disease.

Seems the old adage still holds true — laughter *is* the best medicine.

---

clear resolution of the crisis, no real return to equilibrium as one stressful situation follows another with no respite in between. In this kind of long-term stress, the body never returns to normal between periods of stress. Unrelieved, long-term stress cannot be tolerated, and it generally results in mental or physical illness.

What Causes Stress?

Each of us experiences stress as a result of different stimuli in our environment. Because of our individual biological heritage and our unique emotional and intellectual background, each of us reacts differently to the same situation.

The word *stress* is too often darkly colored with negative connotation — we almost always think of stress as a result of bad events in our lives, such as death, divorce, illness, bad luck, or the loss of a job. But it is important to realize that stress also comes from the positive, happy experiences in our lives — the birth of a new baby, marriage, a promotion at work, or being recognized for an outstanding achievement. Negative stress *(distress)* produces a decrease in health and performance; positive stress *(eustress)* usually produces just the opposite.[7] The problem is this:

your mind can distinguish between the two, but your body cannot. Your body reacts the same whether the stress comes from a positive or a negative event. In some cases, you develop anticipatory stress just thinking about an upcoming event; most of the time, the stress that you get from anticipating the event is worse than the stress that you would suffer from the actual event.

What Stress Does to the Body

Whenever you are threatened in any way, your body prepares for "flight or fight" — it gets ready to protect itself. As part of the general adaptation syndrome (see insert), you experience rapid pulse, increased perspiration, a pounding heart, a tightened stomach, tensing of the muscles in the arms and legs, shortness of breath, gritting of the teeth, clenching of the jaw, racing thoughts, and inability to sit still.[8]

As your body adapts to the threatening situation, it undergoes certain changes that allow you to lift a fallen tree off a child, chase a bus, fight off an attacker, or avoid bleeding severely from a crushing internal injury. You are literally thrown into overdrive and are able to escape the perceived danger.

The problem is this: ancient man had the "fight or flight" reaction to enable him to escape from a savage tiger stalking the forest in search of a meal. Today, the same bodily reactions take place in the executive who did not get an expected pay raise or the woman who argues persistently with her mother-in-law. Most of the time, we have no physical outlet for our stress; we do not run across the forest and climb a tree as did the man escaping from the tiger. We simply sit and stew — and the stress takes an incredible toll in wear and tear on our bodies.

When the stress becomes chronic — lasting for weeks or months or even years — the body systems literally breakdown. You lose your appetite, feel nauseated, and experience heartburn; you cannot seem to cry (or, on the other hand, you burst into tears for no obvious reason). You experience high blood pressure, frequent headaches, chronic diarrhea, and dizziness, to name only a few physical symptoms. Mentally, you feel anxious, irritable, frustrated, depressed, and, in the extreme, self-destructive.

A young divorcee struggling to rear and support her children as a single parent may face stress for many years. A man born without legs

FEELING THREATENED?
HERE'S HOW YOU REACT

Do you feel threatened — by a relationship, a situation, or even by yourself? Human beings react in three distinct stages to any threatening situation — and the set of signs and symptoms that occurs is called the general adaptation syndrome. The three stages of the syndrome are:

1. ALARM. The body automatically prepares to defend itself, and the results can be seen or felt throughout the body. The muscles — especially those in the face, neck, and back — tense up. The stomach muscle also contracts, and feels like it is tied in knots. (If stress is unrelieved, ulcers result.)

   The adrenal glands — one sitting on top of each kidney — begin to pour adrenalin into the blood. The adrenalin production acts like a red alert to the body warning it to prepare for "flight or fight" — blood pressure increases, heart rate speeds, breathing gets faster, and blood is diverted from other body systems to the muscles. Palms sweat, and the mouth gets dry. Noradrenalin and lactate, a substance formed when muscles contract, appear in the blood.

2. RESISTANCE. Here your body reacts to protect itself again — almost like easing a racing engine by putting in the clutch before the brakes are applied. During resistance, body resources are mobilized to overcome the flight or fight response: internal systems return to normal, requiring total energy, and the individual switches his energy focus from the physical to the mental.

   Resistance is a form of adjustment, and it lasts until the stressor ceases. If the stressor continues over a long period of time, however, the body's ability to resist is lost, and exhaustion sets in.

3. EXHAUSTION. If days, weeks, or even months pass without relief from the feeling of peril — a state of jeopardy that can accompany extended financial problems, for example — the original signs and symptoms of the alarm stage return. The resulting storm can be devastating, since the body's resources were depleted during the original syndrome. Even a small amount of stress at this point is crucial. If the stress cannot be stopped or relieved, sickness or even death may result; the individual suffers a physical and psychological breakdown.

Studies of animals under stress conducted by Dr. Hans Selye at the University of Montreal showed that continued stress resulted in enlarged adrenal glands with loss of steroids, decreased level of salt in the blood, and malfunction of the kidneys. As the animals died from exhaustion, it seemed they had been killed by an excess of hormones their bodies had produced in defense. (See Hans Selye, *The Stress of Life,* New York, New York: McGraw-Hill, 1956.)

faces a personal Gethsemane every day fighting the physical barriers that his handicap hurls in his way while he tries to win acceptance and understanding from others; he may labor a lifetime under stress factors. In instances like these, where stress is extremely prolonged, it can literally wear out the body.[9]

Who Is Most Prone to Stress?

Each of us experiences an individual response to stress; you do not react to it in the same way that your roommate does. Researchers have found that people with certain personality traits cope more poorly with stress, while other personality traits enable people to cope more effectively with stress. As a result, researchers have stretched the human race along an axis from the poles of two general personality types: Type A and Type B.[10]

Many of us exhibit a combination of traits along the continuum between each personality extremity; studying the extremes, however, teaches us about stress and about the ways in which we can learn to cope with it.

Type-A Personality

The Type-A individual copes poorly with stress and is most likely to develop a stress-related illness. But there is an additional, more serious problem: a Type-A individual actually *creates* stress for himself by the way in which he lives and through his behavior patterns.

The individual with a Type-A personality exhibits the following traits:

- Is extremely competitive; likes to win
- Is schedule- and time-oriented
- Tries to cram too much work into too little time
- Is extremely concerned with success and social acceptance
- Is numbers-oriented (counts successes, possessions, achievements)
- Is a rapid talker
- Is not content with working on one project at a time

69

IDENTIFYING THE TYPE A PERSONALITY

Type A personalities, according to Drs. Friedman and Rosenman, come in three varieties: the fully developed, hard-core type; the moderate; and the borderline. The hard-core type is presumably in greatest jeopardy of developing coronary artery disease. The identifying signs listed here describe this highest risk person.

- A major sign is a chronic sense of time urgency; if he could stretch indefinitely the number of hours in the day, he still wouldn't find time enough to do all the things he's planned. He's locked in an endless struggle to do more and more in less and less time.
- Another major sign is his free-floating hostility. He may keep his hostility hidden — he's probably not even aware he has it — but there's a hint of rancor and angry competitiveness in virtually all his activities. He can never play a game of tennis, for example, without treating his opponent as an enemy he must beat at all costs. He can't converse on a controversial subject without bristling, fuming, and insulting his "opponents."
- He's utterly convinced that the key to success lies in the ability to get things done faster than others; he's afraid to pause in his frenetic activities, lest his competitors surpass him.
- He has certain characteristic mannerisms: an explosive speech pattern and a tendency to accelerate on the last few words of his sentences (he's even too impatient to speak); he always walks, talks, and eats rapidly, and he has a bagful of nervous tics — habitually clenching his fists or jaws, grinding his teeth, jerking the corners of his mouth, and exposing his teeth.
- He's chronically impatient with the sluggish pace of everything surrounding him. People talk too slowly for him; he's always rushing them along by finishing their sentences. The car in front of him is holding up progress. He's furious at having to stand in lines. And he has no time to read anything except condensations and summaries.
- His head spins with a dozen different thoughts at once. While shaving or having breakfast, he's reading a business or professional journal, mulling over business problems, and thinking about what he should have said to so-and-so.
- He can't talk to anyone about anything except what interests him. If he can't turn the conversation to suit him, he pretends to listen and then drifts off into his own world.
- He feels vaguely guilty — not simply uncomfortable — when he relaxes or does nothing for several hours or days.
- He has no time, it seems to do the things really worth doing because he's up to his neck trying to grab for things worth having.

- Sets several goals at once (often unrealistic)
- Is punctual and is intolerant of those who are not
- Appears outwardly confident but is inwardly insecure
- Is impatient, hates to wait
- Has a tendency to tackle several activities at once (dictates into a tape recorder while driving, eats lunch while working at desk)
- Feels guilty while relaxing or slowing down
- Dominates or interrupts conversations
- Has nervous gestures or tics
- Is easily upset by others
- Is hostile and aggressive toward those whom he perceives as "competition"

These natural pushers and go-getters, with their overabundance of ambition, suffer. They pace themselves, rising quickly through the ranks, experiencing real success early in their careers. But then comes the tragedy: the Type-A personality burns up from his high degree of involvement. He literally crashes and flames out.

Why?

Because his mind and his body simply cannot keep up with the pace; the stresses that he has suffered on his way to the top has literally torn up his body. He is exhausted and depressed; he loses interest in activities outside of work, but his enjoyment on the job disappears, too. He tries harder but even then cannot achieve what he did before.

Soon the physical problems set in. The Type-A personality often develops headaches, muscle spasms, lethargy, increase in appetite, sluggishness, fatigue, and inability to relax. Because they tend to hurry to finish jobs more quickly, Type-A individuals are more prone to accidents on the job. Type-A individuals have also been isolated as those more likely to develop heart disease.

Type-B Personality

The Type-B personality is opposite the Type-A personality: he copes better with stress, partly because he does not create stress for himself. Type-B personalities have the following characteristics:

- Is easygoing

- Is seldom impatient; is content waiting for the bus, the bank teller, or success
- Is able to make decisions easily, without undue influence from others
- Is realistic about what he can achieve
- Is realistic about time schedules
- Does not worry much, especially about the future
- Is much less critical of himself and others
- Is not concerned with petty irritations
- Accepts the fact that he cannot achieve everything at once

The Type-B person is not necessarily lazy or lacking in force — he simply moves ahead through a relaxed, patient, and methodical application of technique, while the Type-A person moves ahead through sheer drive and energy. While the Type-A person pushes frantically forward, working harder and harder and jamming in more assignments as he gives up his leisure time, the Type-B person patiently plods toward

---

WHO'S HAPPY — AND WHY

Happiness. It's something everyone wants; some people have it, and a few never seem to get it. No one has a secret formula for obtaining it, but it's available to everyone without bias.

Ever wonder how to obtain happiness? It doesn't come with youth or wealth. A recent survey of 100,000 Americans does tell us that most of us are happy, and it gives some hints about who seems to be the happiest.

People who love, and who are loved in return, seem to be the happiest; those who are married seem happier than those who are single (especially true with women) or divorced — an explanation for the fact that most people eventually remarry.

Those who are satisfied with their jobs rate high on the happiness scale; working wives, too, seem on the whole to be less worried about their own self-worth. Income and education may be related — and it seems that those with little education who earn a lot are the happiest.

It helps to have a happy childhood and adolescence — but survey results seem to bear out the fact that we are infinitely changeable creatures. To put it simply, you *can* be happy now — no matter how miserable you have been up until now.

---

achieving his goals. While the Type-A person is sitting in his ashes, the Type-B person is enjoying life.

Neither personality type has a corner on intelligence or ambition. Each category includes company presidents, truck drivers, carpenters, fashion models, attorneys, beauticians, and college students. Some doctors believe that Type-B individuals make the better executives: they do not rush decisions, make snap judgments, or antagonize subordinates. In short, they know their capabilities and limitations; Type-A individuals often do not know their own limitations — and do not want to.[11]

Because of the overload of stress that they take upon themselves, Type-A individuals are much more prone to develop a stress-related disease, such as high blood pressure, heart disease, or diabetes.

STRESS AND DISEASE

Originally, disease meant simply a lack of ease — not an illness. Medical researchers unraveled a great puzzle when they discovered that germs cause illness, but a more critical riddle lay in the controversy about what causes the onset of disease. Today, researchers have discovered that life events can help trigger illness: the effort that it takes to cope with certain life events weakens resistance against disease.[12] Emotions have a vast effect on us — they alter the body's hormonal balance, change blood pressure and supply, inhibit digestion, and change our breathing patterns and skin temperature. In other words, our emotions — and the stress that they bring — can cause disease.

How?

Disease development requires three conditions:

1. The presence of bacteria, a virus, or some other disease-causing agent.
2. A host tissue in the body that can be affected by the disease-causing agent (the lung tissue, for example, can be affected by tuberculosis bacteria).
3. An external or internal factor that lowers the body's resistance to the disease-causing factor.

In the presence of bacteria or viruses, stress provides the third critical key: it lowers the body's ability to resist disease and infection.

INFECTION—ALLERGY—STRESS SYNDROME

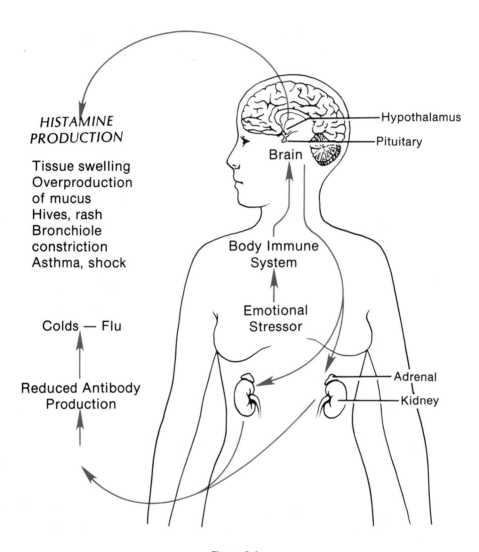

HISTAMINE PRODUCTION

Tissue swelling
Overproduction
of mucus
Hives, rash
Bronchiole
constriction
Asthma, shock

Colds — Flu

Reduced Antibody
Production

Hypothalamus

Pituitary

Brain

Body Immune
System

Emotional
Stressor

Adrenal

Kidney

Figure 3-1.

This decreased resistance renders the body susceptible to an entire range of communicable diseases and to certain other diseases such as heart disease, cancer, and respiratory illness.

Psychosomatic Illness

A number of illnesses are directly related to the amount of stress created by a particular life-style. Those illnesses are psychosomatic: gastric and duodenal ulcers, migraine and tension headaches, colitis, allergic reactions, gum disease, rashes, chronic low back pain, and a number of other diseases.

The origin of the word "psychosomatic" describes it precisely: it is derived from the word *psyche,* meaning mind, and *soma,* meaning body. A psychosomatic illness, then, is one that results from the mind's influence over the body. There is a huge difference between a psychosomatic illness and an illness suffered by a hypochondriac: a psychosomatic disease is caused by the mind, but the symptoms are very real. A gastric ulcer, for instance, is an actual sore in the stomach lining. A hypochondriac, on the other hand, only *thinks* that he is sick. He will suffer the same ulcer symptoms as the psychosomatic victim: heartburn, sharp pains after eating, and stomach discomfort. Examination (including x-ray), however, reveals no ulcer; the hypochondriac's stomach lining is normal. While the hypochondriac suffers symptoms and is convinced that he is ill, the laboratory tests come back negative: he has no illness.

That is where the difference lies. A hypochondriac's illness is imaginary; a psychosomatic illness manifests real tissue damage or dysfunction. Research suggests that all diseases are, in part, influenced by stress — so we are all, at times, victims of psychosomatic disease. But remember — that does not mean that we are all hypochondriacs!

━━━━━━━━━━━━━━━━━━ **TIPS FOR COPING WITH STRESS**

No one can completely escape stress; stress is necessary to life, and it is around us every day. Since you cannot elude stress completely, you need to learn how to manage it instead of letting it manage you.

The most obvious way of coping with stress is to identify all the

BREAKING OUT OF THE TYPE-A RUT

Do you feel so tightly wound up that you're afraid you'll break under the pressure? Colorado State University psychologist Richard M. Suinn contends that you can take steps to eliminate most of your stress by changing your Type-A habits. Here's how:

1. **Learn to relax.** There are as many ways to relax as there are people who need to relax. You can do it almost anywhere — as long as it's quiet, free of interruption, and comfortable. Try listening to some soothing music. Or try deep breathing for ten minutes as you let the tension flow from your body. You might try deep muscle relaxation: alternately tense and then relax the muscles of your arms, legs, chest, stomach, feet, hands, shoulders, and face.

   Once you learn a method that works for you, use it when you feel stressed — retreat to a quiet place for a few minutes, and regain your equilibrium.

2. **Slow down.** You'll feel pressure if you're acting rushed. Make a conscious effort to slow down in every way — walk more slowly, talk at a more relaxed rate, eat more slowly — try putting your fork down between each bite. Be better organized, and allow yourself a few extra minutes to get to class or work. You'll find yourself relaxing when you stop rushing.

3. **Take control of your environment.** You'd be surprised at how much of your stress you create yourself: you set unrealistic goals, you try to please too many people, you schedule your time too tightly, you fail to accomplish what you want to. Allow yourself enough time during the day to get from one activity to another — don't commit to being at a play rehearsal across town ten minutes after your last class is dismissed, for example, or you'll just get upset in the traffic. When you wake up each morning, decide which activities are your priority ones — those things that *have* to be done — and then accomplish them first. Don't move on to other things until you have done what is necessary for the day. And learn how to say "no" — if you don't have time to reasonably accomplish something, don't commit to it. If you do commit, make clear how much you can do by when — in other words, let people know how much they can expect from you. And, perhaps most importantly, schedule some time during the day when you can have a quiet period of relaxation, free from telephone calls and interruptions.

4. **Learn to react differently.** We all face situations that make us tense — and most of us react with some degree of tension. Learn to retrain your reactions — you will need to start with a pencil and paper. Think of a situation that normally makes you tense — perhaps you always get stuck in traffic as you hurry to get to your part-time job downtown. Write down how you normally react; now, re-evaluate. What could you do to make the situation better? How could you react differently to avoid getting so uptight? "Practice" this way with a number of situations until you have a definite set of plans for reducing your tension.

sources of stress in your life. Some you cannot avoid; you cannot change the fact that your mother died last semester. But you *can* eliminate or avoid other sources of stress — do not try to take three difficult physics classes in a single semester, and try finding a new apartment if your room-mate is hopelessly driving you crazy. If you know that certain people start your heart pounding and your blood pressure skyrocketing, avoid them if you can. (If you are related, just try to cut down the number of encounters; no one said that you have to call your sister every day.)

Take some time to relax every day. If you cannot force yourself to live without a schedule, then schedule in a "free" period — a time when you can sit back and do something spontaneous just because you enjoy it. You need an idle period every day, a time to gather your thoughts and your energy. Instead of watching the clock nervously, learn to live by the

---

RELAXATION EXERCISES

There are many breathing exercises that will help you relax. The important thing is to breathe properly and not too hard. Avoid tight clothing and make yourself comfortable.

Exercise #1. Inhale through your nose. Try to take the air all the way down to your stomach. Expand your stomach so that you fill your lungs completely. Exhale slowly through your mouth. Try to completely empty your lungs and stomach. As you exhale, your stomach should contract. Relax, and then repeat.

Exercise #2. Inhale slowly through your nose to the count of 3. Hold your breath to the count of 3. Exhale through your nose to the count of 3. Relax to the count of 3. Repeat this pattern for several minutes. You may find that using a count of 4 or 5 may be best for you.

Exercise #3. After you've done one of the preceding exercises, try this one: lie down, get comfortable, and close your eyes. Think about your body. Imagine that you are transparent and filled to the top of your head with orange drink (or one of your favorite beverages). The liquid represents tension in your body. Imagine the liquid beginning to drain out through your finger tips and your toes. The level will begin to drop, from the top of your head, past your eyes, nose, etc. Feel the tension draining with it. Watch the level of the liquid drop. As it drains out of your body, so does the tension. Let the liquid drain down past your neck, shoulders, torso, thighs, knees, legs, right out the bottom of your toes. Are there any puddles of liquid (tension) left? Imagine you soak them up with a paper towel. Lie there and enjoy the feeling of total relaxation.

Source: American Hospital Association.

---

larger picture: concern yourself with what will be important next week, next month, or next year instead of what you need to be doing in an hour. Designate a place in your apartment or near your home where you can retreat for peace and quiet.

Learn to enjoy other people. Look for their qualities, and forget about their faults; try cultivating a few new friendships by really taking the time to get to know some people who have always just "been

---

GET OUT OF THE CLASSROOM: A "B" IS BETTER THAN AN "A"

With our lifelong academic orientation, we've been conditioned to believe that "A" is better than "B." That's true in the classroom — but not necessarily outside it.

If you're a victim of a Type-A personality — with its accompanying stress and tendency toward disease — you can help yourself break out of the rut. You can take three basic steps that will help you come closer to the control of stress found in a Type-B personality.

1. **Honestly appraise yourself.** This is a tough one — it requires you to dig deep in picking apart your feelings, your thoughts, your moral principles, your personal relationships. Once you've assessed your strengths and your weaknesses, make the most important of all appraisals: figure out what your primary goal in life is. Now figure out what you are doing to work toward that goal — and what you can do better. Get rid of all the clutter that stands between you and attainment of your goal.

2. **Establish a new life-style.** If you're really a Type-A personality, you've probably spent lots of time rushing around in pursuit of trivial goals. Take the time now to determine what is important in your life, and get rid of all the unimportant things you are doing so you'll have time to spend on what is truly important to you. An important part of this change will be learning to relax: set apart a certain amount of time each day and refuse to spend it studying or working. Instead, spend it simply relaxing — or find a fascinating hobby to devote your time to. At least once each day, take some time to relive some pleasant memories; remember how you felt when you were less pressured, less hectic.

3. **Recognize the need to always hurry as a sickness.** Think of it this way: Your race against the clock is simply a race for death. Remind yourself constantly that you can't do everything at once — some things must be left undone to be finished at a later time (or not finished at all). Remind yourself that you can work better if you are calm instead of frenzied. Think of where you'll be ten years from now, and you'll realize that plenty of your racing around is for pursuits that won't matter at all then. Clean everything up — get back to the basics. Sit back, take a breath, and relax. You're on your way.

---

around." Learn to appreciate others, and learn to slow down in conversation — set a goal to listen to others without interruption.

Do some activities just for you: read a good book that you have always meant to tackle. Lose yourself in a new hobby (how about crafting a needlepoint cover for that antique rocker?), or become proficient in a new sport. Take some interesting classes — not those required for graduation, but a few that just sound intriguing. Learn to cook a new ethnic specialty, and have those new friends over for an evening around the wok.

In a nutshell, take it easy. Nothing was ever spoiled because its creator worked too carefully and too slowly. Sit back and take a few breaths of fresh air — you will find plenty to enjoy.

DEPRESSION

Depression is a little bit like stress: it is a universal experience. Everyone who is alive has felt depressed at one time or another — depression is a natural, normal reaction to the disappointments and frustrations that we all encounter from day to day. Most of the time, depression is brief, and it gives way to new hope and determination; in those few instances where the depression becomes all-consuming, however, it can cripple and debilitate for life.

Most of the time, the length and intensity of the depression are directly related to the event that caused the depression. For example, a student who scores poorly on a midterm would probably be depressed for a weekend or a few days; as the course work continues, she would probably become engrossed and look forward to the next exam. She would not be depressed to the degree nor for the length of time as her roommate, who scored poorly on the Law School Admission Test — the roommate's failure has much greater implications as she is forced to plan for an alternative career.

While some cause/effect relationships are quite obvious, others can be extremely elusive; sometimes depression can develop over a period of months or years without its cause being apparent even to the victim.[13]

There are three basic kinds of depression:

1. **Mild depression.** Mild depression usually cures itself with time — it is the normal, brief kind of depression that everyone experiences every once in a while. Feelings of grief are an essential part of life and are critical to the healing process. By experiencing mild depression, we can emerge to work at a higher, more productive level than before. The best medicine for mild depression is a comforting shoulder to cry on — discussing your feelings with a sympathetic friend can often do wonders.

2. **Moderate depression.** When depression moves beyond the mild stage, the victim can begin to feel withdrawn; as he turns inward, he tends to exaggerate his own problems. A small failure can become, in his jaded eyes, a strong indication of doom. A victim of moderate depression literally slows down — he cannot think as quickly as he wants to, and he becomes unable to make even small decisions. He begins to lose his self-worth; at this stage, he begins to question whether life is worth living.

3. **Severe (clinical) depression.** Severe depression ranks as one of the nation's leading health problems; it strikes about one in eight Americans between the ages of eighteen and seventy-four.[14] Depression is the most common of the mental illnesses, and some experts believe that it causes more suffering than any other ailment affecting mankind.[15] Unfortunately, there are no clear-cut symptoms and no definitive laboratory tests that can enable a physician to accurately diagnose serious depression. It is confusing: "I am depressed" may be

---

"A third of a physician's office practice is almost entirely physical, a third almost entirely psychological, and the middle third a mixture of the physical and psychological. Of the latter two-thirds, I would wager that most of these patients are depressed."

— Anonymous Physician

---

uttered with equal conviction by the businesswoman who had a bad lunch meeting and by her neighbor, who is on the verge of committing suicide. While there is no absolute list of symptoms, certain behavior trends hallmark severe depression. While an individual only rarely exhibits all of these behavior trends, more than a few of them can signal severe depression:[16]

- An aura of gloom and sadness with a seeming inability to experience pleasure
- Spells of crying without provocation
- Feelings of uneasiness (often escalating to panic)
- Dramatic loss of self-esteem
- Feelings of guilt and remorse
- Excessive irritability
- Altered mental abilities (inability to concentrate, indecisiveness, loss of memory, lack of interest)
- Obsessive fear of death
- Change in sleep habits (inability to fall asleep, inability to stay asleep, tendency to wake up too early)
- Change in sexual needs

Most victims of severe depression develop physical symptoms, which may include loss of appetite, indigestion, fatigue, loss of energy, headaches, visual hallucinations and/or disturbances, dizziness, and pounding of the heart. Some victims of severe depression become hypochondriacal: they become convinced that they are suffering from a serious or deadly disorder.

Remember — a victim of severe depression is not sad and withdrawn by choice; he *cannot* return to normal simply by heeding the well-intentioned urgings of friends or family members. He cannot return to normal by exercising his own willpower.[17] A victim of severe depression must have professional help, usually including psychotherapy and drug therapy, to overcome the depression. (In some cases, victims of moderate depression must also undergo professional treatment, at least from skilled lay counselors.)

What Causes Depression?

Most illnesses are caused by a specific agent: polio, for example, is a result of a specific organism invading the body. Knowing the cause of a number of diseases makes it easy to begin treatment and, in some cases, to develop a cure.

Such is not the case with depression. The origins of depression are diverse, and the disease does not affect one part of the individual — biological, psychological, and environmental forces all combine to result somehow in the shroud of depression.[18]

Sometimes depression accompanies a specific disease or deterioration of the body — it has been associated with hypertension, myocardial infarctions, electrolyte imbalances, and disorders of the endocrine system.[19] Long-term illnesses such as hepatitis and infectious mononucleosis often breed depression, as do influenza and hypoglycemia. Patients recovering from surgery generally suffer depression, as do women following the birth of a baby (called "postnatal depression"). Organic brain syndrome in the elderly (including the occurrence of cerebrovascular accident) can lead to depression.[20]

In some cases, there might even be a genetic link: research offers evidence that a specific genetic defect may predispose an individual to some kind of depression. Even with a hereditary factor, though, it does not mean a sure affliction — apparently the interaction of several factors is necessary to precipitate the episode of depression.[21]

In addition to possible physical causes, there are a host of psychological causes of depression — most common among them being a reaction to loss. Loss of a loved one, loss of a job, loss of a valuable material possession, loss of health, loss of opportunity, or loss of a cherished value or belief can result in mild to severe depression. (We humans are not the only ones who experience depression as a result of loss — cows have been known to bellow sorrowfully for days after their calves who have been weaned into distant pastures.) The phenomenon of loss is especially critical to the elderly, who lose much with advancing years. They experience loss of independence, loss of loved ones and friends, loss of status in the community, loss of jobs, and loss of a feeling of usefulness. Depression among children, on the other hand, is almost always linked with a poor family environment.[22]

Some unique aspects of our society may also contribute heavily to the incidence of depression. Our high mobility results in people who leave jobs, homes, and familiar surroundings to move to a new place and start all over again. As a result, children change schools frequently; neighbors lose track of the people on the block. We have entered a society where an individual living in a high-rise apartment complex may not know another person in the entire building. Changing sex roles may also contribute to the increase in depression as men and women alike adjust to new jobs, new social demands, and new role identification.

One of the most crucial causes of depression is a loss of self-esteem or self-worth. A taxi driver who has skillfully maneuvered the traffic-choked city streets for eight years loses his job when he is involved in a serious accident. A woman who has rehearsed for months finds that her play has been closed. A young executive feels a desperate sense of loss when she learns that her husband has lost interest in the relationship and wants a divorce. A six-year-old feels incredible sadness when his father moves to a distant city following a divorce. After thirty years at the local steel mill, a foreman is laid off as part of a drastic cutback. Any of these individuals might interpret the temporary set of events as a personal failure — and any of them is therefore a prime candidate for depression.

Overcoming Depression

If you have ever suffered a mild case of the blues (and who hasn't?), then you probably have a collection of remedies stashed away for a rainy day — taking a hot bubble bath, listening to some favorite music, taking a leisurely walk, buying something special, or getting away for the week-end. These techniques probably work for you — if so, great! If you can do a few simple things to overcome your depression, then you can feel reasonbly certain that your depression will never get out of hand. You should be concerned only when your depression is of unusual intensity or duration — when the Monday blahs are still there a couple of Fridays later, or when a bad week stretches into a couple of months.

As long as your depression is mild to moderate, consider taking some of the following steps to manage it:

1. **Try to understand the cause.** Maybe it is readily identifiable (you just found out that your brother is dying of cancer), or maybe you have no idea why you are feeling so depressed. Search deeply. Have you recently suffered some kind of a loss (it may be as subtle as a long-held belief that was disclaimed in a philosophy class)? Are you dissatisfied with your living conditions? Do you have needs that are not being met? Once you figure out why you are depressed, you can

---

HOW TO SAY "I'M SORRY"

You've made a mistake — a bad one. You've hurt someone you care for, and you wish it had never happened.

You want things to be right again — but it's so hard to say "I'm sorry" — so hard to take the first step.

Take that first step, now! It's never easy; admitting you're wrong hurts. But you'll find out that once you swallow your pride and make yourself face up to the situation, saying "I'm sorry" can be a wonderfully healing thing.

Maybe you've never been good at apologies. Maybe you don't even know how to apologize. Dr. Norman Vincent Peale, minister of New York City's Marble Collegiate Church, offers some hints that will help you say those marvelous words:

- Make sure you're sincere. Don't confuse regret with the need to apologize; you might have done something necessary that you hated to do, but it probably doesn't call for an apology.
- When an apology is due, offer it promptly. If you delay, the apology will be more difficult, and it may become impossible.
- Maintain your dignity — don't go crawling on your knees.
- Don't apologize just to keep the peace if you really don't think you were wrong. That kind of spinelessness hurts everyone.
- If you can't speak up and apologize, try something that will speak for you: send flowers or a little note; tuck a small gift under a pillow. You might even try touching — it's the language of the heart, and it never lies.

What if you feel like someone owes you an apology, and it never comes? Try to forget about it. If you can't, let the person know why you are upset, and tell him that you'd like to be free of your bad feelings. Make it easy for the other person to apologize, and he usually will. Whatever you do, don't fume or brood — it only builds barriers and widens gaps.

---

work on attacking the problem at its roots. You may even discover that the cause is really pretty trivial and that, in the course of daily living, it got blown out of proportion.

Do not get too concerned if you cannot discover a cause. Remember that in many cases of depression, a number of factors combine to result in feelings of hopelessness and sadness.

2. **Concentrate on what you do well.** Depression is often the result of a lack of self-esteem, so skip activities that you know you aren't good at. If your roommate beats you at tennis every Friday afternoon, challenge him instead to a game of chess — which you know you can win — or go swimming by yourself. Take time off to pursue a hobby that gives you satisfaction and that you do well.

3. **Participate regularly in physical exercise.** You are probably angry at yourself; try smashing a racquetball for half an hour after classes tomorrow. Many depressed people complain of fatigue — but it is usually emotional in origin, not physical. Exercise has plenty of benefits. First, it helps to release pent-up tension. Second, it helps to get your mind off of your problems and your depression. Third, good physical health has a positive effect on mental and emotional health. So go ahead — jog, bowl, or work in your garden. Whatever you decide to do, make sure to have some physical activity on a regular basis.

4. **Talk about your feelings.** Find a confidante (or two), and talk about your feelings. Make sure that you choose someone who you can trust, and take care not to alienate him or her with outbursts of anger or impatience. Remember, if you choose to share your feelings with someone else, he will probably offer suggestions. Use the opportunity to discuss your feelings so openly that you, too, have a chance to view them as for the first time — you might discover something that did not even occur to you before.

5. **Get a physical checkup.** If your depression persists, ask your doctor for a good physical exam — there may be a physiological reason why you are feeling blue. Once the physical problem is corrected, your depression will likely vanish.

6. **Avoid using drugs and alcohol.** It is tempting to reach for a bottle (whether full of pills or alcohol) to ease away your problems. It will not help. You might feel better temporarily, but in the long run, your problems will be made worse.

7. **Change your routine.** If you always go to the campus cafeteria for lunch, try going to the pizza parlor across the street instead. Walk to

campus by a different route than the one you usually take — and ask a different friend to walk along. Go somewhere for the weekend — or just for the evening. Or try doing something kind for someone else. One student who was depressed from a family quarrel over the Christmas holidays went with his roommate to take portraits of some elderly people at a local rest home. He was buoyed up by their childlike enthusiasm as they saw the photographs; in return, the older people filled some of the void that the student had felt from his family.

Remember, a certain amount of depression is normal — it is part of being human, and it happens to everyone. Give yourself time to heal, and be patient with yourself. You are probably harder on yourself than anyone else is. If your own efforts do not seem to help after a fair amount of time, and if the efforts of friends and family members seem to be in vain, you should consider seeking professional help. Remember, depression is one of the most treatable mental disorders. Help *is* available, and it can make you feel happy and whole again.

What if you are faced with helping a friend or family member who is suffering from depression? Keep in mind the tips listed above, and try these four suggestions:

1. **Do not be a know-it-all.** It is difficult enough for professionals to ascertain the cause of depression sometimes; do not think that you can diagnose emotional difficulties just because you were the top in your Psychology 101 class. Provide support, but do not try to diagnose or tell the depressed person what to do.
2. **Do not force cheerfulness.** It is a common mistake: you encounter a friend who is depressed, and you do everything that you can to force him to cheer up. First of all, it does not work; second, it can cause the person to put up defenses. Most of the time the depressed person just needs someone to listen.
3. **Be empathetic — not sympathetic.** Never try to belittle the person's feelings; do not tell them that it is not that important, or that it will just "go away." Let the person know that you really are trying to understand how *he* feels. But do not swing to the other side — do not be sympathetic. Do not go into gruesome detail, explaining all the terrible things that could happen if the depression is allowed to go on. Do not minimize the individual's feelings, but do not give him an excuse to sink even deeper.

4. **Just listen.** You will probably feel a bit uncomfortable, and you will worry about how to react and what to say. Do not worry too much about what to say: the individual may not even be interested in your comments. He may just want to talk, while you listen. Make sure that you listen kindly; do not shove him away with the attitude that "It's your problem, buddy." Nod, touch his arm, smile; he will let you know how you should react.

It Is Not the Same as Anxiety

Maybe you have confused depression and anxiety — but they are a world apart. Depression is a feeling of loneliness or sorrow; sometimes the depressed individual feels hopeless or helpless. Anxiety, on the other hand, is a sense of impending doom, a feeling of nameless dread. An anxious person often feels overwhelming panic of something unknown.

Anxiety and depression can be differentiated in a number of ways:

1. A depressed person moves and speaks slowly; an anxious person moves and talks rapidly or at a normal pace.
2. A depressed person is not eager to talk about himself, his feelings, or his behavior; talking about his depression does not bring about improvement in his condition. An anxious person, on the other hand, gains relief by talking in animated tones about his problems, fears, and symptoms.
3. A depressed person tends to lose interest in his usual activities, and it is difficult for him to enjoy things; an anxious person enjoys things and actually regains interest in some of his previous activities.
4. A depressed person usually suffers from constipation, while an anxious person suffers diarrhea.
5. Depression is relieved by antidepressant drugs and worsened by tranquilizers; anxiety is relieved by tranquilizers and worsened by antidepressants.
6. An anxious individual's thoughts tend to center on troubling ideas, and the thoughts are usually the same over and over. His movements, as well as his thoughts, tend to be repetitive.

While anxiety and depression are two completely different disorders, a depressed person may also occasionally become anxious.

SUICIDE ▬▬▬▬▬▬▬▬▬▬▬▬▬▬▬▬▬▬▬▬

When twenty-year-old Larry arrived home for Christmas vacation, his parents were worried. There was a lot to talk about — his C grades, for instance. It was not easy to get into Harvard Law School these days. And then there was the problem with his girlfriend. Larry's father did not mind him having a fling — everyone does now and then — but this girl was kind of wild. Even Larry admitted that. Larry's parents told him that it was about time to settle down.

The tensions ran high during most of the vacation, and Larry's parents were worried that nothing they had said would sink in. But their worries dissolved as they waved goodbye to Larry at the airport — he seemed more relaxed. He smiled.

"See you in June," his father called out. His mother sighed with relief. They had managed to overcome a potentially unpleasant situation. They felt sure that Larry's grade point average would improve and that he would sever relationships with his girlfriend.

The next day, Larry was dead. His girlfriend found him hanging from her shower rod.[23]

Suicide — a deliberate act of self-destruction — has fascinated and frightened man from antiquity until the present. And it is a major human problem: more than 25,000 people kill themselves each year in the United States alone. Sadly, that number may be a gross underestimate, since many suicides go unreported or become covered up or disguised. Some estimate that figures may be closer to 100,000 each year. Even more shocking is the fact that there are more than five million attempts to commit suicide each year.[24]

Suicide is in the top-ten causes of death in the United States. In the fifteen- to nineteen-year-old group, suicide is surpassed as a cause of death only by accidents. On some college campuses, *it is the leading cause of death!*

Who Commits Suicide

Suicide is no respector of persons: it is not limited to any one age or social group. People of all ages and colors and members of all occupations and professions kill themselves. In some cases, the victims seem

88

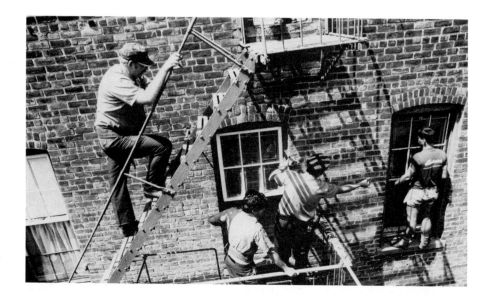

depressed, hostile, and withdrawn; those around them are not surprised at the news of self-destruction. Other times, the victims of suicide seem popular, happy, well adjusted, and at ease with themselves; their act of self-destruction comes as a shock, and acquaintances often deny the obvious, claiming a homicide or illness as the thief of life.

While suicide cuts across all socioeconomic and racial groups, some patterns occur in the following categories:

1. **Sex.** Women attempt suicide ten times as often as men do, but more than two times as many men as women actually succeed. Men commit suicide most often during adolescence, college, and during the middle years when they realize that their high career goals will not be met. Many men also commit suicide during old age or after retirement due to boredom, loneliness, and poor health. Suicide for women is highest during the same periods, with middle-age suicide being linked to menopause and the inability to bear children.

2. **Age.** Suicide is highest among two age groups: college students and the elderly. Some have suggested that the crushing stresses of college contribute to suicide, since the rate for young adults enrolled in college is much higher than among non-students of the same age. The greatest suicide risk among the elderly is the white

male, partially due to a feeling of uselessness following a full and busy career.

3. **Race.** The suicide rate is three times greater among whites than non-whites. While suicide is still more common among whites, an alarming increase has been seen among blacks who are twenty to thirty-five years of age and who live in high-concentration urban areas. An increase has also occurred among non-white women of all ages, especially those fifteen to twenty-four years of age. Suicide among the young adult (fifteen to thirty years of age) has increased alarmingly over the last few years in all racial groups; the increase has been as high as 185 percent in one decade.

4. **Social Status.** Only the poor commit suicide, right? Wrong. Suicide is more frequent at both extremes of the socioeconomic scale — the very rich and the very poor both suffer high suicide rates. In any given year, those with high incomes commit suicide more frequently than those with lower incomes.

5. **Profession.** White-collar workers have a higher suicide rate than laborers, and professional people commit suicide more frequently than do non-professionals. Psychiatrists have the highest rate of suicide of any occupation in the United States.[25] Other highly educated professionals, including doctors, lawyers, dentists, and mental health workers, have suicide rates three times the national average. Stresses associated with work and with great changes in status contribute to these suicidal tendencies, as do the stresses that accompany a loss of status or failure to perform on the job. In addition, many professional people, even in times of recession, tend to live beyond their means, with the heavy burden of debt causing an increase in suicidal behavior.

6. **Education.** Each year, approximately 1,000 students commit suicide, and another 9,000 attempt suicide; more than 100,000 threaten suicide. Among those who attempt suicide unsuccessfully, about one-third will try again within six months. The highest rate of suicide is among graduate students, and suicide is the third leading cause of death among high school students.

    Suicide is higher at Ivy League colleges and the highly prestigious universities throughout the nation. Most suicides occur during the first five weeks of the semester and during final examination time.

7. **Geography.** The rate of suicide is highest in the western mountain

regions and on the Pacific coast. More suicides occur in urban areas than in rural areas.

8. **Time of Year.** Suicides are more frequent at Christmas time and during the spring and summer seasons. The overly high expectations of the holiday season and the hope for help that sometimes does not come from family at this time may be contributing factors. Suicides occur most often on Friday or Monday.

9. **Religious Affiliations.** Suicides are more frequent among individuals of non-Catholic faiths.

10. **Marital Status.** In general, suicide rates tend to be lower among married individuals than among single individuals. People who are separated, divorced, or widowed commit suicide more frequently than do single people who never married. Married people who have children tend to commit suicide less frequently than those who do not have children. However, those who marry before the age of twenty-four and have many children have a higher tendency to commit suicide.

11. **Methods.** The most common suicide method in the United States is the use of a firearm. Men most often use a firearm, followed by hanging, gas fumes, and poison. Women most frequently use poisoning (including overdoses of medication), gas, firearms, and hanging, in that order.[26]

Characteristics of Suicide Victims

Before you finish reading this page, someone in this country will have tried to kill himself. At least sixty Americans will have succeeded in taking their own lives by this time tomorrow. Nine times that number will have tried and failed. And here is the irony: except for a very few, most of those who try to kill themselves (and most of those who succeed in doing so) desperately want to live.[27]

So why do people try to kill themselves? Everyone has problems and burdens to bear; some people persevere, and others kill themselves.

Most people who kill themselves come from families that stress success and competition and the ability to win. These individuals choose death rather than face impossibly high expectations and failure. Many come from broken homes; many others feel that their own family members do not understand them. Most feel unappreciated and unloved by family members.

Among college students, the most prominent characteristic is withdrawal and isolation; most suicide victims are shy, have few social contacts, and have no close friends in whom they can confide. Many are heavily influenced by the opinions of others, and they lack reinforcement from people whose opinions are important to them. Many have suffered an early loss of one or both parents.

Suicide Warning Signs

Whatever the reason for self-destruction, a suicide rarely occurs without warning. The warning might come in the form of verbal clues: "I'm going to kill myself." "You won't have to worry about me anymore." "Life isn't worth living." "That won't matter where I'm going."

Even if the individual does not offer a verbal clue, he will generally manifest one or more behavioral clues to the impending suicide attempt. Watch for the following behavioral clues:[28]

1. A dramatic shift in the quality of school performance.
2. Changes in social behavior.
3. Excessive use of drugs or alcohol.
4. Changes in daily behavior and living patterns.
5. Extreme fatigue.
6. Boredom.
7. Decreased appetite.
8. Preoccupation and inability to concentrate.
9. Overt signs of mental illness (hallucinations, delusions, talking to self, and so on).
10. Giving away treasured possessions.
11. Truancy.
12. Failure to communicate with family members and school personnel (adolescents who reach despair enough to lead to suicide often choose to talk to a peer or to some other interested individual outside their own family or school associations).
13. Isolation and morose behavior.
14. Insomnia.
15. Lack of a sufficient father-son relationship (this may have occurred either because the father is absent as a result of death or divorce or

because the father has been so wrapped up in his career that he has not taken time to develop a relationship with his son).

16. Difficult mother-daughter relationship (especially in the absence of a strong father figure).
17. Pregnancy.
18. Excessive smoking.
19. A history of child abuse in the home (early experiences of being battered as a child can spur violence later in adolescence; such violence is usually aimed at self, resulting in suicide).
20. Apparently "accidental" self-poisoning, especially if the behavior is repeated.

Obviously, any one of these symptoms — or even a combination of them — could be present in the life of a very normal teenager who is *not* contemplating suicide. But these signs should never be ignored.

Additional factors present in college-age suicides can give you further clues:[29]

1. A person who talks about suicide is probably serious about committing suicide. Not everybody who commits suicide talks about it first, and not everybody who makes verbal threats follows through, but more than 80 percent of those who commit suicide communicate their intentions first. Someone who talks about committing suicide might be asking for help. *Always* take the person seriously; never treat him lightly or dismiss him. He feels hopeless; by communicating his feelings to you, he is trusting you and asking you for help.
2. The suicide will not occur without warning. Be alert for any signs of mental distress, depression, or isolation.
3. Confront the individual if you think that he might be contemplating suicide. You will not plant ideas in his head; instead, you will probably open the door to further discussion that may serve to lessen the impact of the person's problems.
4. Actual suicide and attempted suicide are not in the same class of behavior. Of ten persons who attempt suicide, only one will go on to eventually complete the suicidal act. Women attempt suicide eight to nine times more often than their male peers (although the men complete the act two times as often). Such attempts are only a way of getting attention, of asking for help.
5. Economic conditions do not affect suicide among college students.

6. Suicide is not a disease of the mentally ill. It is true that those with mental illness have a higher risk of committing suicide, especially if they hear voices commanding them to destroy themselves, but suicide can be committed by those who do not suffer from any mental illness at all.

7. People who attempt suicide are not always intent on dying — but they are always intent on changing something. Many wish simply to escape from an intolerable situation and would be happy to go on living if they could be removed from that particular situation. Even as they decide to kill themselves, most hope for rescue.

8. People can change. Just because a person has attempted suicide once does not mean that he will be suicidal forever. Thoughts of suicide come and go, even among the most healthy individuals.

How can you decide if a friend or family member runs a serious risk? Unfortunately, there is no *sure* way. However, you can *generally* determine seriousness in a couple of ways:

1. **Ask how he plans on killing himself.** A person who plans on using a gun is probably very serious — there is little time for rescue or intervention. Hanging is another highly lethal method. Ingestion of barbiturates may be a highly lethal method, depending on how well thought out the plan is. A person who is planning on slitting his wrists is probably hoping for rescue.

2. **Ask about the plan.** Does he have a specific plan with well-worked-out details and timing? If so, he is a high risk. (Contrary to popular belief, most suicidal persons will openly discuss a plan for suicide if you ask them about it.) On the other hand, a person whose "plan" is vague and not really structured or thought out is probably not as serious.

3. **Has the person attempted suicide before?** If so, he is an extremely high risk. Of special concern are those who nearly died as a result of previous suicide attempts.

Suicide Prevention

If you determine that an individual is at a high risk for attempting suicide, use some specific methods to help:[30]

1. **Listen.** Really listen. Try to really hear what he is trying to say.
2. **Evaluate the seriousness of the situation.** Remember — a person who has formulated a specific plan is probably quite serious.
3. **Evaluate the intensity of the emotional disturbance.** A person who has been depressed and then becomes agitated and restless is usually a cause for alarm. Keep in mind that a person may be extremely upset but not necessarily suicidal.
4. **Take everything that the person says seriously.** Even if he talks calmly, never disvalue what he says in any way.
5. **Ask directly whether he has entertained thoughts of suicide.** Do not worry — you will not plant seeds. He may be relieved at the chance to get it off his chest.
6. **Do not be fooled.** Once the person talks to you about his feelings, he may experience an overwhelming sense of relief. He may tell you that the crisis is over. Do not believe it — the same thoughts will probably recur. Follow-up is critical.
7. **Be affirmative but supportive.** A distressed person needs strong, stable guideposts. Give the impression that you know what you are doing; tell the individual that everything will be done to prevent him from taking his life.
8. **Act specifically.** Give the person something to hang on to. Arrange to see him later, and make sure that someone else is there for him to depend on. Nothing is more frustrating for a person in trouble than to feel that he gained nothing from the confrontation.
9. **Do not treat the individual with horror.** Chances are, feelings of rejection and isolation led to his suicidal thoughts in the first place. The last thing that he needs is to be rejected again — this time by a person in whom he placed his trust and confidence.
10. **Never deny his thoughts.** The individual's suicidal thoughts may seem ridiculous to you, but they are real to him.
11. **Never challenge the individual.** Do not try to shock him out of his ideas. One student crawled out on the ledge of a high building on campus, threatening to jump. A crowd gathered below; a professor, hoping to shock the student back into reality, shouted, "Go ahead! Jump!" The man plunged to his death at the invitation of the professor.
12. **Do not try to argue about the suicide.** A person who has decided on suicide has usually undergone a long process of considering and eliminating various other methods of solving his problem. He is convinced that suicide is the only way out, and he is convinced that

he is right. Instead of getting into an argument, concentrate instead on winning his confidence and trust.

13. **Never leave a suicidal person alone.**
14. **Get help.**

Help the individual realize that if he chooses to die, the choice is permanent — the decision can never be reversed. Help him understand that if he chooses some other way of coping with his problem — hospitalization, counseling, moving to another town, transferring to a different school, taking a semester's leave — he can always change his mind and try something else. But if he chooses to die, he will not be free to change his mind later. Remind him that as long as he is alive, he can always get help and possibly resolve his problems, but that when he dies, he loses all options. Death is final — there can be no resolution of problems after death.

Finally, the most important assistance that you can offer is your friendship and support. Chances are that the suicide was prompted in part by a feeling of isolation, loneliness, and loss — a suicidal person desperately needs to have the support and care of others. And that support and care is even more important after a suicide attempt, when members of his family and others may shun him. He needs people in whom he can trust and who accept and love him despite his attempt at suicide. He needs to feel worthy of affection, worthwhile as a human being. He needs to have a reason to live and to overcome the problems that prompted the suicide in the first place.

The most valuable gift that you can give him is yourself, but anyone seriously considering suicide needs professional help.

MENTAL ILLNESS

It is difficult to define mental illness; some have even campaigned to drop the word "ill," claiming that those with mental problems are simply experiencing "living problems," not illness.[31] The most comfortable definition seems to be one that allows for a continuum of behavior with mental health on one end and mental illness on the other. When an individual moves toward the mental illness end of the spectrum, it is because his coping and adjusting mechanisms have given out; anxiety and conflict have become intolerable. At that point, the individual's life becomes so disrupted that he cannot function normally.

Unfortunately, we concentrate too much on the "symptoms" of mental illness — alienation, aggression, depression, and withdrawal, to name a few — instead of on the *severity* of the symptoms. Any person can feel depressed once in a while or may feel alienated occasionally. It is when these symptoms become severe enough to disrupt normal functioning that the condition is considered serious.

While it is difficult to label an individual according to any precise definition, a number of categories of mental illness describe various inabilities to cope and adjust.

Psychoses

Psychoses are the most serious mental disorders; either physical or emotional in origin, most require hospitalization for treatment.

Psychoses are generally characterized by a loss of contact with reality that involves a departure from the usual patterns of thinking, feeling, and acting. A psychotic individual usually suffers a regression of thought and behavior — a college student may suddenly begin acting as he did at the age of five years. Perception becomes distorted; many experience hallucinations and delusions. There is usually a marked decrease in the ability to control impulses and desires.

There are several major categories of psychoses:

1. **Schizophrenia.** Contrary to popular belief, schizophrenia does *not* describe a split personality — instead, it describes a split between perception and reality that leads eventually to a deranged and distorted mental process. A loss of self-respect and self-esteem often occurs as the personality becomes disorganized. The schizophrenic's fundamental perceptions of reality are seriously fragmented and distorted — a businessman may look at his boss and see the president of the United States instead. Many schizophrenics feel that they are controlled by outside forces (such as the "Son of Sam" murderer in New York City who claimed that a dog gave him the command to kill).

    Schizophrenics vary widely in personality traits. They may be torpid or agitated, verbose or silent, apathetic or cruelly upset, ecstatic or depressed, insightful or vacant. Some symptoms are mild;

WHAT MENTAL ILLNESS IS NOT

There are plenty of myths and misconceptions surrounding mental illness. Lots of people think they know what mental illness *is* — but let's take a look at what mental illness is *not*.

First of all, a person who is mentally ill is not necessarily insane. Sometimes a person can be both mentally ill and insane, but those are not the same conditions. A person who is insane is incapable of determining between right and wrong; he is so unreliable that he is dangerous to himself and to others. While mental illness is a medical term, insanity is a legal one, usually used to judge whether or not an individual should be held responsible for a criminal act.

Except in rare instances, a mentally ill person does not "lose his mind." It's common for a person to *temporarily* suffer the loss of some mental functions, such as concentration and memory, but almost never are these losses permanent.

There's a big difference between mental illness and mental deficiency (or "feeble-mindedness," as it is often called): while a mentally defective person never develops average intelligence, a mentally ill person is one of normal intelligence. Many people who develop mental illness, in fact, are far above average in intelligence.

Some of the most common myths about mental illness are the most hurtful. Mental illness is *not* a punishment for sin or for some other wrongdoing. Mental illness is *not* a result of masturbation. Most importantly, mental illness is *not* directly inherited. If more than one case of mental illness develops in a single family, it is probably because members of that family have been exposed to the same stress, the same cultural heritage, the same social factors, and the same environment — not because mental illness was passed through the germ plasm of the gene.

—. Adapted from Justus J. Schifferes,
Family Medical Encyclopedia (New York, New York:
Pocket Books, 1977), p. 306.

others engulf the entire personality. Schizophrenia may come on suddenly and hit hard, or it may take years to develop (and it may seem a natural part of the personality).

2. **Paranoia.** A paranoid person seems normal in most ways, but he has delusions of persecution. Sometimes these delusions are singular ("Everyone is out to get me!"). At other times, the persecution complex is combined with delusions of grandeur ("They are betraying me. I am Hitler, and I can trust no one!"). Some paranoid

individuals even believe that certain groups — the Communists, the Mafia, or the CIA — are trying to eliminate them.

3. **Manic Depression.** A manic-depressive individual experiences massive swings in mood. At one moment he is extremely elated, and at the next he is suffering severe, incapacitating depression. In some cases, the swings in mood occur over the course of several weeks or months; in serious cases, the swings can occur within hours or minutes of each other.

4. **Organic Psychoses.** In the case of organic psychoses, a literal brain disease or illness — such as a brain tumor, brain infection, or head injury — causes a major personality disturbance. Once the disease or injury is corrected, the personality disturbance is eliminated.

Neuroses

Less serious are neuroses — situations in which individuals try to cover up problems or conflicts in inappropriate ways. Although thinking and judgment are generally impaired, very little loss of contact with reality and very little distortion of perception occur. Everyone displays some neurotic behavior at some time in his or her life; only those behaviors that are persistent or severe are cause for concern.

Conflicts and problems can be covered up with a variety of neurotic reactions:

1. **Anxiety Reaction.** Probably the most common neurosis, this reaction causes the individual to feel uneasy and apprehensive toward even daily problems. In other words, the apprehension is inappropriate in degree. The apprehension and worry linger on long after the dreaded event has passed.

2. **Conversion Reaction.** Unresolved conflicts that trouble the individual are converted to bodily symptoms; many are serious, and they can include blindness, deafness, or paralysis. A woman who witnessed the murder of a younger brother when a child may be afraid of viewing such a scene again, so she reacts by becoming blind.

3. **Depressive Reaction.** When conflicts result in a severe and a prolonged depression, the individual suffers all of the problems associated with depression — yet he can rarely pinpoint the cause.

4. **Dissociative Reaction.** When the conflict is deeply troubling or

painful, the individual tries to separate himself from the conflict through sleepwalking, the development of multiple personalities, or continual dream states. In the extreme, the individual develops amnesia — a total loss of memory. Separation from reality is pronounced.

5. **Obsessive Compulsive Reaction.** Obsessive compulsive individuals are generally inflexible, rigid, and highly critical of others. To compensate for the conflict that they feel, they engage in repeated ritualistic behavior. For instance, a homosexual who is made to feel guilty about his sexual identity and who feels dirty as a result may resort to compulsive showering and bathing in a frenzied attempt to "make himself clean."

6. **Phobic Reaction.** A phobic individual has an irrational fear toward some object. This fear is actually a reaction to an unrelated source or conflict. For example, a woman who has a severe conflict with her mother may transfer that conflict and develop an irrational fear of water or of heights. Some of the most common are claustrophobia (fear of closed places), acrophobia (fear of heights), and xenophobia (fear of strangers).

Prevention of Mental Illness

Mental illness is not just an individual concern — it is a concern of the family and the community and is a focus of public health. As an individual, you can try for balance in your life: work, worship, love, and play, and, appropriately, cry and laugh. Try to understand yourself, and accept the fact that you, too, have faults — we all do.

As families and as individuals, we can rear children in an environment of acceptance, love, and concern. Children need to be taught to be tender and caring toward others. And we can all do a great deal to break down the misconceptions regarding mental illness. We need to teach our children — and ourselves — that, just as our physical health can sometimes break down (as with the flu or a cold), so can our mental health temporarily become disabled. We need to learn that mental illness is just that — an illness. It is not a source of shame and humiliation. When we correct our own attitudes and the way in which we treat others, we can take a massive step in preventing many of the stresses that lead to a breakdown in coping.

Seeking Professional Help

As discussed earlier, every healthy, normal individual suffers some symptoms of neuroses at some time in his life. How, then, do you discern when things have gotten out of hand?

A good rule of thumb is this: if your concerns or conflicts are interfering with the way in which you want to live your life, and if you cannot seem to solve the problem by yourself, it is time to seek professional help.

PSYCHOQUACKERY

More and more Americans are paying increasing attention to their emotional needs. By exercising self-reliance and self-control, most people are able to handle their emotional health problems. Still, thousands are seeking professional aid from psychiatrists, psychologists, marriage counselors, sex therapists, and other emotional health practitioners. Many are turning to mental health quacks because of the lack of skilled therapists, loss of confidence in existing practitioners, or lack of knowledge.

Dangers of mental health quackery include financial loss and prolonging the absence from qualified assistance. Be wary of the psychological practitioner who does any of the following:

1. He advertises his services flamboyantly.
2. He offers quick or guaranteed solutions to your problems.
3. He charges excessive fees.
4. He makes a hasty diagnosis — perhaps over the telephone — without first sifting the essential facts.
5. He resents any request for his credentials or inquiries into his training and experience.
6. His approach to you is intimate or obscene.
7. He is unwilling to refer you to someone else, claiming to be all things to all people.
8. He professes to use only one therapeutic approach for all problems.
9. He harps on sex as the underlying cause of all problems.
10. He claims to provide services for which his training and experience are clearly inadequate.
11. He makes excessive claims without good evidence (whereas caution typifies the honest professional).
12. He claims (without evidence) that his treatment is more "natural" than other's.

TAKE TEN THIS YEAR!

It's a new year, a new beginning. Try these ten tips from the National Retired Teachers Association for making this your best year ever:

1. **Assess your needs.** Maybe you need more creativity; maybe you yearn for more independence. Make a list of your basic needs, and then develop a plan of action. Your solution might be as simple as trying out a new recipe or as complex as a year-long reading and discovery program.
2. **Learn something new.** You might have some excellent skills that you consider a source of pride. But you can always learn something new. If you're an excellent cook, sign up for a course in Chinese cooking. Like to sew? Learn how to tailor like a pro.
3. **Unclutter your life.** Start with the physical — sort out your belongings, clean out your drawers, shovel out your closet. Give away your old clothes (anything you haven't worn in two years), or host a yard sale to get rid of all that stuff out of the basement. Then get rid of the emotional clutter — anything that's burdening you. You might try forgiving someone who has offended you.
4. **Set your priorities.** Every morning when you first wake up, ask yourself the question, "What is the most important thing I need to do today?" Then make that your first activity of the day. Don't let yourself get distracted; don't start other projects until you finish. Even if you spend the whole day on just that one thing, at least you'll have the satisfaction of knowing it was the most important one.
5. **Complete some unfinished projects.** We all have them — the oil painting half-done, the basket full of yarn to be hooked into a rug, the novel half-read and shoved under the bed. Do yourself a favor: get up an hour earlier each morning and use the time to work on your unfinished projects. There's just one steadfast rule: only one project at a time. Stick with it until it's done this time!
6. **Do something new and different.** Try visiting a place you've never been before; pack a picnic lunch and climb to a favorite lookout spot to watch the sunset. If you haven't read much, pick something from the bestseller list and dive in. There's a whole world of new and exciting things to try!
7. **Put some beauty into your life.** There are many ways to bring some beauty into your life — and into the lives of others. Write a thank you note to someone who has been kind to you; make it a point to tell someone each day that you love him or her. If you're handy with a brush, paint something colorful and bright for your dorm wall; crochet a pillow to toss on your bed.
8. **Enhance your appearance.** Rare is the person who couldn't stand some improvement. Want to lose a few pounds? Try munching on raw vegetables instead of raiding the vending machine: Tired of the way your hair looks? Save

your money and visit a really good stylist. Feel tired after a semester of studying? Grease your gears and go on a good bike trip.

9. **Do something you've always wanted to do.** We all have unfulfilled dreams. Go on — dare to do what you've always wanted to do this year! Write a book, arrange to ride in a helicopter, or learn to play the violin. It's never too late to try.

10. **Keep a journal.** A journal can be your best friend; if you read it frequently, you can identify roadblocks that stand in your way. You can use it to dream up detours and alternatives that will help you get where you want to go.

A number of health care professionals are trained specifically to help in cases of emotional trauma brought on by a breakdown in the ability to cope and adjust:

1. **Psychiatrist.** The most expensive alternative, a psychiatrist is a medical doctor who has completed specialized training in psychiatry. A psychiatrist is especially trained to treat the mind and the body as a unit — to consider any physical problems that may accompany (or cause) mental and emotional ones. A psychiatrist is permitted by law to prescribe drugs. Most psychiatrists use clinical interviews to work with patients.

2. **Psychologist.** A psychologist has done clinical and often doctoral course work in psychology and has served an internship; most states require that psychologists take a licensing examination before they can practice. Many psychologists use diagnostic testing as a part of treatment.

3. **Psychoanalyst.** A psychoanalyst generally has a private practice and is usually a medical doctor who has specialized in psychiatry. Psychoanalysts often prescribe to Sigmund Freud's theory of personality development.

4. **Psychiatric Social Worker.** After completing the usual training for social work, the psychiatric social worker also completes specialized training in psychiatric casework. He is best equipped to handle counseling, rehabilitation, and follow-up care; psychiatric social workers are most often used for marital, family, or group therapy. They cannot prescribe drugs or conduct psychological testing.

5. **Psychiatric Nurse.** Best suited to group and individual therapy under the supervision of a psychiatrist, a psychiatric nurse has completed specialized training beyond that of a registered nurse.

If you have questions concerning a professional's credentials, ask to see them; psychiatrists and clinical psychologists are both subject to stringent licensing procedures, and either should be able to show you a license. A number of good directories (including the *American Medical Directory* and *The Directory of Medical Specialists*) also list credentials.

Once you have made sure that the professional is qualified and licensed for practice, you should keep these four guidelines in mind:

1. Remember that the counselor is human; he should be believable and honest.
2. Remember that not every counselor can help every client; a counselor who does not help you is not necessarily a bad counselor. He may extend excellent support to other clients with similar or different problems.
3. If you want to find out what a particular counselor is like, talk to some of his clients. Ask them if they received help from the counselor and if their lives are better because of it.
4. Try to find out how the counselor is living his own life. A counselor who is grappling with a number of serious personal problems is probably short-fused and unable to offer help and support to others who are troubled.

Visit a therapist who is appropriate to your problem. A mild case of depression would best be treated by a counselor or therapist, while a case of schizophrenia should probably be treated by a psychiatrist or psychologist in a hospital, where medication can be administered in a controlled environment. You will probably have the best success with a counselor who comes from your own cultural, ethnic, or socioeconomic group.

Notes

1. Curriculum Concepts, Inc., *Stress,* (Chicago: American Hospital Assoc., 1977), p. 4.
2. Daniel Johnson, "Crisis Intervention, Part II," *Journal of Practical Nursing,* February 1978, p. 20.
3. Ralph Hirschowitz, "Crisis Theory: A Formulation," *Psychiatric Annals* 3, No. 12 (December 1973), p. 36.

4. Ibid.

5. Donald B. Ardell, *High Level Wellness* (Emmaus, Pennsylvania: Rodale Press, 1977), p. 134; also cited in *Stress Without Distress* (New York: Lippincott, 1974), p. 111.

6. Matthew J. Culligan and Keith Sedlacek, *How to Kill Stress Before It Kills You* (New York: Grosset and Dunlap, 1976).

7. Daniel A. Girdano and George S. Everly, Jr., *Controlling Stress and Tension: A Holistic Approach* (Englewood Cliffs, New Jersey: Prentice-Hall Publishing Company, Inc., 1979), p. 68.

8. Philip Goldberg, *Executive Health* (New York: McGraw-Hill Book Company, 1979), p. 39.

9. *Feel Younger — Live Longer* (New York: Rand McNally, 1976), p. 80.

10. Curriculum Concepts, Inc., *Stress!* (Chicago, Illinois: American Hospital Association, 1977), p. 12; *Feel Younger — Live Longer*, pp. 82-83; and Richard M. Suinn, "How to Break the Vicious Cycle of Stress," *Psychology Today*, December 1976, pp. 59-60.

11. Meyer Friedman and Ray H. Rosenman, *Type-A Behavior and Your Heart*.

12. Thomas H. Holmes and Minoru Masuda, "Psychosomatic Syndrome," *Psychology Today*, April 1972.

13. "When Depression Strikes," *Depression: Dark Night of the Soul* (West Point, Pennsylvania: Information Services, Merck, Sharp, and Dohme, 1977), p. 3.

14. "Depression: When the Blues Become Serious," *Changing Times*, March 1978, p. 37.

15. "When Depression Strikes," p. 3.

16. "Recognizing Depression: Symptoms and Disguises," *Depression: Dark Night of the Soul*, op. cit., p. 7.

17. "Depression: When the Blues Become Serious," p. 37.

18. Marilyn Mercer and Edward J. Sachar, "The Complete Book of Depression," *Good Housekeeping*, October 1979, p. 91.

19. Frederick K. Goodwin, "What Causes Mental Depression and How to Cope," *U.S. News and World Report*, October 8, 1979, p. 39.

20. Wilfred Dorfman, "Depression: Its Expression in Physical Illness," *Psychosomatics*, November 1978, p. 702.

21. Goodwin, "What Causes Mental Depression," p. 39.

22. Naomi Richman, "Depression in Mothers of Young Children," *Journal of the Royal Society of Medicine*, July 1978, p. 493.

23. Mary Susan Miller, "Teen Suicide," *Ladies' Home Journal*, February 1977, p. 68.

24. Jan Fawcett, "Before It's Too Late," (West Point, Pennsylvania: Merck, Sharp, and Dohme), p. 2.

25. Richard H. Seidan, "The Problem of Suicide on College Campuses," *Journal of School Health* 41 (May 1971):245.

26. Laurence C. Calhoun, James W. Selby, and H. Elizabeth King, *Dealing with Crisis* (Englewood Cliffs, New Jersey: Prentice-Hall, Inc., 1976), p. 222.

27. Edwin S. Shneidman and Philip Mandelkorn, *Suicide — It Doesn't Have to Happen* (West Point, Pennsylvania: Merck, Sharp, and Dohme, 1967).

28. Susan A. Winickoff and H. L. P. Resnik, "Student Suicide," *Today's Education, NEA Journal*, April 1971, p. 32.

29. Donald E. Berg, "A Plan for Preventing Student Suicide," *School Health Review* 8 (1969): 206-211.

30. Calvin J. Frederick, "Self-Destructive Behavior Among Adolescents," reprinted from *Keynote* 4 (May 1976):3-5.

31. Arlene Eisenburg and Howard Eisenburg, *Alive and Well: Decisions in Health* (New York: McGraw-Hill Book Company, 1979), p. 41.

Self-Evaluation

Determining Your Personality

Below is a list of personality traits. After each trait description, circle the word in either Column A or Column B that best describes you. (If you feel that you fall somewhere in between the two columns, circle the word that comes *closest* to describing you.)

	Column A	Column B
I get impatient when things move slowly.	often	rarely
I am generally interested in what is going on around me.	no	yes
I am eager to compete.	yes	no
I can accomplish many different things at the same time.	yes	no
I bring work home from my job.	often	rarely
I set deadlines and schedules.	at least once a week	rarely
I feel guilty if I relax and "do nothing."	yes	no
I have a driving, forceful personality.	yes	no
I speak and move quickly.	yes	no
I eat quickly.	yes	no
I am achievement-oriented.	very	slightly
I am constantly striving for advancement in my career or for success in a hobby or sport.	yes	no
I have a strong need for success.	yes	no
I like to finish jobs quickly and move on to something else.	yes	no
I am anxious while speaking, and do not finish my sentences.	yes	no
I need public recognition.	yes	no
I get angry easily.	yes	no

	Column A	Column B
I am number-oriented — I like to **count** my achievements and possessions.	yes	no
I have aggressive or hostile feelings toward others who are competitive.	yes	no
I am observant.	yes	no
I accomplish many things.	yes	no
I am anxious about social advancement.	yes	no
I try to do more than one thing at once.	yes	no
I get upset if things do not happen on schedule.	yes	no

Scoring: If you circled the majority of traits in Column A, you are a Type-A personality and are much more apt to develop stress-related illnesses than if you circled more traits in Column B (Type-B personality traits).

Note: The Self-Evaluation that follows is *not* designed to predict or to diagnose. It is designed only to pinpoint areas of *potential* trouble. If you take the test and answer honestly, and if your test score indicates that you may be prone to high stress levels, you should accept that as a *suggestion* and should consider ways of altering your life-style so that you are less likely to suffer from stress. A test score indicating that you may be prone to high stress levels does *not* mean that you will get ill, that you will develop fatal diseases, or that you will suffer sudden death. It does not even necessarily mean that you will be unhappy. Use this test as a positive tool, a help in pinpointing areas of potential trouble — not as a stress-invoking subject of worry and concern.

Are You a Victim of Chronic Stress?

Read both the lists below; circle any sign or symptom that you have had for more than two weeks.

Physical Signs and Symptoms
    high blood pressure
    rapid pulse

loss of appetite
increase in appetite
nausea or queasiness
frequent heartburn
tightened muscles in the jaw and neck
clenched jaw
grinding of the teeth
cold hands and sweating palms
excessive perspiration
tightness of general body muscles
irregular or shallow breathing
strained voice, often high-pitched
frequent headaches
chronic diarrhea
chronic constipation
chronic indigestion or belching
chronic weakness or fatigue
dizziness
tendency to faint easily
insomnia
inability to sleep through the night
inability to cry
tendency to burst into tears at slight or no provocation

Mental/Emotional Signs and Symptoms

depression
feelings of anxiety (vague or ill-defined)
constant irritability
desire to escape
impulsive behavior incompatible with normal
strong urge to cry
inability to think clearly
inability to make decisions
feelings of self-destruction
tendency to perfectionism
meticulousness about self and surroundings
inability to physically relax
concern over personal health
tendency to lose temper more quickly
fear of death or disease
feeling of distance from people and things
inability to freely express emotion

inability to freely express anger
inability to laugh or cry
feelings of rejection
inability to confide problems or concerns
tendency to live mostly in the past
tendency to punish self with guilt feelings
overly critical of others while unable to accept criticism of self

Scoring: Look back at each list. If you circled two or more physical signs and symptoms, four or more mental/emotional signs and symptoms, *or* a combination of four or more from both lists, you may be exerting a high risk on your health from stress. If you circled many of the items on each list, you may want to consider seeking professional help.[9]

Your Personal Stress Level

University of Washington Medical School Professors Dr. Thomas H. Holmes and Dr. Richard H. Rahe developed the following index of forty-three life events that enable an individual to measure the amount of stress that he or she is suffering and the likelihood of becoming ill as a result.

To find out where you stand, check any of the following events that you have experienced during the past twelve months:

1.	_____	Death of spouse	100
2.	_____	Divorce	73
3.	_____	Marital separation	65
4.	_____	Jail term	63
5.	_____	Death of close family member (other than spouse)	63
6.	_____	Major personal illness or injury	53
7.	_____	Marriage	50
8.	_____	Fired at work	47
9.	_____	Marital reconciliation	45
10.	_____	Retirement	45
11.	_____	Change in health of family member other than yourself	44

Reprinted with permission of Microform International Marketing Corporation, exclusive copyright licensee of Pergamon Press Journal back titles.

12.	_____	Pregnancy	40
13.	_____	Sexual difficulties	39
14.	_____	Gain of new family member	39
15.	_____	Business readjustment	39
16.	_____	Change in financial state	38
17.	_____	Death of close friend	37
18.	_____	Change to different occupation	36
19.	_____	Change in number of arguments with spouse	35
20.	_____	Taking on mortgage of over $10,000	31
21.	_____	Foreclosure of mortgage or loan	30
22.	_____	Change in responsibilities on the job	29
23.	_____	Son or daughter left home	29
24.	_____	Trouble with in-laws	29
25.	_____	Outstanding personal achievement	28
26.	_____	Spouse begins or quits work	26
27.	_____	You begin or quit school	26
28.	_____	Change in living conditions	25
29.	_____	Change in personal habits of self or family	24
30.	_____	Trouble with boss	23
31.	_____	Change in work hours or conditions	20
32.	_____	Change in residence	20
33.	_____	Change in schools	20
34.	_____	Change in recreation	19
35.	_____	Change in church activities	19
36.	_____	Change in social activities	18
37.	_____	Mortgage or loan less than $10,000	17
38.	_____	Change in sleeping habits	16
39.	_____	Change in number of family get-togethers	15
40.	_____	Change in eating habit	13
41.	_____	Vacation	13
42.	_____	Christmas	12
43.	_____	Minor violation of the law	11

Scoring: Now add up your score by finding the value attached to each life event. If your score is between 150 and 200, you stand a 33 percent chance of developing a serious illness within two years. If your score is between 250 and 300, your chance of getting seriously ill within the next two years climbs to 53 percent. If your score is greater than 300, you suffer an 80 percent chance of getting seriously ill in the next two years.

Want to avoid such illness? Go back over the stress scale and examine the life events that you checked. Some, of course, cannot be avoided — you cannot change the fact that a close friend died or that you were fired from your part-time job. Some of the factors you *can* change. You might also use the Holmes scale as a way of helping you decide what you can and cannot adapt to within a certain time. If you were recently divorced, for example, you should not move to a new city, start a new job, enroll in evening classes at the local university, and start on a diet — doing all of those things within a short time would literally short-circuit your stress adaptors.

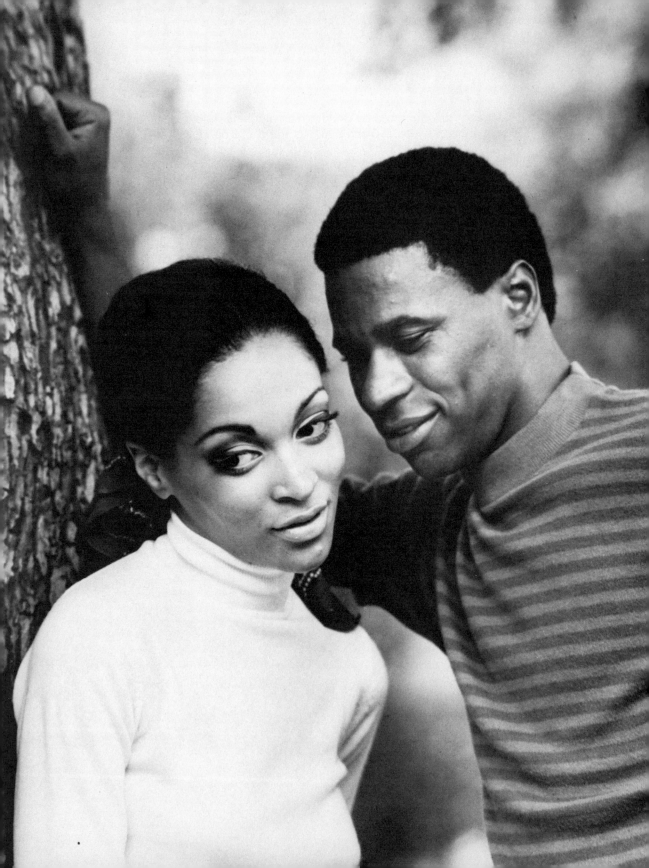

4
Human Sexuality: His and Hers

The word *sexuality* engenders all kinds of images — most of them physical. We too often consider only the biological aspects of sexual reproduction.

But human sexuality is much more. In the broad focus, it is the sum total of the qualities of behavior, thought, and feelings that enable an individual to find identity in society. Simply put, it is a way of relating to life. You might be a student, a machinist, a psychiatrist, or a homemaker — but those are secondary. First and foremost is your personal perception of maleness or femaleness — a perception that permeates your entire life and rules the way in which you relate to every other person in your life.

The concept of sexuality, then, is a total one. Your position on your family tree is perceived in terms of where you fit with respect to the malés and females who have gone before (and who will go after). The whole social fabric is woven around the complex, sometimes erroneous, occasionally malignant, but nevertheless cherished differences between men and women.

As a child develops, the search for identity affects all dimensions of his or her life. That search for identity includes the search for a sexual identity — indeed, one of the major jobs for a child is finding out what it means to be a boy or a girl. Before a baby is born, we guess at whether it will be a boy or a girl — and all of its experiences throughout its life will provide what is usually an overwhelming direction toward maleness or femaleness in every facet of its life.

While the process of sexual identity may seem natural and simple, it is becoming more and more confusing. The women's liberation movement and other movements that seek to minimize sexual distinction are contributing to children's confusion and concern over sex roles.[1] A child who finds that his biological and social genders are in conflict suffers deep and enduring pain as a result.[2]

Actual gender is determined, of course, biologically. Gender identity, on the other hand, is a product of socialization; it can occur as early as fifteen months of age and is usually establshed by the age of five years. Once established, that gender identity is extremely difficult to change. In one study of children whose physical gender was anomalous at birth, researchers determined that it would be much easier to change the child's physical structure and functioning through surgery than to change his or her psychosocial sense of gender once it had been established.[3]

Social learning contributes largely to a sense of sexuality, but it is not the only factor.[4] There may be innate psychological differences between males and females, but a person's sexuality might not conform to those differences — due usually to sociological pressures in another direction. There might even be physical influences: female fetuses exposed to excessive male hormones become little girls who demonstrate many characteristics of the opposite sex (a "tomboy," as they are often called).[5]

INFLUENCE OF THE HOME

The home is the original source of a child's notions about maleness and femaleness and about where he or she fits into the picture. Sex-role learning takes place throughout childhood, but the period between the ages of five and six seems to be critical.[6] A child of this age becomes aware that mother and father are different in many dimensions: femaleness is associated with a higher voice, gentler touch, food provision, pain relief, and more frequent presence; maleness, on the other hand, is associated with a lower voice, rougher touch, and different clothing. These

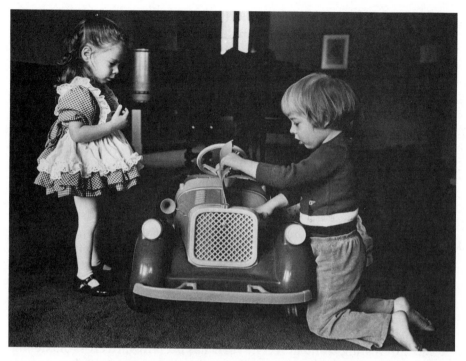

Role stereotypes are established early and are learned behavior.

characteristics — mannerisms and clothing — become so reliable that the child uses them to quickly judge the gender of a new acquaintance. Later, a child finds that gentleness — which he has always associated with his mother, a female — may not always indicate a female; there is too much overlapping in human behavior.

A critical consideration in the development of sexuality is identification. Specific factors help to determine which role a child will emulate. Present evidence seems to indicate that a child is more likely to identify with the parent who they think has greater power to give rewards, an ability that fathers more often display.[7] But the importance of other forces is evident from the observation that girls are more likely to imitate males than are boys to imitate females when parental roles are crossed. The reason may be that society still reinforces the masculine role.[8]

Parents in the home encourage the development of what they believe are gender-related characteristics and behaviors, and most of the time they serve as appropriate models. Having a model is not as necessary as having encouragement, though. Even a boy who is reared in a fatherless home can establish a male identity if his mother encourages and reinforces his "masculine" behavior.[9]

A study of hermaphroditic children points out the importance of home influence on role identity. Some children were assigned sexual roles based on external genitalia; later in life it was discovered that internal reproductive structures were different, necessitating a change in sex-role identity. The change was generally successful in children younger than four years of age — possibly because the parents, the chief figures in a young child's life, helped with the adjustment by defining new behaviors and roles. In children older than four, significant mal-adjustment was suffered.[10]

At least in the early years of life, then, a child's sex identity stems from two factors: the ability to tell parents apart on the basis of gender, and the gender assignment and reinforcement of the parents. Once a child enters school, the influence of the home is lessened, but it lingers: a little boy maintains the masculine behavior that his parents taught him even though he has a female teacher who rewards him for feminine activities.[11] As the child grows older, peer pressures become more significant in sex-role development.[12]

An interesting trend in recent years has been toward cross-modeling: the tendency of a child to pattern his or her behavior after the opposite sex. Some crossover may be desirable, since certain traditionally "feminine" traits tend to make life easier for everyone (tact, intuitiveness, willingness to compromise, appreciation of the arts, interest in people, sympathy, sweetness).[13] While some cross-identification is harmless, it can become detrimental to social and personal health if carried to the point of confusion and confict.

PROBLEMS IN GENDER IDENTITY ━━━━━━━━

Gender identity is important. A society with sex stereotypes is more interesting and productive than a society without them.[14] And, the home will probably continue to be the most important source of their development.

During the earliest period of a child's development, the home is central — and the attitudes of the parents in the home toward a child's

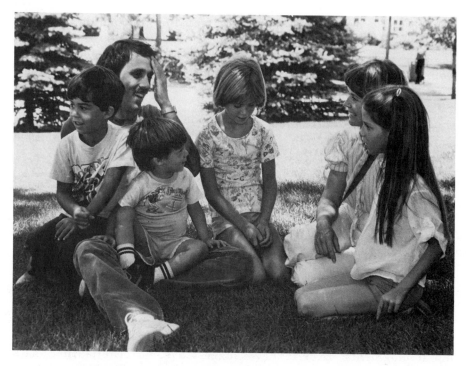

Gender identity is the product of parent-child interaction.

emerging sexuality will influence the child's own attitudes. A parent who reacts with disgust at a child's early sexual explorations teaches a child some important lessons: he should be ashamed of his body and of his pleasurable feelings. A positive parent, on the other hand, will teach by his or her behavior that a child should have self-respect — and that sex is an important and gratifying component of responsible behavior.

The key word, of course, is *responsible.* A child needs to be helped to manage his feelings and his behavior in all dimensions of his life — including the sexual one. To manage does not mean to suppress them altogether. Parents should guide children to control and express feelings and impulses in ways that will enhance the childrens' growth and the growth of others.

The importance of early training is obvious — the older a child gets (especially as he or she approaches adolescence), the greater the influence of peers, books, movies, magazines, and other sources outside the home.

There is a big problem with these sources: the information that they provide is usually inaccurate and confusing. Even though the information is misleading, it will not be as disruptive to a child who has been well schooled in the appropriate integration and use of his capabilities.

Several problems must be overcome in helping a child attain a mature, responsible sexuality:[15]

First, parents must evaluate and analyze their own perspectives and standards before they can help their children toward responsible sexuality.

Second, childhood and early adolescence is a period of limited cognitive development. It is difficult for a child to think in conceptual, future-oriented terms; it is difficult for the child to consider others outside himself. The idea that behavior involves and affects others is sometimes difficult for the young teenager to grasp.

Third, communication skills are poorly developed in the adolescent. This is bad enough when a teenager is unable to talk to his parents — but it is compounded when discussions crop up between teenagers ("the blind leading the blind"). Too often, teenagers will turn to sexual activity because they are frustrated about a lack of interpersonal communication.

Fourth, adolescents need help in establishing the criteria for making moral judgments. Experts have suggested some criteria that mark attitudes, decisions, and actions that are moral (or right):[16]

1. They cause an appreciation of the worth of the individual.
2. They lead to cooperative attitudes.
3. They lead to increased trust among people.
4. They enhance self-respect.
5. They promote greater integrity in relationships.
6. They help to dissolve the barriers that separate people.

The same criteria can be used to determine decisions, actions, and attitudes that are immoral (or wrong) — they exploit others, lead to uncooperative or resistant attitudes, lead to increased distrust among people, cause diminished self-respect, lead to deceit and duplicity in relationships, and cause barriers between persons and groups of people.

There is a big difference between simply getting bigger and growing up: everyone gets bigger, but some people never manage to grow up. A healthy interpersonal relationship between parents and children is more

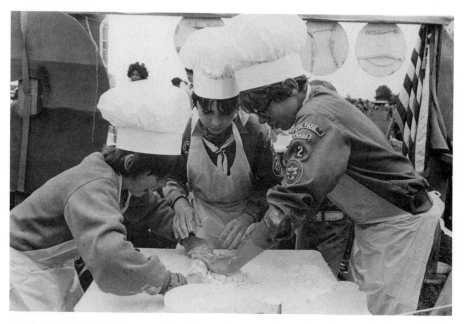

Boys and girls often enjoy participating in activities that have traditionally been associated with the opposite sex.

responsible than any other factor for the healthy "growing up" of children.

SEXUAL BEHAVIOR

A person who truly grows up is one who is capable of expressing unneeding, unselfish love for another person.[17] That kind of an orientation is critical to sexual behavior. Sexual behavior is healthy when it is an expression of the kind of love for another that is unselfish and undemanding. Sexual behavior is unhealthy, on the other hand, when it is used as a tool of personal gratification, of exploitation of another person, or when it occurs with total disregard for — or even worse, at the expense of — another person.

Masturbation

Almost all children explore their genitals early in their lives; at that point, a parent should teach a child that the pleasurable feelings that accompany genital exploration (and all sexual feeling) can be used either in caring ways or in selfish ways. Later, an older child or teenager may be prompted by erotic thoughts, literature, or pictures to masturbate — a way of inducing orgasm through self-stimulation.

We do not know the significance of masturbation to sexual development. The few studies that have been conducted have not been based on a coherent theory, and they have not followed the criteria of adequate sampling, data collection techniques, or statistical analysis.[18] Contemporary writing treats it as a common, acceptable, and harmless practice; some believe that it is really a negative behavior that has been so widely spread and accepted that it is no longer recognized as unhealthy.[19]

Obviously, personal and professional views regarding masturbation differ vastly, but among those differences is an important question: Is masturbation a growth-promoting behavior, or is it motivated by self-gratification with the potential for dependency that tends to block self-actualization and the necessary growth and development so critical to a fulfilling marital relationship?

As a parent, it is best to respond to masturbation without overreacting. Try to casually and gradually focus the child's interests away from himself — something you can best accomplish by developing a healthy relationship that provides security and allows the child to approach you with all sexual questions, including those about masturbation.

Masturbation is more likely to be a symptom of problems than a problem itself. Poor social and psychological adjustment may lead a person to use sexual arousal as an escape mechanism from problems with which he cannot cope. Other signs of trouble include preoccupation with self-centered behavior at the expense of other-oriented activities; blunting of emotional and heterosexual maturation; feelings of self-devaluation and guilt (a common reaction among those who regard masturbation as a degrading or immoral act). Relieving the root problem usually takes care of the masturbation problem.[20]

Masturbation is definitely a problem for those who feel that it conflicts with healthy social and emotional growth or is morally unacceptable. The following may be helpful to those who are motivated to stop:

1. Develop many channels in which to direct your interests. There are plenty of physical activities or social activities that can consume your energy.
2. Avoid contacts (literature, movies, conversation) that focus on sexual activity or promote arousal.
3. Keep yourself occupied — avoid idle hours.
4. Resolve tensions as quickly as possible. Frustration leads to diversion through both excessive masturbation and excessive heterosexual activity. Even young children resort to genital play when they are under stress or tension.
5. Keep involved with other people, and avoid solitude. When you are with other people, your interests tend to be focused on them instead of on yourself.
6. Eliminate or minimize those antecedent behaviors or situations that lead to masturbation.

Normality and Abnormality

When you are being evaluated, there is probably no more comforting word than *normal;* to be judged as *abnormal* — whether it is in regard to your weight, blood pressure, behavior, or desires — provokes anxiety and fear.

It is extremely difficult to arrive at a universal definition of what is normal and abnormal, especially in an emotionally charged area such as sexual behavior. One solution to the dilemma is to define "normality" in terms of consequences: a behavior might be classified as "abnormal" if its consequences are disabling, resulting in inefficiency or failure in adaptation.[22] But there is a problem even with this definition — who decides which consequences are "desirable?" Some feel that sexual expression is profoundly good and should be a continuing source of entertainment and satisfaction.[23] If the consequences are "positive" merely because you enjoy the activity, then could not any behavior (manipulative, seductive) from which you derive satisfaction be deemed "normal?" Perhaps a more responsible definition of "normal" would be one that included consequences in a more selfless context.

In a desire to make sex and sexual expression seem "normal," some parents try to create an atmosphere in the home that regards sex as ordinary. They try to develop lines of communication that allow discussion of sex in as casual a context as discussions of nutrition or table manners.[24] Emotionally, though, sex and table manners, for example, do not equate — we do not even think that they could, nor should they. Consider the difference in impact between a decision to use a salad fork and the decision to engage in premarital sex.

Under the vast heading of "abnormal" are a number of sexual problems that can develop during any stage of a person's life. Some of these are merely perplexing, while others are clearly deviant.

Homosexuality

The word *homosexual* — meaning a person who is attracted sexually to members of his or her own sex — is derived from the Greek root *homo*, which means sameness. (Female homosexuals are often called "lesbians.") Pure homosexuals — those who engage exclusively in homosexual relationships — are relatively rare; there are as many variations in homosexuality as in heterosexuality. Most homosexuals also engage in heterosexual relationships part of the time — a variation known as *bisexuality*.[25]

Whether heterosexual or homosexual, our choice of a sexual object is not based on instinct. It is a learned behavior, and it depends on the culture, experiences, and environment impacting on us throughout our lives. Some people believe that homosexuality is a by-product of malfunctioning glands or hormones. However, experts believe that homosexuality results from disturbed psychosexual development, probably as a result of adverse life experiences.[26]

Just as the home is the basis for early sexual attitude development, it also plays a critical role in determining the development of homosexual behavior. In fact, one expert calls parents the "architects of the homosexual pattern." Studies have revealed that specific patterns of family life tend to influence homosexual behavior in both males and females.

Male Homosexuals and the Home

Homosexuality in men most often results from a disturbed father-son relationship; this disturbed relationship provides the basis for the complex relationships that the son will have with other males.[27] Fathers of homosexual men show a classic pattern of being disinterested in the son, detached from him and others in the family, competitively hostile

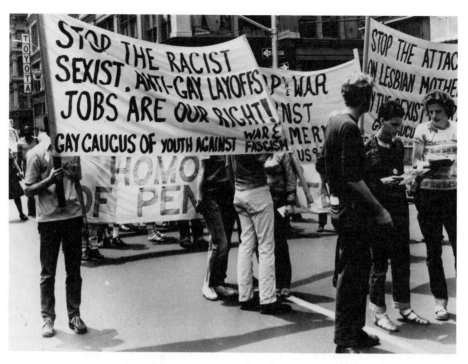

The homosexual life-style has many disadvantages.

with the son, and minimizing. In many cases, the father is extremely harsh and suppressive when his son displays masculine behavior. As a result, fears of such masculine behavior (and the "punishment" that accompanies it) have a serious impact on healthy sexual development.

In the classic family pattern, the mother of a homosexual male is often inappropriately intimate with the homosexual son — and he is her favorite child. The mother is overprotective, overcontrolling, and infantilizing toward the son, preventing him from growing to become an independent and self-assertive individual.

Together, the parents are uncomfortable about and unable to accept their own sexual identities and behaviors. A child who sees that his father is uncomfortable about being a man actually starts to wonder about the advantages of being male. In addition, a child who inspires anxiety and guilt in his parents when they discover his innocent first genital play will find his own sexual interest suppressed. This inhibition becomes an actual pattern in his life. In some cases, a boy may even

123

respond more to the way in which his parents rear him than to his own biological sex.

Female Homosexuals and the Home

As with male homosexuals, female homosexuals are usually the product of a distorted parent-child relationship. The habits, character, and personality of a girl's parents literally shape the way in which she will relate to other women as an adult. Any heterosexual relationship that is unacceptable to the girl — even her feelings toward her own father — may cause her to later reject men and be drawn toward women.[28]

Research has revealed two primary kinds of mothers whose behavior leads to female homosexuality in their children.[29]

1. The first kind of mother is highly possessive, controlling, and demanding. She interfers with her daughter's normal heterosexual development as the daughter becomes devoted and bound to the mother. In essence, and usually subconsciously, the mother wants a slave — and the daughter fits the bill.
2. The second kind of mother never shows warmth or affection for her daughter. She is critical, competitive, and defeminizing. In a very real way, she rejects her daughter. She shows no enthusiasm toward the girl, and she becomes extremely jealous of the girl's relationship with her father and brothers. The mother openly prefers her sons to her daughters. She does not encourage her daughter to develop feminine skills or pursuits.

There are also two basic kinds of fathers of homosexual women:[30]

1. Like the close, binding mother of a male homosexual with her inappropriate intimacy, the first kind of father may form a sexual alliance with the daughter — an alliance that exlcudes the mother. He is jealous of his daughter's sexual attention toward other males, but he tries to hide his feelings of jealousy and intimacy by treating the girl as a boy. As a result, the girl is defeminized.
2. The second kind of father is often the companion of the second kind of mother. He is rejecting and detached, and he seldom expresses tenderness toward the daughter. He cooperates with his wife in

alienating the daughter. Interestingly, this kind of father often suffers from sexual frustration and is afraid to express his affection for his daughter — especially physically.

Not all experts agree with these theories — not all believe that a faulty parent-child relationship is at the root of homosexual behavior. Study results in one sample prove to be confusing and lack supportive evidence for the parent-child theory. All of the homosexuals in the study had loving, affectionate mothers — but so did 75 percent of the heterosexuals. While about three-fourths of the homosexuals had emotionally detached fathers, so did 54 percent of the heterosexuals.[31]

Disadvantages of Homosexuality

Whatever may ultimately prove to be the cause (or causes) of homosexuality, the idea that homosexuals cannot change or be effectively treated is a damaging myth. Those who have a strong desire to be rid of homosexuality, particularly those who experience guilt, anxiety, or depression about their impulses or practices and have tried on their own to fight homosexual thinking and behvior, are very treatable, and their prognosis is favorable with competent help.[32] And it would seem that help is distinctly desirable in the light of several problems faced by the homosexual.

1. Society tends to be negatively influenced by homosexuality, a reality with which the homosexual must continually cope. The homosexual who feels that it is easier to change society than to change himself may be a bit naive, particularly if he assumes additionally that his moral or ethical stance is somehow superior.
2. The homosexual is frequently in personal conflict. He has grown up in a heterosexual home with heterosexual values. Pursuing a homosexual life-style perpetuates and may augment the conflict.[33]
3. Although society may come to tolerate their orientation, homosexuals will always constitute a variant group. While several observers note that homosexuality in a society is associated with an increase in birth rate it should be patently obvious that there is no cause and effect relationship. Since homosexuality is antiprocreative, it is as malignant in its extreme as irresponsible childbearing, a

phenomenon lamented by many students of population dynamics.

4. In general, the rate of companionate satisfaction is lower among homosexuals than among heterosexuals. Although this may be an artifact of the antagonistic milieu in which the homosexuals find themselves, it is nevertheless a fact of life and a problem incurred by pursuing the homosexual life-style.[34]

5. The homosexual Christian is on particularly shaky ground. Scriptural references (Gen. 19:3-5; Levit. 18:22; Romans 1:26-27; Corin. 6:9) condemn homosexual behavior in both sexes. Although some have attempted to rationalize their position and explain away the biblical references, their arguments smack more of convenience than of conviction.[35]

The homosexual orientation has been granted some relief from the deviance stigma by the American Psychiatric Association, which officially removed homosexuality from its list of mental illnesses in December 1973. However, as Altschuler states:

> Some confusion still exists about the decision of the APA to remove homosexuality from its list of mental illnesses. That the decision was made after debate and referendum attests to the influence of social and humanitarian forces rather than the pure burden of scientific evidence. The illness label has been misconstrued by the general public and was misused as the basis for scapegoating of homosexuals. To counter this trend, the APA by acclamation changed the label. However, you don't vote a scientific decision; you either have the data or you don't. It's foolish to claim a more positive or preferential status for homosexuality because of this decision.[36]

Voyeurism and Pornography

Voyeurism is broadly regarded as the attainment of sexual gratification or arousal from sexually related visual stimuli.[37] More specifically, however, the term is usually applied to individuals who receive gratification from the danger and excitement of the act rather than simply viewing nudity, which, through pornography, satisfies the latent "voyeurism" in many individuals. The difficulty in attaching the label is related to the different types of activities that seem to be variations of the practice.

Pornography (unfortunately, perhaps) lacks precise definition. Generally speaking, it is verbal, written, or visual material depicting sexual activity or related anatomy. (Some use the term "pornography" to refer to "sick" material, reserving the term "erotica" to refer to arousing material depicting more normal sexual activity.) In the United States, at least, such material is primarily produced to make money through sexual arousal. The social and psychological implications of pornography are evaluated at extremes. For example, much has been made of the research suggesting that violent sex crimes do not increase in the presence of pornography. Not all evidence is supportive of that contention, however, and studies can be quoted to support a variety of relationships between pornography and sexual activity.

In general, there seem to be several negative aspects of pornography:

1. The emphasis is on sexual activity and arousal rather than on caring relationships.
2. People, particularly women, tend to be depicted as objects for personal gratification rather than personalities.
3. Sexual activity is often presented obsessively and in abnormal contexts, such as in sadomasochistic relationships or child pornography.
4. Pornographic representations of sex emphasize genitalia and eroticism rather than human relationships that are fulfilling.
5. Because pornography sells well, it displaces other material from the market — material that appeals to rather than offends the asthetic senses.
6. The emphasis of pornography is on body function rather than on the positive qualities of dignity, nobility, and rationality.
7. Much pornography attacks the basic family structure, with its cohesive characteristics of responsibility, fidelity, affection, trust, and commitment.

The proponents of pronography seem more preoccupied with rights of a free press than with responsibility to its clientele and may even be found extolling unproven virtues, hailing its ability to increase knowledge about sexual activity and functioning. Some even say that it acts "as a nucleus for the developmental socialization of the adolescent and adult."[38]

Despite such glowing excesses, several important questions remain: Does pornography present realistic models for growth-oriented relationships? Does it help a person become less self-centered and more concerned for others? Does it enhance family and personal stability? Does it indirectly contribute to sexually transmitted diseases and unwanted pregnancies? Doesn't it seem odd that a society so concerned about exploitation of women would condone pornography? Does present "evidence" that pornography is unrelated to delinquent or criminal behavior grant it redeeming social value or warrant the approbation of a responsible citizenry?[39]

RAPE AND SEXUAL ASSAULT

This subject is placed here because it represents a violent and distorted adjustment involving sexual behavior. However, the motivation for rape must be clearly understood.

Legally, rape is described as "the carnal knowledge of a female by a male without her consent by compulsion through force, threats, or frauds." There are three general categories of rape:

1. **Forcible — intercourse is forced.** There may or may not be ejaculation; intromission may be completed or only attempted. The intromission may be vaginal, oral, or anal but must be forcible and against the woman's will.
2. **Statutory — sexual intercourse with a female who is under legal age,** who is inebriated, who is mentally retarded, or who is for some other reason unable to use her proper judgment constitutes statutory rape — even if no force is involved and even if the woman seemingly consents.
3. **Forcible situations preceded by limited consent** — sexual intercourse that results from force used to complete the sexual act even after the woman desires to terminate the act or the relationship.

Seven out of ten rapes are committed by people whom the victim knows. Only 10 percent of those rapes are reported. Half of the rapes committed involve the use of some weapon (usually a knife), and more than half of them result in some physical sign of violence. Ten percent are severe enough to require medical treatment. About 1 percent of the rape victims die.

Some large cities report an average of one rape victim every eight hours, and statistics increase every year — often much more markedly than for other crimes.

Most rapes occur in the victim's house or automobile; others occur in hidden or deserted places where police are usually not seen.

Because rape involves a sexual act, many mistakenly think that the rapist is out to satisfy his sexual desires. Rape is *not* primarily a sexual act. It is a crime of violence that uses sex as a weapon. The physical violence is only a part of the crime — the rapist is trying to destroy the separate ego of the victim. That ego destruction is the most damaging aspect of the rape; it persists for years beyond any physical damage.

Many rapists start out as "Peeping Toms," and a few are exhibitionists before they commit rape. More than half are married, and most have children. Most rapists rape women at least once a week — some three and four times; many report that when they are not actually raping a woman, they are thinking about it. But the crime is not predominantly a sexual one: most rapists report that they become more violent as time passes, and many carry weapons. Many eventually kill a victim.

Rapists act to satisfy the desire for power. A few plan the crime in advance, but about 82 percent choose the victim spontaneously because she is "available," and about 72 percent choose the victim because she is "defenseless." Less than half choose a victim because she is attractive.

The rapist is expressing rage, contempt, and hatred. Many use more force than is necessary to subdue the victim. The rapist is not an oversexed he-man. He is usually a loner.

Most rapists are between fifteen and twenty-four years of age; many rape after they have suffered repeated sexual rejection, and a few rape to prove their sexual prowess. Many rapists have mental problems. They cannot enjoy relations with voluntarily submissive women but have to take advantage of women by force and physical violence. Many rapes are committed by "opportunists": men whose primary motive was some other kind of crime, such as burglary, but who end up taking advantage of women who they find alone or defenseless. The motivation behind the most brutal rape/murders is hinted at in all rape cases: inability to tolerate feminine beauty combined with a vicious drive to erase it. The "despoiler complex" seems to encompass an enjoyment and compulsion for destruction.

The Best Protection Against Rape — Prevention

The best protection from sexual assualt is to recognize and avoid situations that are conducive to sexual assault. The most common denominator in rape attempts is the fact that the woman is alone. Women, and especially those who reside or must travel alone, can protect their vulnerability by observing a few simple precautions.

In General

Many rapes are committed by strangers, but the majority are committed by persons known to the victim. A woman's actions are important deterrents to sexual crime:

- Say what you mean, and mean what you say (with voice *and* body language) to friends, dates, relatives, and strangers.
- Do not dress or act in a sexually provocative way at bars and parties.
- Do not accompany a man to his apartment late at night. Many assume that this is a tacit agreement to sexual activity.
- Avoid pickups of or by "nice" strangers.
- Do not go bar-hopping.
- Do not remain at parties alone after other women have gone home.
- Rely on your "sixth sense" or feelings of impending danger; acting on fears of robbery or assault is important, even if you do not realize that rape is imminent.
- Give children, and yourself, adequate education concerning sexuality.

Away From Home

- If you work at night, know your neighborhood. Check for places where you can get help if needed. Vary the route that you take home.
- Carry dimes or quarters for emergency calls.
- Carry identification.
- Let friends know where you are going and when you expect to return.
- Know where your children are, who is chaperoning their parties, etc.

At Home

About half of all rapes in many large cities take place in the victim's home — an afterthought of burglars or planned attacks on sleeping victims. Apartment building laundry rooms, parking lots, and elevators are also frequent scenes of crimes.

- Keep window shades down, especially when dressing and undressing.
- Securely lock all doors and windows. Always lock the door, even if leaving for only a few minutes.
- Do not broadcast that you live alone or with women only. List an initial and last name on the mailbox, not a first name.
- Do not invite salesmen, repairmen, or delivery boys inside if you are alone or not expecting them. Ask for identification. Act businesslike and not too friendly.
- If you find a door or window open, a light on, or something amiss, do not enter. Call the police at a neighbor's home. Act on intuitive feelings of danger.
- Know who is knocking at the door before you open it. If you are alone and not expecting anyone, answer the door with, "I'll get it, John."
- Do not get on an elevator with a suspicious man. Pretend that you have forgotten something and get off. It is better to play it safe and offend someone than to take a chance.
- Do not go to the laundry room alone, especially late at night when the area is deserted.
- Ask your building superintendent to accompany strangers to your room.
- Keep porch, back door, and lawn light on when home alone.
- When your husband is away on business, do not lock the car in the garage if it is usually kept in the driveway.
- If you receive an obscene phone call, hang up without response.
- Call police to investigate prowlers. They can at least frighten trouble away.

On Foot

- Do not hitchhike.
- Do not walk alone at night.
- Never accept rides from strangers.
- Look confident when you walk (rapists expect passive victims).
- Keep your hands free when walking on the street (not overladen with packages). Always be aware of your surroundings.
- Walk in the middle of the sidewalk, not near buildings, alleyways, or close to the curb.
- Do not take shortcuts through deserted alleys, abandoned buildings, or dark areas.
- Take the bus instead of the subway at night. Sit in the front near the driver, and remain awake and alert.

- Avoid drivers pulling to the curb for directions.
- Wear a comfortable pair of shoes (platform shoes are good for kicking but are hard to run in).

By Car

- Always lock doors and roll up windows in a parked car.
- Leave a car key only with parking attendants — never house keys.
- Walk with a friend to the parking lot. Be sure that you see each other leave.
- Have keys in hand when approaching your car or home.
- Check the back seat before entering your car.
- Keep doors locked and windows rolled up while driving.
- Avoid stopping to give directions or converse with pedestrians.
- Keep your car in good running order. If your car is disabled on the road, lock the doors and remain inside. Wait for identifiable help to arrive. If an unknown motorist stops, roll down your window slightly and ask him to phone the police.
- If you come upon a motorist needing help, do not stop. Continue to a well-lit area, and phone the police to send aid.
- If someone follows you, do not drive home. Drive to a busy, well-lit area, and phone the police.

LOVE AND SEXUALITY ▄▄▄▄▄▄▄▄▄▄

Sexual feelings enjoy a confusing relationship to love: when a couple is in love, their feelings about each other are a complex mixture of emotional attachment, sexual arousal, caring, and respect all wrapped up in one excitingly comfortable package. There are three basic kinds of love:[40]

1. **Romantic love** is a strong emotional attachment to a member of the opposite sex; romantic love includes strong physical attraction and idealization.
2. **Conjugal love** is an affection that is characterized by feelings of spirituality, respect, and contentment.
3. **Agape love** is a love borne out of concern for the welfare of another

person — it is marked by a spontaneous, selfless, giving kind of love most concerned with the growth of another person.

Mature love should be a composite of all of the above. But in the naive, "love" is rarely analyzed. Unfortunately, the term "love" carries connotations of something pure, selfless, and lasting, thereby imparting a spiritual and unselfish quality. Under such circumstances, the term is deceptive, convincing the individual that the relationship has a lasting quality that in fact may not exist. Delora states that "Young people use 'being in love' to legitimate their sexual activities."[41]

A classic example is the unmarried couple that is engaging in sexual activities. The woman knows that it would hurt her parents tremendously if they knew; the man dissuades her from telling them, saying that it is more immoral to hurt someone else than to enjoy sexual activities. The woman, though, is burdened with guilt — not only about the illicit sexual activities, but about deceiving her parents.[42] The man's attitude brings up some important questions. Would it be alright to participate in extramarital sexual activities as long as the spouse did not know?

Establishing criteria for the governance of sexual behavior must be an individual enterprise developed after a careful evaluation of many sources of information. In contemporary literature, the prevailing thrust seems to be one of responsible hedonism, the essence of which is personal gratification without hurting others.[43] Unfortunately, this orientation eludes the point that personal behavior should be viewed positively — not "Does it hurt others?" but rather, "Does it help them?" Furthermore, others can be and frequently are hurt when you hurt yourself. In the above classic example, the women's behavior was perceived as hurting someone else, a perception that hurts her because she may now see herself as a source of hurting behavior. You are left to conjecture whether she further hurts herself by behaving (with the man) in a way contrary to her own expectations or perceptions of herself.

An additional question prompted by consideration of a hedonistic viewpoint is: Does self-gratification promote a preoccupation with self? Does it encumber growth toward becoming a caring and concerned individual to the degree that there is encouragement to be more concerned about self? Is self-gratification more akin to "what can I get out of it?" than "what can I contribute to it?" in relationships?

Some contemporary experts believe that people who say they are capable of dispensing love with no thought of return are simply deceiving

133

themselves.[44] Such a philosophy endangers a society that should be dedicated to greater selflessness and a concern for the welfare of others.

Current emphasis on sex — with a proliferation of manuals describing techniques for attaining the ultimate in sexual gratification — has had the opposite effect intended. Instead of serving to revitalize a marriage, this emphasis on sex can lead to new frustration and pressure. Overemphasis on sex, ignoring the more important and fulfilling aspects of the relationship, tend instead to debase and dissolve companionate relationsips rather than to strengthen them.[45]

MATURE LOVE

The high rate of marital failure and divorce is a brazen testimony to the error that many people make when they get married: they think that their marriage is permanent, that their feelings for each other will last forever. Too late they discover that their feelings were, indeed, romantic or erotic.

Many experts believe that the greatest threat to marriage is the unrealistic expectations entertained by those entering the relationship.[46] More realistic expectations come with maturity — and maturity brings with it better emotional control, coping skills, and selflessness, all contributors to more stable marriage relationships.

While it is difficult on a short-term basis to predict success in a marriage relationship, certain criteria seem most highly predictable of success. They include: good childhood relationships with both parents, wholesome early acquisition of sexual knowledge, willingness to postpone the final marital decision until both partners know each other thoroughly, absence of sharp differences in attitudes about matters emotionally important to both, the presence of considerable similarity in social background, a reasonably good (but not too close) relationship with both sets of in-laws, openness in expression of affection and readiness to confide in the partner, good psychological adjustment in general, and — most important — realistic awareness that marital success is based on "friendship love," not the Hollywood glamour myth of perpetual romantic bliss.[47]

Those who naively perceive the sexual aspect of marriage as the peculiar cement of a lasting relationship are confusing romantic or passionate love with "friendship love," which has a greater binding

134

power. Sometimes called companionate love,* it is much more characteristic of satisfying, long-term relationships. As Walster put it:

Although passionate love loses its fight against time, companionate love does not. The friend/lover who shored up our self-esteem, shared our attitudes and interests, kept us from feeling lonely, reduced our anxiety, and helped us get the things we wanted early in the relationship continues to be appreciated many years later.[48]

With a commitment to friendship love in mind, we can isolate certain elements that, while they vary from person to person, can help identify a good partner:[49]

1. **Friendly** — He should get along well with people and feel comfortable in group settings.
2. **Responsive** — He should be able to perceive and even anticipate your needs and respond to them in helpful and fulfilling ways.
3. **Affectionate** — He should like you and be able to express freely and frequently his love for you.
4. **Orderly** — Is neat and well organized as demonstrated by his appearance and behavior.
5. **Intelligent** — Seeks and assimilates new information; exercises wisdom in decisionmaking.
6. **Grateful** — Recognizes his indebtedness to others and expresses gratitude for their contributions to his life.
7. **Thoughtful** — Remembers special occasions and important events in your relationship.
8. **Tolerant, Supportive** — Accepts and respects the uniqueness of others; allows you to be yourself and encourages you in the pursuit of activities that fulfill your needs and interests.
9. **Even-Tempered** — Demonstrates good emotional control, does not take himself or situations too seriously, is not given to excessive mood swings, is congenial in his interpersonal relationships.
10. **Involved** — Takes an active part in the lives of others; shares their burdens; listens, contributes, encourages, and sustains.

---

*Not to be confused with "companionate marriage," which is usually defined as a form of marriage in which legalized birth control would be practiced, the divorce of childless couples by mutual consent permitted, and neither party would have any claim on the other.

Now comes the hard part. Look in the mirror, and see how you stack up against the list above. Remember — it is just as important to *be* the right person as to *find* the right person!

Notes

1. Kenneth L. Woodward, "Do Children Need Sex Roles?" *Newsweek*, June 10, 1974.
2. Richard Green, "Children's Quest for Sexual Identity," *Psychology Today*, February 1974.
3. John Money and Patricia Tucker, *Sexual Signatures* (Boston: Little, Brown & Co., 1975), Chapter 4.
4. Tom Alexander, "There are Sex Differences in the Mind Too," *Fortune*, February 1971.
5. Richard Green, "Children's Quest," op. cit.
6. O.R. Matteson, *Adolescence Today* (Homewood, Ill.: Dorsey Press, 1975), p. 12.
7. Helen Gum Westlake, *Children, A Study in Individual Behavior* (Lexington, Mass.: Ginn and Co., 1973), p. 208. *See also* A. Bandura, D. Ross, and S. Ross, "A Cooperative Test of the Status Envy/Social Power and the Secondary Reinforcement Theories of Identification Learning," in *Human Learning*, Arthur Staats, ed. (New York: Holt, Rinehart and Winston, 1964), p. 382.
8. "Sex-role Development in a Changing Culture," *Psychology Bulletin* 55 (1958): 232-42. *See also* K. Vroegh, "Masculinity and Femininity in the Elementary and Junior High School Years," *Developmental Psychology* 4: 254-62.
9. H. B. Biller, "Father Absence, Maternal Encouragement, and Sex Role Development in Kindergarten-Age Boys," *Child Development* 40 (1969): 539-46.
10. J. Money, Joan G. Hampson, and J. L. Hampson, "Imprinting and the Establishment of Gender Role," *Archives of Neurology and Psychology* 77 (1957): 333-36.
11. B. J. Fagot and G. R. Patterson, "An In Viva Analysis of Reinforcing Contingencies for Sex Role Behaviors in the Preschool Child," *Developmental Psychology* 1 (1969): 563-68.
12. Ibid.
13. Westlake, *Children*, p. 211.
14. Rosenberg and Sutton-Smith, *Second Identity* (New York: Holt, Rinehart and Winston, 1972), p. 90.
15. Catherine S. Chitman, *Adolescent Sexuality in a Changing American Society*, DHEW, 1979, p. 94.
16. Lester A. Kirkendall, *Premarital Intercourse and Interpersonal Relations* (New York: Julian Press, 1961).
17. Abraham H. Maslow, *Motivation and Personality* (New York: Harper & Row, 1954).
18. Chitman, op. cit., p. 95.
19. Abraham H. Maslow, *Toward a Psychology of Being* (Princeton, N.J.: D. Van Nortrand, 1962), p. 15.
20. Harrison S. Evans, "What Do You Tell Parents Who Are Concerned About Their Child's Masturbation," *Medical Aspects of Human Sexuality*, vol. 1, no. 3 (November 1967).

21. Frederick Kilander, *Sex Education in the Schools* (New York: The Macmillan Company, 1971), p. 305.
22. Warren R. Johnson and Bruce R. Frotz, "What is Sexual Normality?" *Sexual Behavior*, June 1971, p. 72.
23. Denn Byrne and Lori A. Byrne, *Exploring Human Sexuality*, (New York: Harper & Row, 1972), p. 508.
24. Ibid., p. 509.
25. Jack Sandler, et. al., *Human Sexuality: Current Perspectives* (Tampa, Flor.: Mariner, 1980), p. 138.
26. Charles W. Davenport, "Homosexuality: Its Origins, Early Recognition, and Prevention," *Clinical Pediatrics*, January 1972, pp. 7-10.
27. Irving Beiber, "Homosexuality," *American Journal of Nursing*, December 1969, pp. 2637-41.
28. Harold K. Bieber, "A Phenomenological Inquiry into the Etiology of Female Homosexuality," *Journal of Human Relations*, 1969, pp. 570-80.
29. Harold K. Bieber, "Homosexuality," pp. 2637-41.
30. Ibid.
31. David R. Kissler, "What Causes Homosexuality," *Patient Care*, September 15, 1980, p. 56.
32. Lawrence J. Hatterer, "Nine Myths About Homosexuality," *Medical Opinion*, January 1973, p. 46; and "New Light on Homosexuality," *Medical World News*, April 3, 1979, p. 8.
33. David F. Shope,, *Interpersonal Sexuality*, (W.B. Saunders, 1975), p. 118; and Kenneth Z. Altshuler, *in* "What Causes Homosexuality," *Patient Care*, op. cit., p. 53.
34. Martia Hoffman, "Homosexual's Attitudes Toward One Another," *in Medical Aspects of Sexuality*, op. cit., p. 280.
35. Brian McNaught, "Dear Anita," *Human Sexuality*, 1980/1981, Dushkin Publishing, Gailford, Connecticut, 1980, p. 210.
36. Altshuler, 2, loc. cit.
37. David Barton, "Voyeurism," *in Medical Aspects of Human Sexuality*, op. cit., p. 294.
38. Shope, *Interpersonal Sexuality*, p. 70.
39. Commission on Obscenity and Pornography, "Report of the . . .," Superintendent of Documents (Washington, D.C.: Government Printing Office, 1970), p. 27.
40. B. F. Marstein, *Love, Sex and Marriage Through the Ages* (New York: Springer, 1974), p. 378.
41. J. S. DeLora, and C. A. B. Warren, *Understanding Sexual Interaction* (Boston: Houghton Mifflin, 1977), p. 509.
42. Shope, *Interpersonal Sexuality*, p. 261.
43. H. T. Christensen, *Sex, Science and Values*, SIECUS Study Guide No. 9 (New York: SIECUS, 1969b), p. 10.
44. Elaine Walster, and G. William Walster, *A New Look at Love* (Reading, Mass.' Addison-Wesley, 1978), p. 134.
45. Natalie Shainess, "How 'Sex Experts' Debase Sex," *World*, January 2, 1973, p. 21.
46. Shope, *Interpersonal Sexuality*, p. 132; and David A. Schulz and Stanley F. Rodgers, *Marriage, The Family, and Personal Fulfillment* (Englewood Cliffs, N.J.: Prentice Hall, 1980), p. 8.
47. Harold I. Lief, *Medical Aspects of Human Sexuality* (Baltimore, Md.: The Williams and Wilkins Co., 1975), p. 111.
48. Walster and Walster, *A New Look at Love*, p. 126.
49. Ibid., p. 130.

Self-Evaluation

Too frequently, we fail to make a serious in-depth inquiry into our own attitudes and feelings in many areas of life. We frequently fail in relationships because we lack understanding of our own values and feelings, let alone those of others. Respond to the following questions as honestly as you can:

What is the relationship between sex and love?

Are there things which you do that are unrelated to your gender? Give examples.

Is it easy for you to express love to people?

Is it wrong for a girl to ask a boy for a date?

Do you feel comfortable with the idea of males doing the dishes, doing the laundry, changing diapers, etc. in a marriage?

Should a marriage be patriarchal, matriarchal, democratic, other?

Could you feel comfortable associating closely with a known homosexual?

Is it appropriate to use sex for reasons other than to express love for your spouse or have babies, i.e. relieve tension, recreation?

Is it easy to tell whether your feelings are mature love or infatuation, romantic, or erotic love?

Should you encourage gender behavior stereotypes in your children?

Are there health implications to pornography or erotica?

Are there health implications to masturbation?

Do you think males and females generally differ in their feelings about the items below? If so, how do they differ? Why do they differ?

	Males	Females
1. Pornography		
2. Sex in marriage		
3. Extramarital sex		
4. Masturbation		
5. Homosexuality		
6. Rape		
7. Virginity at marriage		
8. Marital fidelity		
9. Having and rearing children		
10. Swearing		

What characteristics, roles, or activities done by the opposite sex do you think you would like or not like to have or do yourself?

Your answers to these questions reflect feelings and attitudes which permeate your relationships with others and will have particular relevance in marriage.

How many cigarettes a day does your child smoke?

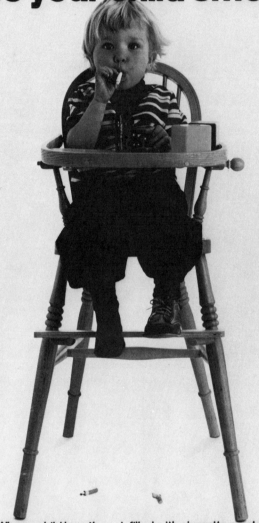

When a child breathes air filled with cigarette smoke
it can be as bad as if he actually smoked the cigarette himself.
Don't smoke when there are children present.

5
Substance Abuse: The Crutches That Cripple

Drug dependency is not a new problem in this country. Dangerous or habit-forming drugs, particularly alcohol and tobacco, have been a problem since colonial days. The increase in drug abuse during the last twenty years, however, has created an entirely new situation. The number and kinds of mood-altering drugs has multiplied, and drug abuse has spread to segments of the population that had had limited experience with drugs — school children, college students, and young people in the armed forces.

Of course, not all of the individuals who use these drugs experience negative health or social consequences, but many do. Three definitions describing the parameters of the problem have come into common usage:

- **Drug Abuse:** The nontherapeutic use of any psychoactive substance, including alcohol and tobacco, in such a manner as to adversely affect some aspect of the user's life.
- **Drug Misuse:** The inappropriate use of drugs intended for therapeutic purposes.
- **Drug Problem:** The sum of the negative medical, social, and economic consequences of drug abuse and misuse as they affect the user, the user's family, and the community at large.

Photo courtesy World Health Organization.

HIGH-RISK POPULATIONS ━━━━━━━━━━━━━

Four population groups appear to be at an extremely high risk for drug and alcohol misuse or abuse:

1. Youth, who are far more likely to experiment with drugs than older Americans or than youth in the past. Drug use by adolescents has been correlated with poor school performance; with low levels of self-esteem, social responsibility, coping ability, and psychological well-being; and with ego deficiencies, regressive tendencies, rebelliousness, and lack of ambition. (Most studies also indicate that these personality traits precede drug use.)

   In any case, early or excessive drug use is of great concern because it keeps young people from dealing effectively with the challenges of adolescence. It impedes judgment, motor coordination, and social performance. In the long run, drug use may rob a young person of the skills and maturity necessary to cope with adult responsibilities.

   In addition, early or excessive drug use may have a detrimental effect on the adolescent's changing physiology. Some reports suggest that marijuana use is associated with lung disease. Also, many questions remain unanswered concerning the relationship between most drugs and reproductive functioning, the immunization system, and basic cell metabolism.

2. Women, especially pregnant women and women of childbearing age, whose special needs have often been ignored by the drug abuse treatment network. The individual and social costs of drug abuse by women are complex and far-reaching. Because the vast majority of women who use, misuse, and abuse psychotropic drugs and alcohol are of childbearing age, the implications are profound. Recent scientific findings indicate that illicit drug abuse by women leads to problems in female physiological functioning, poor pregnancy outcomes, and inadequacies in fulfilling the parental role. Thus, drug dependencies in women between fifteen and forty years of age may seriously affect not only this generation of adult women, but also future generations.

3. Ethnic and racial minorities, for whom drug dependency is often a means of coping with socially imposed cultural and economic disadvantages. The health consequences of drug abuse for minority group members are determined more by the user's age, sex, and drug

history than by the minority status, per se. It is with respect to social and economic consequences that minority groups suffer the most serious disadvantages.

4. The elderly, who consume a disproportionate number of prescription and over-the-counter drugs. As a group, the elderly are at risk because of their increasingly frail physiology. With aging, the human body undergoes significant alterations that affect body use. The aged show greater variation in clinical response and in side effects to drugs.

DRUGS OF RECENT CONCERN

The variety of psychoactive (mood altering) substances abused today in the United States is extensive. Although abuse of all substances is of grave concern, particular attention has been focused recently on nine drugs that are the focus of greatest public concern:

1. **Alcohol.** In terms of numbers, disability, death, economic cost, family disruption, and loss of human potential, alcohol is the number-one drug problem in the United States.
2. **Tobacco.** The effect of cigarette smoking on the nation's health is tragic and staggering in its significance. It is clearly the largest preventable cause of illness and premature death in the country.
3. **Heroin** continues to be the number-one priority drug (by the government) because of its strong addictive potential and its relationship to crime.
4. **Marijuana** is of major public concern, because its use continues to rise, especially among young people.
5. **PCP (Phencyclidine)** — a potent veterinary tranquilizer classed as a hallucinogen — has come to public attention only recently but is of concern because of its association with a sizable number of violent and bizarre deaths, especially among young people.
6. **Barbiturates** share the number-one priority designation with heroin, largely because they account for 20 percent of the drugs mentioned in medical examiner reports and because they are highly addictive.
7. **Amphetamines,** which often lead to tolerance and psychological

Health Consequences of Six Major Clusters of Abused Drugs

Drug cluster	Most Common Drug of Abuse	Consequence of Abuse
STIMULANTS AND APPETITE SUPPRESSANTS	AMPHETAMINES Caffeine Cocaine Ephedrine Methylphenidate Nicotine Over-the-Counter Preparations	Moderate dosages cause increased alertness, excitation, euphoria, increased pulse rate and blood pressure, insomnia, loss of appetite. Overdoses can cause agitation, increase in body temperature, hallucinations, convulsions, possible death. Although the degree of physical addiction is not known, sudden withdrawal can cause apathy, long periods of sleep, irritability, depression, disorientation.
CANNABIS PRODUCTS	Hashish Marijuana THC (Tetrahydrocannabinol)	Moderate dosages cause euphoria, relaxed inhibitions, increased appetite, disoriented behavior. Overdoses can cause fatigue, paranoia, possible psychosis. Although the degree of physical addiction is not known, sudden withdrawal can cause insomnia, hyperactivity, and decreased appetite is occasionally reported.
DEPRESSANTS — NARCOTICS AND OPIATES	Codeine Heroin Methadone Morphine Opium	Moderate dosages cause euphoria, drowsiness, respiratory depression, constricted pupils, nausea. Overdoses can cause slow and shallow breathing, clammy skin, convulsions, coma, possible death. Sudden withdrawal results in watery eyes, runny nose, yawning, loss of appetite, irritability, tremors, panic, chills and sweating, cramps, nausea.
DEPRESSANTS — SEDATIVES AND TRANQUILIZERS	Alcohol Antihistamines Barbiturates Chloralhydrate, Other Non-Barbiturate, Nonbenzodiazepine, Sedatives, Over-the-Counter Preparations, Diazepam and Other Benzodiazepines, Other Major Tranquilizers, Other Minor Tranquilizers	Moderate dosages can result in slurred speech, disorientation, drunken behavior without odor of alcohol. Overdose can result in shallow respiration, cold and clammy skin, dilated pupils, weak and rapid pulse, coma, possible death. Sudden withdrawal results in anxiety, insomnia, tremors, delirium, convulsions, possible death.
PSYCHEDELIC DRUGS	DET (N, N-Diethyltryptamine) DMT (N, N-Dimethytryptamine) LSD (Lysergic Acid Diethylamide) Mescaline MDA (3, 4 Methylenedioxyamphetamine) PCP (PHENCYCLIDINE) STP (DOM-2, 5-Dlmethoxy, 4-Methylamphetamine)	Moderate dosages can result in illusions and hallucinations, poor perception of time and distance. Overdose can result in intense "trip" episodes, psychosis, and possible
INHALANTS	Medical Anesthetics Gasoline and Kerosene Glues and Organic Cements Lighter Fluid Lacquer and Varnish Thinners Aerosol Propellants	Moderate dosages cause excitement, euphoria, giddiness, loss of inhibitions, aggressiveness, delusions, depression, drowsiness, headache, nausea. Overdoses can cause loss of memory, confusion, unsteady gait, and erratic heart beat and pulse are possible. Sudden withdrawal results in insomnia, decreased appetite, depression, irritability, headache.

dependence, have been of concern since their introduction as appetite suppressants in the 1930s.

8. **Inhalants** are of vital concern because they are so readily accessible, are used mostly by the young, and are believed to be responsible for serious brain damage in chronic users.

9. **Cocaine,** a high status drug, is of serious concern because it is the most powerfully reinforcing of all illicit drugs used today.

To illustrate the magnitude of the problem associated with these nine drugs, their particular health and social consequences, a discussion of each drug appears on the following pages.

ALCOHOL

Alcohol is classed pharmacologically as a depressant drug. Many people drink alcoholic beverages to get feelings of pleasure or relief from tension and attribute such feelings as stimulant effects. This is why some people believe alcohol to be a stimulant. Actually, these feelings result from the depressant effects of alcohol on the brain.

Drinking larger amounts of alcohol over long periods of time seems to change the sensitivity of the brain to the effects of alcohol. This means that increasing amounts of alcohol are required to produce the same effects. This adaption is called "tolerance." It shows up in the chronic use of all addictive drugs and is believed to be the basis of addiction or dependence.

Drugs used in combination with alcohol can grossly exaggerate the usual responses expected from alcohol or from a drug alone. For example, alcohol and barbiturates, when combined, multiply each other's effects; taking both drugs in close order can be dangerous and may result in death. The use of alcohol with any drug that has a depressant effect on the central nervous system is hazardous to health and safety and, in some cases, to life itself.

The projected total number of drinkers in the United States eighteen years of age and over is about 101 million — nearly 48 million women and 53 million men. A recent national survey indicated that 81 percent of tenth through twelfth grade students reported having had at least one drink in the previous year, and 27 percent reported drinking at least once a week.

If we accept estimates that 10 to 12 million adults in this country are problem drinkers (including alcoholics), and that 3.3 million youth are problem drinkers, then the average drinker with no alcohol-related problems actually drinks less than the national average of 2.68 gallons of alcohol. Thus, as surveys confirm, this nation has millions of occasional and very moderate drinkers.

Health and Social Consequences

1. Alcohol misuse has a potentially detrimental effect from its point of entry at the mouth through the entire gastrointestinal tract and to related organs, such as the liver and the pancreas. The liver is often seriously damaged by chronic alcoholism, the most common disorders being hepatitis and cirrhosis.

2. Alcohol abuse contributes to nutritional deficiency and has been suggested as the most common cause of vitamin and trace element deficiency in adults in the United States.

3. There is an association between alcoholism and depression in both men and women. Alcoholics often have high levels of depression, and alcohol can increase depression.

4. Compared to the general population, a disproportionately high number of people with drinking problems commit suicide. Approximately one-third of suicides involve alcohol. A propensity for suicide is thought to be associated with certain conditions such as depression, anxiety, mood fluctuations, and a decreased ability to interact socially, which are related to alcohol abuse.

5. Heavy alcohol consumption has been associated with a number of adverse effects on the cardiovascular system, including a specific deterioration of the heart muscle, diminished cardiac output, and decreased contractibility of the heart muscle. On the other hand, moderate alcohol consumption has been associated with lower rates of coronary heart disease than those observed for abstainers. Further research is warranted.

6. Heavy consumption has been related to degeneration of skeletal muscle.

7. Heavy drinking increases the risk of developing cancer of the tongue, mouth, oropharynx, hypopharynx, esophagus, larynx, and liver. In the United States, these sites represent 6.1 to 9.1 percent of all cancers in the white population and 11.3 and 12.5 percent in the

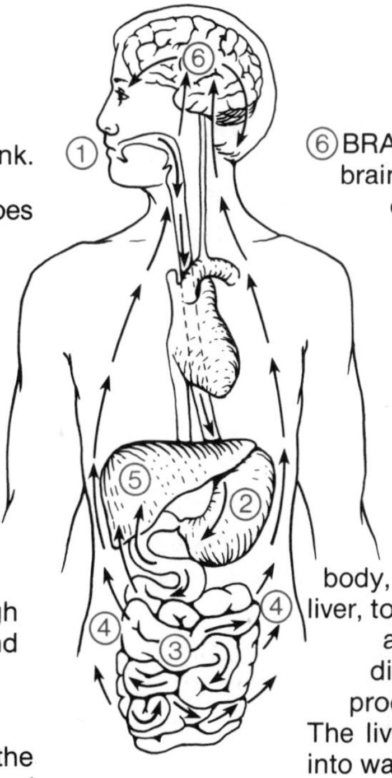

ALCOHOL'S EFFECTS
ON THE MIND AND BODY

① MOUTH. Alcohol is drunk.

② STOMACH. Alcohol goes right into the stomach. A little of the alcohol goes through the wall of the stomach and into the bloodstream. But most of the alcohol goes down into the <u>small intestine</u>.

③ SMALL INTESTINE. Alcohol goes from the stomach into the small intestine. Most of the alcohol then goes through the walls of the intestine and into the <u>bloodstream</u>.

④ BLOODSTREAM. The bloodstream then carries the alcohol to <u>all</u> parts of the body, such as the brain, heart, and <u>liver</u>.

⑥ BRAIN. Alcohol goes to the brain almost as soon as it is drunk. The bloodstream carries it there. Alcohol keeps passing through the brain until the liver has had time to change (oxidize) all the alcohol into carbon dioxide, water, and energy.

⑤ LIVER. As the bloodstream carries the alcohol around the body, it carries it through the liver, too. The liver changes the alcohol to water, carbon dioxide, and energy. This process is called <u>oxidation</u>. The liver can oxidize (change into water, carbon dioxide, and energy) only about one-half ounce of alcohol an hour. This means that until the liver has time to oxidize all of the alcohol, the alcohol <u>keeps on</u> passing through all parts of the body, including the <u>brain</u>.

Figure 5-1.

black population. Alcohol appears to interact with tobacco to increase the risk of cancer.

8. Laboratory experiments have shown that body sway, a motor function, shows significant impairment at fairly low blood alcohol levels of 0.04 percent. This is less than half the level (0.10 percent) that most states require as evidence for driving under the influence of alcohol.

9. Traffic deaths are the major cause of violent death in this country. One-half of all traffic fatalities are alcohol-related. Drinking by drivers also plays a greater role as the severity of the crash increases. Alcohol is especially involved in accidental death and injury among young people.

10. A significant number of industrial accidents, drownings, burnings, and falls have been attributed to alcohol misuse.

11. Alcohol is a central nervous system depressant. Chronic exposure can result in tolerance and physical dependence.

12. Alcohol consumption can affect both the pharmacologic and therapeutic actions of prescription drugs, over-the-counter drugs, and illicit drugs. Alcohol-drug interactions are reported to be the second most frequent cause of drug-related medical crises in the United States.

13. Mortality rates for alcoholics continue to be higher than for the general population; one recent longitudinal study reported a mortality rate in a group of alcoholics 2.5 times greater than normal.

14. Studies show that, regardless of race or sex, regular consumption of large amounts of alcohol is associated with substantially higher prevalence of high blood pressure.

15. Loss of brain cells is one of the major consequences of alcoholism; brain atrophy is reported in 50 to 100 percent of alcoholics. New evidence suggests that heavy social drinking may also result in brain atrophy.

16. Numerous studies have shown that acute or chronic ingestion of alcohol results in lowered testosterone in the serum of males of all species. This reduced level may cause sexual impotence, loss of libido, breast enlargement, loss of facial hair, and testicular atrophy in many male alcoholics.

17. Fetal Alcohol Syndrome (FAS) has been identified among some children of women who drink heavily. It is characterized by central nervous system disorders, growth deficiencies, a specific cluster of facial abnormalities, and other malformations, particularly skeletal, urogenital, and cardiac. FAS is suspected to be one of the leading causes of birth defects associated with mental retardation.

18. Decreased birth weight, frequently associated with increased risk to the newborn, has been observed among the children of women averaging one ounce of absolute alcohol (two standard drinks) per day during pregnancy.

EXCESSIVE ALCOHOL CONSUMPTION
AND COMMON SIDE-EFFECTS

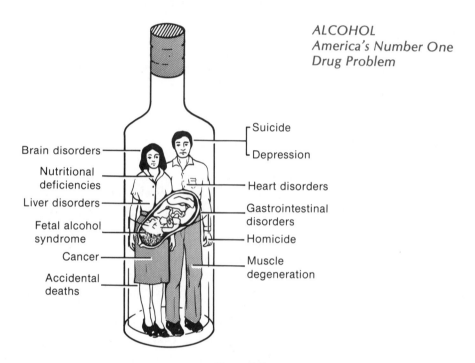

ALCOHOL
America's Number One
Drug Problem

Brain disorders

Nutritional deficiencies

Liver disorders

Fetal alcohol syndrome

Cancer

Accidental deaths

Suicide

Depression

Heart disorders

Gastrointestinal disorders

Homicide

Muscle degeneration

Figure 5-2.

19. In one study, evidence points to an association between consumption of two standard drinks a week and spontaneous abortion.

20. For some drinkers, alcohol releases violent behavior that might be unlikely or even unthinkable in a sober state. Half of all homicides are alcohol-related. Evidence of alcohol consumption is estimated as high as 50 percent for rape offenders and 31 percent for victims. Although estimates vary widely, alcohol involvement in reported assaults has been calculated to as high as 72 percent for offenders and 79 percent for victims. Studies have indicated that 19 to 77 percent of child molesters were drinking at the time of the offense. Researchers question whether the role of alcohol, if any, was a

contributing factor, or if the use of alcohol was given as an excuse for the offense. One study has indicated that almost four out of every ten child-abusing parents have a history of drinking problems. Estimates of drinking prior to committing a robbery range from 7 to 72 percent.

21. Alcohol also contributes to criminal behavior of a less violent nature. For example, more than one-third of the 10.2 million arrests in a recent year in the United States were related to the misuse of alcohol.

Problem Drinking and Alcoholism

Distinctions are sometimes made between people with drinking problems and those suffering from alcoholism — alcoholics being considered the more uncontrolled and injured group. In practice, however, the two are often hard to distinguish. Within our society, problem drinking is usually recognized whenever anyone drinks to such an excess that he loses ability to control his actions and maintain a socially acceptable life adjustment. A problem drinker has been more specifically defined as:[1]

1. Anyone who must drink in order to function or cope with life.
2. Anyone who by his own personal definition, or that of his family and friends, frequently drinks to a state of intoxication.
3. Anyone who goes to work intoxicated.
4. Anyone who is intoxicated and drives a car.
5. Anyone who sustains bodily injury requiring medical attention as a consequence of an intoxicated state.
6. Anyone who, under the influence of alcohol, does something that he contends he would never do without alcohol.

Other warning signs that often indicate problem drinking are the need to drink before facing certain situations, frequent drinking sprees, a steady increase in intake, solitary drinking, early morning drinking, and the occurrence of blackouts. For a heavy drinker, a blackout is not "passing out," but a period of time in which he walks, talks, and acts, but does not remember. Such blackouts may be one of the early signs of the more serious form of alcoholism.

150

Alcoholism is addiction to alcohol. When expanded to include symptomatology, characteristics, and sociological manifestations of the illness, no definition satisfies everyone. The World Health Organization defines it as:

A state, psychic and usually also physical, resulting from taking alcohol, characterized by behavioral and other responses that always include a compulsion to take alcohol on a continuous basis in order to experience its psychic effects, and sometimes to avoid the discomfort of its absence; tolerance may or may not be present.

The following is another widely accepted definition:

Alcoholism is a chronic disease, or disorder of behavior, characterized by the repeated drinking of alcoholic beverages to an extent that exceeds customary dietary use or ordinary compliance with the social drinking customs of the community, and which interferes with the drinker's health, interpersonal relations, or economic functioning.[2]

By whatever definition used, there are an estimated 10 to 12 million adults in the United States with drinking and alcoholism problems.

SMOKING

Until the early years of the twentieth century, cigarettes were neither a major article of consumption nor an important threat to health. Tobacco was used mainly for chewing and for cigars, pipe tobacco, and snuff. As late as 1915, only about 18 billion cigarettes were consumed annually in this country, as contrasted with more than 600 billion today.

The sudden and enormous increase in the use of cigarettes came about for a variety of reasons. Cigarettes are inexpensive and are less offensive than other forms of tobacco to many people, and they are the only form of tobacco that has been taken up by large numbers of women. Cigarette smoke is milder than smoke from pipes and cigars, making inhalation easier and thus nicotine absorption into the bloodstream more rapid. Once a person begins smoking cigarettes, addiction in the sense of

DEATH RATES FOR SMOKERS AND NONSMOKERS

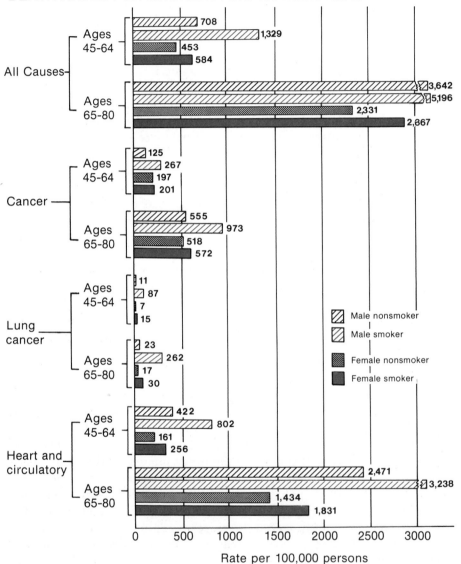

Figure 5-3.

building up a physiological and psychological dependence can quickly follow. Cigarettes are also profitable to manufacture, which has permitted the cigarette companies over the years to invest immense sums in advertising and promotion.

Scientists became suspicious of cigarettes as a cause of illness and death as early as the 1930s. One reason for their concern was an increase in the incidence of lung cancer. In 1930, less than 3,000 Americans were listed as dying from this disease; by the 1950s, this number had grown to 18,000 annually. Estimates put the number of deaths for 1980 at over 100,000.

Since the 1930s, medical evidence has grown stronger, until cigarette smoking can now be identified as a major cause of death and disability in this country and throughout the world. Cigarettes are linked not only to lung and other cancers, but to heart disease, chronic lung disease, and other diseases as well.

As measured by per capita consumption and the percent of people smoking, cigarette use in the United States reached its peak in the early 1960s. Since then, in the face of medical evidence, consumption has decreased. What has been called the "epidemic" of cigarette smoking — the chief preventable cause of death in our society — may now be waning.

Who Smokes Cigarettes?

About 37 percent of adult men and 31 percent of adult women smoke cigarettes. This is the lowest figure for men since the government began collecting this information in 1955. Women started smoking later as a group than did men. Their smoking increased from 1955 to 1975, but since then, their percentage, too, has declined.

Education, income, and race all play a role in deciding who smokes and who does not. College graduates of both sexes are less likely to smoke than those with less education. Among men, the percentage of smokers generally drops as income increases, although for women the opposite tends to be true. Blacks are more apt to be smokers than whites, but on the average, they smoke fewer cigarettes.

About 13 percent of females and about 11 percent of males under the age of nineteen are regular smokers. This is a marked decline from smoking levels five years ago, when the percentages were 15 and 16. Teenage smoking patterns are similar in many ways to those of adults.

PERCENT OF ADULTS WHO SMOKE, BY SEX:
1965, 1974, and 1980

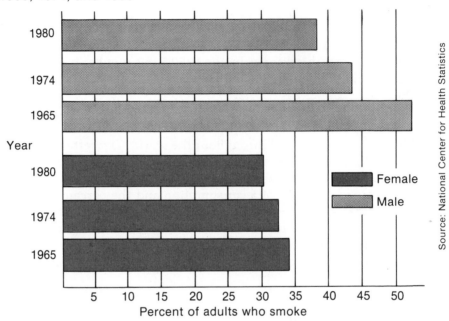

Figure 5-4.

There are fewer smokers among adolescents coming from higher socioeconomic backgrounds and among adolescents taking college preparatory
courses in high school.

Health and Social Consequences of Smoking

The effects of cigarette smoking on the nation's health are tragic and
staggering. Although new information continues to appear, here is what
is already known:

1. Cigarette smoking is clearly the largest preventable cause of illness
    and premature death in the United States.
2. Cigarette smoking is a causal factor for coronary heart disease and

154

PERCENT OF TEENAGERS WHO SMOKE, BY SEX:
1968, 1974, and 1980

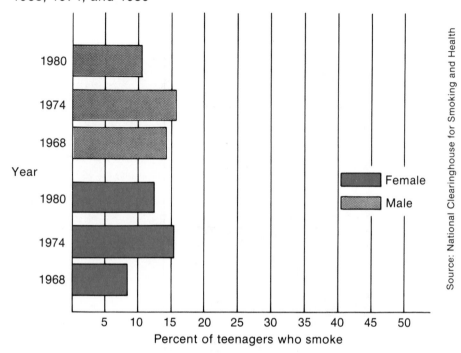

Source: National Clearinghouse for Smoking and Health

Figure 5-5.

arteriosclerotic peripheral vascular disease; cancer of the lung, larynx, oral cavity, and esophagus; and chronic bronchitis and emphysema.

3. Cigarette smoking is associated with cancer of the urinary bladder and pancreas, and ulcer disease. Maternal cigarette smoking is associated with retarded fetal growth, an increased risk for spontaneous abortion and prenatal death, low birth weight, and slight impairment of growth and development during early childhood.

4. Cigarette smoking acts synergistically with oral contraceptives to enhance the probability of coronary and some cerebrovascular disease; with alcohol to increase the risk of cancer of the larynx, oral cavity, and esophagus; with asbestos and some other occupationally encountered substances to increase the likelihood of cancer of the lung; and with other risk factors to enhance cardiovascular risk.

5. The effect of smoking is most serious for those who smoke two or

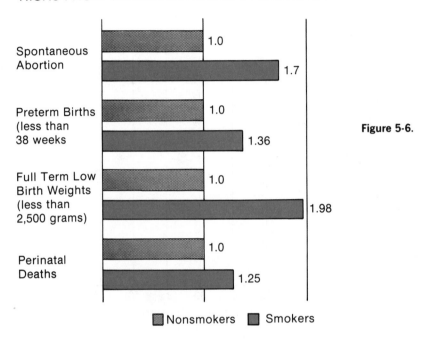

RISKS FROM SMOKING DURING PREGNANCY

Spontaneous Abortion
Nonsmokers: 1.0
Smokers: 1.7

Preterm Births (less than 38 weeks
Nonsmokers: 1.0
Smokers: 1.36

Full Term Low Birth Weights (less than 2,500 grams)
Nonsmokers: 1.0
Smokers: 1.98

Perinatal Deaths
Nonsmokers: 1.0
Smokers: 1.25

Nonsmokers   Smokers

Figure 5-6.

more packs a day. Those who begin smoking as adolescents also have expectancies much shorter than those who begin smoking later. Those who smoke pipes and cigars have life expectancies only slightly less than those who do not smoke, but their mortality rates from cancer of the oral cavity, larynx, pharynx, and esophagus are elevated over those of nonsmokers.

Passive Smoking

Passive or involuntary smoking occurs when nonsmokers find themselves in a smoke-filled atmosphere — for example, elevators, offices, restaurants, or automobiles. For most people, passive smoking is a discomfort and nuisance, and for some people — those with lung and heart problems — it can aggravate symptoms of those diseases.

Researchers have also shown that, for one aspect of pulmonary

AGE-ADJUSTED CANCER DEATH RATES FOR FEMALES, SELECTED SITES, 1930 - 1983

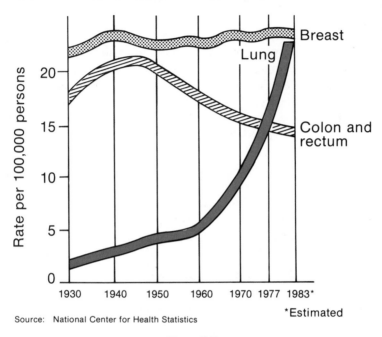

Source: National Center for Health Statistics

*Estimated

Figure 5-7.

function, healthy nonsmokers who work in a smoky environment show the same amount of abnormality as do smokers who inhale between one and ten cigarettes a day.

Because of these health factors, more than thirty states and hundreds of communities now have ordinances restricting smoking in public places.

HEROIN

Heroin accounts for 90 percent of the illegal narcotic abuse in the United States. Heroin is a white crystalline narcotic powder, derived from morphine (a natural alkaloid found in opium). It is a strong analgesic and produces an intense state of euphoria.

Heroin is the most addictive of all drugs, although it is possible for some people to use it and not become addicted. Unfortunately, very little is known about who can and cannot use heroin safely. Also, the length of time and amount of use required to produce addiction vary. Most studies find that users experiment with the drug for between five and eighteen months before a long-term physical dependency develops.

For those who do become addicted, heroin creates a very powerful dependency. The drug is usually administered intravenously, and, because it is short-acting, must be taken every few hours if withdrawal is to be avoided. Because of its strong addictive potential, heroin is among the most stringently controlled drugs in the United States today. Manufacture and importation of heroin are prohibited by law, and severe penalties are used to discourage smuggling and dealing.

Recent large-scale household surveys indicate that about 1 percent of all youth (twelve to seventeen years of age) have tried heroin, compared to 4 percent of young adults (eighteen to twenty-five) and less than 1 percent of adults over twenty-five.

Health and Social Consequences

Since addicts tend to become preoccupied with the daily round of obtaining and taking drugs, they often neglect themselves and may suffer from malnutrition, infections, and unattended diseases or injuries. Among the hazards of narcotic addiction are toxic reactions to contaminants such as sugar and talcum powder, as well as unsterile needles and injection techniques, resulting in abscesses, blood poisoning, and hepatitis.

Because there is no simple way to determine the purity of a drug that is sold on the street, the potency is unpredictable. A person with a mild overdose may be stuporous or asleep. Larger doses may induce a coma, with the victim experiencing shallow respirations. The skin becomes clammy and cold, the body limp, and the jaw relaxed; there is a danger that the tongue may fall back, blocking the passage of air. If the condition is sufficiently severe, convulsions may occur, followed by respiratory arrest and death.

When a heroin-dependent person stops taking the drug, withdrawal begins within four to six hours after the last injection. Full-blown withdrawal symptoms — which include shaking, sweating, vomiting, running nose and eyes, muscle aches, chills, abdominal pains, and diarrhea —

begin some twelve to sixteen hours after the last injection. As withdrawal progresses, restlessness, irritability, loss of appetite, insomnia, goose flesh, tremors, and, finally, yawning and severe sneezing occur. These symptoms reach their peak in forty-eight to seventy-two hours. Weakness and depression, nausea, vomiting, stomach cramps, and diarrhea are common. Heart rate and blood pressure are elevated. Chills, alternating with flushing and excessive sweating, occur. Pains in the bones and muscles of the back and extremities occur as do muscle spasms and kicking movements, which may be the source of the expression "kicking the habit."

Without treatment, the syndrome eventually runs its course, and most of the symptoms will disappear in seven to ten days. For a few weeks following withdrawal, the addict will continue to think and talk about heroin and be particularly susceptible to an urge to use it again.

Death rates among heroin addicts are a great deal higher than rates for the general population. The excess deaths are attributed chiefly to drug overdose and to suicides, accidents, and homicides. Many of the overdose deaths are not caused by the heroin itself, but by the drugs used to dilute it in the street market.

Finally, the relationship between heroin addiction and crime has engendered much discussion. Some believe that the association between crime and heroin use is entirely explained by the fact that criminals are especially vulnerable to addiction. Others, who concede that addicts steal to support their habits, blame this entirely on the illegal status of heroin, which creates a black market and high prices. Nonetheless, it is known that certain crimes — forgery, conning, prostitution, and theft —increase in proportion to addiction. There seems to be little increase in violent crime with addicts, but a definite increase among promoters.

Thus, while it is true that the kinds of people who use heroin are also likely to commit crimes, and that committing crimes makes them especially likely to come to public attention as addicts, the fact that the number of property crimes does seem to fluctuate with the use of heroin suggests that addiction directly increases the frequency of theft and other crimes designed to provide money for drugs.

MARIJUANA

Marijuana is a common plant with the biological name of *Cannabis sativa*. The psychoactive ingredient in marijuana is delta-9-tetra-hydrocannabinol, or THC. Plant strain, climate, soil conditions, time of harvesting, and other factors determine the strength of marijuana. The plant that grows wild in the United States is usually lower in THC than cultivated marijuana, especially Mexican, Lebanese, Southeast Asian, or Indian varieties.

Marijuana is usually smoked, although some people eat it after baking it into cookies or brownies. It produces feelings of euphoria, relaxation, and altered sense of identity, and bouts of exaggerated laughter are commonly reported at social dose levels. Other physical changes associated with marijuana use are an increase in heart and pulse rate, reddening of the eyes, and dryness in the mouth and throat. Many feel that their hearing, vision, and skin sensitivity are enhanced by the drug, although these reports have not been objectively confirmed by research.

Who Uses Marijuana?

Marijuana use has increased dramatically during the last decade. Between 41 and 47 million Americans have tried marijuana, and between 16 and 20 million use it regularly (once a month or more). Marijuana is used increasingly by the young, more frequently, and at a greater strength than ever before. Evidence suggests that marijuana use is age-related and that large numbers of people who once used marijuana heavily or regularly are no longer doing so.

Health and Social Consequences

There is an emerging consensus among leading experts that marijuana is not a "safe" drug. Research has proven that marijuana intoxication impairs motor coordination, reaction time, and visual perception that would affect driving ability. The National Safety Council has found an alarming incidence of marijuana use linked to highway traffic accidents. A recent study of 300 fatal car accidents in the Boston area also discovered an increased presence of marijuana: at the time of the fatal crash, 30 percent of the drivers had used alcohol and 16 percent had used marijuana. Many marijuana smokers readily admit that their driving skills are impaired by marijuana intoxication, and there is reason to believe that more marijuana users drive today while "high" than in the past.

Marijuana is also widely used by adolescents and young adults — a time of rapid physiological and psychological change. Chronic marijuana intoxication can impair physical and emotional maturation and impede the individual's acquisition of intellectual and social skills. Marijuana intoxication interferes with immediate memory and intellectual performance and impairs thinking, reading comprehension, and verbal and arithmetic problem-solving abilities. Less familiar, more difficult tasks are interfered with more than well-learned tasks, and the effect depends on the amount used and the tolerance levels of the individual. Heavy marijuana use can inhibit good study habits and can have a detrimental effect on an individual's motivation to strive for long-term goals.

Recent clinical studies show that heavy marijuana smoking may be harmful to lung functioning. Like tobacco, marijuana is usually smoked and inhaled deeply. Marijuana may interfere with lung function and may produce bronchial irritation in habitual users. One study has found that smoking four or more "joints" per week decreases the lung's vital capacity as much as, or more than, smoking nearly a pack of cigarettes a day. Evidence also indicates that, under conditions of ready availability, the number of marijuana cigarettes consumed (up to ten "joints" daily) may approach that of tobacco cigarettes. In another study, rats were forced to inhale active marijuana smoke daily for up to one year. The dosages corresponded to the amount smoked by a chronic marijuana user, and the period of exposure corresponded to between one-eighth and one-half of the human's normal life span. The exposed rats developed extensive lung inflammation and other damage not found in animals exposed to tobacco or to inert marijuana smoke.

There is some evidence that marijuana smoking may cause lung cancer. Researchers have discovered that marijuana smoke contains more carcinogens than tobacco, that smoke residuals produce skin tumors in experimental animals, and that human lung tissue exposed in vitro to marijuana smoke shows more cellular changes than tissue exposed to tobacco smoke. Very heavy marijuana smoking by healthy young male subjects under controlled experimental conditions has been demonstrated to cause mild but statistically significant airway obstruction.

So far, research on the effects of marijuana on heart functioning have shown it to be benign, except in people with preexisting heart conditions or the elderly. Preliminary research has shown possible adverse impact of marijuana on other bodily functions, such as the immune response, basic cell metabolism, and sexual functioning. Although several

CONTROLLED SUBSTANCES:

	Drugs	Schedule	Trade or Other Names	Medical Uses	Physical Dependence
NARCOTICS	Opium	II, III, V	Dover's Powder, Paregoric, Parepectolin	Analgesic, antidiarrheal	High
	Morphine	II, III	Morphine, Pectoral Syrup	Analgesic, antitussive	
	Codeine	II, III, V	Codeine, Empirin Compound with Codeine, Robitussin A-C	Analgesic, antitussive	Moderate
	Heroin	I	Diacetylmorphine, Horse, Smack	Under investigation	High
	Hydromorphone		Dilaudid	Analgesic	
	Meperidine (Pethidine)	II	Demerol, Pethadol	Analgesic	
	Methadone		Dolophine, Methadone, Methadose	Analgesic, heroin substitute	
	Other Narcotics	I, II, III, IV, V	LAAM, Leritine, Levo-Dromoran, Percodan, Tussionex, Fentanyl, Darvon*, Talwin*, Lomotil	Analgesic, antidiarrheal, antitussive	High-Low
DEPRESSANTS	Chloral Hydrate	IV	Noctec, Somnos	Hypnotic	Moderate
	Barbiturates	II, III, IV	Amobarbital, Phenobarbital, Butisol, Phenoxbarbital, Secobarbital, Tuinal	Anesthetic, anticonvulsant, sedative, hypnotic	High-Moderate
	Glutethimide	III	Doriden	Sedative, hypnotic	High
	Methaqualone	II	Optimil, Parest, Quaalude, Somnafac, Sopor		
	Benzodiazepines	IV	Ativan, Azene, Clonopin, Dalmane, Diazepam, Librium, Serax, Tranxene, Valium, Verstran	Anti-anxiety, anti-convulsant, sedative, hypnotic	Low
	Other Depressants	III, IV	Equanil, Miltown, Noludar Placidyl, Valmid	Anti-anxiety, sedative, hypnotic	Moderate
STIMULANTS	Cocaine†	II	Coke, Flake, Snow	Local anesthetic	Possible
	Amphetamines	II, III	Biphetamine, Delcobese, Desoxyn, Dexedrine, Mediatric	Hyperkinesis, narcolepsy, weight control	
	Phenmetrazine	II	Preludin		
	Methylphenidate		Ritalin		
	Other Stimulants	III, IV	Adipex, Bacarate, Cylert, Didrex, Ionamin, Plegine, Pre-Sate, Sanorex, Tenuate, Tepanil, Voranil		
HALLUCINOGENS	LSD		Acid, Microdot	None	None
	Mescaline and Peyote	I	Mesc, Buttons, Cactus		
	Amphetamine Variants		2,5-DMA, PMA, STP, MDA, MMDA, TMA, DOM, DOB		Unknown
	Phencyclidine	II	PCP, Angel Dust, Hog	Vet. anesthetic	Degree unknown
	Phencyclidine Analogs		PCE, PCPy, TCP		
	Other Hallucinogens	I	Bufotenine, Ibogaine, DMT, DET, Psilocybin, Psilocyn	None	None
CANNABIS	Marihuana	I	Pot, Acapulco Gold, Grass, Reefer, Sinsemilla, Thai Sticks	Under investigation	Degree unknown
	Tetrahydrocannabinol		THC		
	Hashish		Hash		
	Hashish Oil		Hash Oil	None	

Source: National Institute of Drug Abuse
Note: The lower the Schedule Number — The more severe the penalty for possession or sale.

USES & EFFECTS

Psychological Dependence	Tolerance	Duration of Effects (in hours)	Usual Methods of Administration	Possible Effects	Effects of Overdose	Withdrawal Syndrome
High			Oral, smoked			
			Oral, injected, smoked			
Moderate		3 - 6	Oral, injected	Euphoria, drowsiness, respiratory depression, constricted pupils, nausea	Slow and shallow breathing, clammy skin, convulsions, coma, possible death	Watery eyes, runny nose, yawning, loss of appetite, irritability, tremors, panic, chills and sweating, cramps, nausea
	Yes		Injected, sniffed, smoked			
High						
		12 - 24	Oral, injected			
High-Low		Variable				
Moderate	Possible	5 - 8	Oral			
High-Moderate		1-16				
High	Yes	4 - 8	Oral, injected	Slurred speech, disorientation, drunken behavior without odor of alcohol	Shallow respiration, cold and clammy skin, dilated pupils, weak and rapid pulse, coma, possible death	Anxiety, insomnia, tremors, delirium, convulsions, possible death
Low						
Moderate						
	Possible	1 - 2	Sniffed, injected	Increased alertness, excitation, euphoria, increased pulse rate and blood pressure, insomnia, loss of appetite	Agitation, increase in body temperature, hallucinations, convulsions, possible death	Apathy, long periods of sleep, irritability, depression, disorientation
High	Yes	2 - 4	Oral, injected			
			Oral			
Degree unknown		8 - 12	Oral	Illusions and hallucinations, poor perception of time and distance	Longer, more intense "trip" episodes, psychosis, possible death	Withdrawal syndrome not reported
	Yes	Up to days	Oral, injected			
High			Smoked, oral, injected			
Degree unknown	Possible	Variable	Oral, injected, smoked, sniffed			
Moderate	Yes	2 - 4	Smoked, oral	Euphoria, relaxed inhibitions, increased appetite, disoriented behavior	Fatigue, paranoia, possible psychosis	Insomnia, hyperactivity, and decreased appetite occasionally reported

studies suggest that subtle changes occur in brain functioning in animals exposed to marijuana smoke, the implications for humans are still unknown.

There is also preliminary evidence that marijuana affects the glands and hormones that control growth, energy levels, and reproduction. The possibility that embryos and fetuses may be adversely affected by heavy maternal smoking is also under serious investigation.

PCP

Phencyclidine (PCP) — or "angel dust" — is a licit veterinary anesthetic and tranquilizer. Although originally developed as an anesthetic for humans, it was abandoned because of its erratic and unpleasant side effects. PCP can cause stimulation, depression, hallucinations, or analgesia, depending on the dosage.

Most street PCP is made in bootleg laboratories (an investment of several hundred dollars yields thousands of dollars worth of street PCP), so quality and purity vary considerably. Because of its bad reputation on the street, PCP is often sold as mescaline or as other drugs more attractive to users. Users can never be sure what they are buying or whether PCP has been mixed with other drugs (such as marijuana) to heighten the effect.

PCP can be snorted, swallowed, or smoked (e.g., in marijuana or other cigarettes). Only rarely are PCP injections recorded. Smoking is the most common method of administration, partly because users have more control over the drug's effects when it is smoked than when it is ingested orally.

Who Uses It?

Despite these limitations, evidence suggests increasing usage. A recent national survey found that 6 percent of youth between twelve and seventeen years of age (an estimated 1,440,000) had used PCP at least once. Among young adults eighteen to twenty-five, the age category in which all drug use peaks, 14 percent (an estimated 4,210,000) reported having used PCP.

164

Compared to nonusers, PCP users are more likely to have been treated for substance abuse or emotional problems, to evidence self-destructive behavior, to be involved with the criminal justice system, to have poor relationships with peers and families, and to be doing poorly in school.

Health and Social Consequences

Depersonalization is the most common effect of moderate doses of PCP. The user feels a sense of distance and estrangement from the environment. Time and body movements are slowed down; the user may stagger as if drunk. Speech is blocked, sparse, and purposeless. Auditory hallucinations may occur (more frequently at higher doses), and feelings of impending doom or death may appear and disappear. Touch and pain sensations are dulled. Unusual behavior, such as nudity in public places and barking while crawling on the floor, have been reported.

PCP users have also reported feelings of strength, power, and invulnerability which sometimes lead to violent and antisocial behavior even in people not otherwise prone to such behavior. Violent actions, directed at themselves or others, often account for serious injuries or death.

Erratic behavior can lead to death through drowning, burns, falls from high places, and automobile accidents. Suicides by self-inflicted trauma or a massive oral overdose of PCP have occurred in chronic users who had become moody or severely depressed. Other individuals have been found dead with high concentrations of PCP in their bodies, apparently having succumbed due to respiratory depression.

The possible role of PCP in precipitating long-term psychosis is poorly understood. It may be that PCP triggers psychosis in latent schizophrenics. Whatever the cause, there is some evidence that individuals who have used PCP in the past later develop a more enduring schizophrenia despite months of abstinence from the drug.

Chronic PCP users develop persistent cognitive and memory problems; speech problems such as stuttering, poor articulation, and difficulty in expressing themselves; and mood disorders, such as depression, anxiety, and violent behavior. These symptoms often appear after PCP use is discontinued and sometimes occur spontaneously after long periods of abstinence.

BARBITURATES

Barbiturates are a class of drugs containing barbituric acid, a strong central nervous system depressant. They belong to a larger family of drugs known as sedative-hypnotics, or, more commonly, sleeping pills or depressants. The most widely used barbiturates are *Nembutal* (phentobarbital), *Seconal* (secobarbital), and *Amytal* (amobarbital). Taken as prescribed by a physician, depressants may be beneficial for the relief of anxiety, irritability, and tension, and for the symptomatic treatment of insomnia. In excessive amounts, however, they produce a state of intoxication that is remarkably similar to that of alcohol.

Depending on the circumstances in which barbiturates are used, they can also bring on increased energy, sadness, irritability, agitation, rapidly fluctuating mood drifts, and hypochondriacal concerns. Barbiturates are among the most widely prescribed psychoactive drugs in the United States and have a high potential for abuse.

Who Uses Them?

A recent national household survey found that 6 percent of all adults had used sedatives (primarily barbiturates) for nonmedical reasons. Compared to all adults, young adults were three times more likely (18 percent) and youth only half as likely (3 percent) to have used barbiturates for nonmedical purposes. Members of the drug subculture (who may be underrepresented in surveys such as those cited above) often resort to the use of barbiturates as self-medication to soothe jangled nerves brought on by the use of stimulants, to quell the anxiety of "flashbacks" resulting from prior use of hallucinogens, or to ease their withdrawal from heroin. Barbiturates also serve as a means of suicide, a pattern particularly common among women.

Health and Social Consequences

Barbiturates used in small therapeutic doses tend to calm nervous conditions, and larger doses cause sleep twenty to sixty minutes after oral administration. Apparently, however, people who have access to barbiturates — through legal or other channels — do not understand their potential dangers.

166

About 50 percent of all the people admitted to emergency rooms as a result of nonmedical sedative use had a legitimate prescription for their drug but deviated from the prescribed dosage levels. Two household surveys of white, middle-class women not employed outside the home found that few of the women taking these sedatives were using them as prescribed and few seemed to recognize the possible danger in what they were doing. At high dosages, the effects of the barbiturates may progress through successive stages of sedation, sleep, and coma, to death from respiratory arrest and cardiovascular complications.

At best, excessive or inappropriate use of barbiturates relieves anxiety or stress and produces a temporary sense of well-being. It may also produce mood depression and apathy. In marked contrast to the effects of narcotics, intoxicating doses invariably result in impaired judgment, slurred speech, and loss of motor coordination. The dangers of disorientation include a high incidence of highway and household accidents.

Tolerance to the intoxicating effects develops rapidly, leading to a progressive narrowing of the margin of safety between an intoxicating and lethal dose. The person who is unaware of the dangers of increasing dependence will often increase the daily dose up to ten or twenty times the recommended therapeutic level. This, and a common practice of mixing barbiturates with alcohol or other drugs, is responsible for the high number of barbiturate-related overdose deaths and emergency room crises each year.

Moderate depressant poisoning closely resembles alcoholic inebriation. The symptoms of severe depressant poisoning are coma, cold clammy skin, weak and rapid pulse, and slow or rapid but shallow respiration. Death will follow if the reduced respiration and low blood pressure are not counteracted by proper medical treatment.

Barbiturates can also create a strong physical dependency. The abrupt cessation or reduction of high-dose depressant intake may result in a characteristic withdrawal syndrome, which should be recognized as a serious medical emergency. An apparent improvement in the patient's condition may be the initial result of detoxification. Within twenty-four hours, however, minor withdrawal symptoms manifest themselves. These include anxiety and agitation, loss of appetite, nausea and vomiting, increased heart rate and excessive sweating, tremors, and abdominal cramps. The symptoms usually peak during the second or third day of abstinence from the short-acting barbiturates; they may not be reached until the seventh or eighth day of abstinence from the long-acting barbiturates. It is during the peak period that the major withdrawal symptoms usually occur. The user may experience convulsions indistinguishable from those occurring in grand mal epilepsy. More than half of those who experience convulsions will go on to develop delirium, often resulting in a psychotic state identical to the delirium tremors associated with the alcohol withdrawal syndrome. Detoxification and treatment must therefore be carried out under close medical supervision.

AMPHETAMINES

The amphetamines are composed of three closely related drugs (amphetamine, dextroamphetamine, and methamphetamine) that stimulate the central nervous system, promote a feeling of alertness, increase speech and general physical activity, and suppress appetite (anoretic). Amphetamines were first used clinically in the mid-1930s to treat narcolepsy, a rare disorder resulting in an uncontrollable desire for sleep. After their introduction into medical practice, amphetamines were prescribed for an increasing number of conditions, and in greater quantities. For a time, amphetamines were sold, without prescription, in inhalers and other over-the-counter preparations, and abuse of the inhalers became popular. Heavy users who injected amphetamines won notoriety in the drug culture for their bizarre and often violent behavior. Whereas a prescribed dose is between two and one-half and fifteen milligrams per day, those on a "speed" binge have been known to inject as much as 1,000 milligrams every two or three hours.

Recognition of the deleterious effects of these drugs and their limited therapeutic value has led to a marked reduction in their use by the medical profession. The medical use of amphetamines is now limited to narcolepsy, hyperkinetic behavioral disorders in children, and certain cases of obesity — as a short-term adjunct to a restricted diet. About 88 percent of amphetamines are prescribed for weight control. In addition, vast quantities of amphetamines, particularly methamphetamine, are produced in clandestine laboratories for distribution in the illicit market.

Who Uses Them?

Nonmedical use of this class of drugs has been increasing, especially among young adults (age eighteen to twenty-five). In a recent year, an

168

estimated 4 million Americans received a prescription for amphetamines, and another 1.8 million illicitly obtained them. In the same year, 21 percent of this age group reported nonmedical use of stimulants.

Some people use or abuse amphetamines to stimulate alertness or suppress appetite. For others, amphetamines are part of a cyclical drug-taking life-style in which the user takes "uppers" in the morning to make it through the day, and "downers" (such as alcohol or sedatives) at night to relieve amphetamine-induced insomnia.

Health and Social Consequences

The consumption of amphetamines and other stimulants may result in a temporary sense of exhilaration, superabundant energy, hyperactivity, extended wakefulness, and a loss of appetite; it may also induce irritability, anxiety, and apprehension. These effects are greatly intensified with administration by intravenous injection, which may produce a sudden sensation known as a "flash" or "rush." The protracted use of these drugs is followed, however, by a period of depression called "crashing" that is invariably described as unpleasant. Since the depression can be easily counteracted by a further injection of more amphetamines, this abuse pattern becomes increasingly difficult to break.

Heavy users may inject themselves every few hours, a process sometimes continued to the point of delirium, psychosis, or physical exhaustion. In scientific tests, rats and monkeys have been found to administer remarkably large amounts of amphetamines to themselves after only a brief experience with the drug. Moreover, they will continue to self-administer the drugs until lethal toxic effects have ensued. Heavy, frequent doses of amphetamines can produce brain damage that results in speech disturbances and difficulty in turning thoughts into words. Taking more amphetamines increases these risks. Users who inject amphetamines intravenously can contract serious and life-threatening infections from nonsterile equipment. Long-term users often have acne resembling a measles rash; trouble with teeth, gums, and nails; and dry, lifeless hair.

Tolerance develops rapidly to both the euphoric and appetite suppressant effects. Doses large enough to overcome the resulting insensitivity cause various mental aberrations, the early signs of which include repetitive grinding of the teeth, touching and picking the face and extremities, performing the same task over and over, a preoccupation with one's own thought processes, suspicion, and a sense of being watched. Continued high doses result in paranoia with auditory and visual hallucinations and can produce what is known as an amphetamine psychosis. People in this extremely suspicious, paranoid state frequently exhibit bizarre — sometimes violent — behavior.

In the absence of medical intervention, high fever, convulsions, and cardiovascular collapse may precede the onset of death. Physical exertion increases the hazards of stimulant use, since accidental death is due in part to negative drug effects on the cardiovascular and body temperature regulating systems. Fatalities under conditions of extreme exertion have been reported among athletes who have taken these stimulants in moderate amounts.

If withdrawn from amphetamines, chronic high-dose users exhibit profound depression, apathy, fatigue, and disturbed sleep for up to twenty hours a day. The immediate withdrawal syndrome may last for several days. There may also be a lingering impairment of perception and thought processes. Anxiety, an incapacitating tenseness, and suicidal tendencies may persist for weeks or months. Many experts now interpret these symptoms as indicating that amphetamines and other stimulant drugs are capable of producing physical dependence. Whether the withdrawal syndrome is physical or psychological in origin is academic, since the stimulants are recognized as among the most potent agents of reward and reinforcement that underlie the problem of dependence.

INHALANTS ━━━━━━━━━━━━━━━━━━━━━

Inhalants are a diverse group of chemicals that produce psychoactive (mind-altering) vapors. Although most people do not think of them as drugs, they are powerful central nervous system depressants and produce a "high" similar to alcohol intoxication but that is of shorter duration.

Glue and coolants first surfaced as inhalants of abuse, but an astonishing variety of common household products are now inhaled: paint and paint thinner, gasoline and transmission fluid, cleaning and polishing agents, and almost anything that comes in an aerosol can — hair spray, vegetable oil, paint, and room deodorizers. Some products with legitimate medical uses are popular inhalants, such as amyl nitrite (used to treat heart patients), nitrous oxide (laughing gas), and halothane (anesthesia).

Methods of inhalation vary, although sniffing rags or the fumes in plastic bags are preferred. Youth groups in different cities prefer particular inhalants, and most inhalants are used in social settings such as parks, school grounds, and shopping centers.

Who Uses Them?

An estimated 7 million Americans have experimented with inhalants. Most are under the age of twenty, and many are as young as seven. Fully 9 percent of all youth under the age of seventeen have used inhalants; in some youth populations, one-fourth have tried them. The majority of chronic users are male and are either white or hispanic, although females and youngsters from other minority groups are rapidly catching up. Inhalant use is a low-status activity in the drug subculture. Chronic users are likely to be delinquent, disruptive, bored, antisocial, involved with the criminal justice system, lacking in self-esteem and motivation, faring poorly in school, and come from troubled families.

Health and Social Consequences

At low doses, inhalant users may feel slightly stimulated. At higher amounts, they may feel less inhibited, less in control. At high doses, a loss of consciousness can occur. Users develop a tolerance for inhalants, which means that higher doses are needed each time to achieve the desired effect. Although some sniffers come to depend on sniffing and the behaviors associated with the practice as part of their life-style, no evidence of physical dependence exists.

Effects of inhalants are immediate and last from fifteen to forty-five minutes. Drowsiness usually follows. Headache and nausea can also occur. Some users experience partial amnesia for the period of intoxication, similar to the effects of several alcoholic drinks. Sniffing moderate amounts of inhalants for even a relatively short time can disturb vision and heavily impair judgment and cognitive skills, reduce muscle and reflex control, and cause acute psychosis, paranoia, and hallucinations. Even just one sniffing episode can provoke such effects. Although disturbances resulting from short-term sniffing are usually temporary, some damage may be difficult to reverse.

Repeated sniffing of concentrated inhalant vapors over a number of years can cause permanent damage to the nervous system. Several recent studies have confirmed that mental impairment and brain damage result from sustained inhalant abuse. All thirty-seven chronic inhalers (over 7,000 inhalations each) tested had brain damage, compared to 60 percent of the moderate sniffers (average of fifty or more inhalations) and 30 percent of the experimental sniffers. It has not been determined whether this brain damage is reversible. Other long-term dangers are liver, kidney, blood, and bone marrow damage; drastic weight loss; impaired memory; and central nervous system disorders.

Inhalants — especially propellants used in aerosol sprays — cause "sudden sniffing death." Large doses cause heart failure or suffocation (especially when inhaled from a bag). As in all drug use, taking more than one drug at a time multiplies the risks. Inhalants in combination with other central nervous system depressants — tranquilizers, sleeping pills, or alcohol — increase the risk of overdose. Loss of consciousness, coma, or death can result.

There is also a consistent and long-standing association between inhalant use and violent or other "antisocial" behavior. Inhalant intoxication can result in accidental injury or death when these aggressive impulses are released.

COCAINE

Cocaine is a strong, naturally occurring stimulant to the central nervous system. It is extracted from the leaves of the coca plant, native to South America. Cocaine is sold as a white, translucent, crystallilne powder and is typically adulterated to about half strength with ingredients such as talcom powder or dry milk. It is usually taken intranasally ("snorted"), but some heavy users inject the drug. The average street dose is twenty to fifty milligrams. The acute effects are: euphoria, confidence, energy, increased heart rate and blood pressure, dilated pupils, constriction of peripheral blood vessels, and rise in body temperature and metabolic rate. Cocaine is considered to be a high-status drug thought to be used in some professional, artistic, and creative circles.

Who Uses It?

An estimated 10 million Americans have tried cocaine. Despite its high cost, it has gained popularity on the "street" faster than any other drug in this decade. Adults surveyed recently reported higher lifetime experience levels (6 percent) than youth (4 percent). Current use of the substance is reported by about 1 percent for both groups. The highest lifetime prevalence rate (19 percent) was found among young adults of age eighteen to twenty-five.

Health and Social Consequences

Until recently, scientific knowledge about cocaine use and abuse was very limited, and most of it was based on studies more than fifty years old. More scientific research on cocaine has been done in this decade than in the preceding forty years. Recent research has involved: controlled experiements on human beings and animals; animal studies aimed at discovering theoretical models of psychosis; studies on medical uses; clinical reports on adverse effects and treatment; survey and sociological reports on illicit use; and chemical detection and identification studies. As a result, our knowledge rests on a sounder base and contains fewer gaps.

Most Americans who use cocaine use it sporadically and in small quantities. Its relatively high cost and unavailability have limited its use. Studies of recreational users suggest that, for the great majority, adverse effects are rare and not serious. Nevertheless, some authorities familar with the street scene insist that both laboratory experiments and surveys tend to underestimate the number and severity of undesirable effects. Despite its street representation as a "safe" drug, cocaine has been associated with a sizable number of hospital emergencies and deaths.

Chronic cocaine users often experience perceptual disturbances (especially pseudohallucinations) and paranoid thinking. Hospitals rarely see cases of cocaine psychosis, but a few have been reported. Cocaine psychosis is qualitatively similar to, but of shorter duration than, amphetamine psychosis. In high doses, cocaine can also cause depression of the medullary centers and death from cardiac or, more often, respiratory arrest. Severe physical poisoning and death from the toxic effects are not common.

What little evidence is available suggests that cocaine is not as conducive to aggression as other drugs like alcohol, barbiturates, and amphetamines. Further research is necessary before its aggression potential is adequately determined. Cocaine does not produce a physical dependence of the type that chronic alcoholics or heroin addicts experience, where severe withdrawal pains and anxiety result if the abuse substance is discontinued. It does, however, engender an extreme craving in people who have constant access to it, particularly in users who administer it intravenously.

ADDICTIVE BEHAVIOR

Addiction does not happen only in cases of drug use (and by drugs, we include alcohol and tobacco); the phenomenon of compulsive drug use, dependence, and addiction has parallels in all other areas of human behavior.[3] Addiction is not caused by a drug or its chemical properties —it has to do with the effect that a drug produces for a given person in a given circumstance, usually an effect that provides a welcome relief from anxiety.[4]

The most powerful addictive drugs in America today are narcotics, barbiturates, and alcohol. The chemical agents of these drugs vary widely; no two are remotely alike. But their effect is similar, if not identical: they depress the action of the central nervous system, reducing the user's sense of pain and his sense of the difficulties in life. Ironically, they also lessen the individual's ability to deal with those difficulties, thus producing *more* anxiety. Thus, the cycle of addiction begins: a person uses drugs to combat anxiety; the drugs lessen his ability to overcome stressful situations, thus creating more anxiety and increasing the individual's need for the drug. As the addiction strengthens, the individual's contemplation of having to cope *without* the benefit of the drug becomes more and more frightening.

Soon the individual — now an addict — turns increasingly to the drug to gain the rewards that he used to gain elsewhere but that he is no longer capable of gaining from life. At some point in the addiction process, the main rewards in the individual's life are actually coming from the drug itself.

Here is a truth basic to an understanding of all addiction: people can resist addiction to *any* substance when they gain enough satisfaction from their life that they do not have to seek out *one* thing that alone must provide them with contentment. As long as an individual's life is rich with rewarding activities and associations, he gains that contentment

174

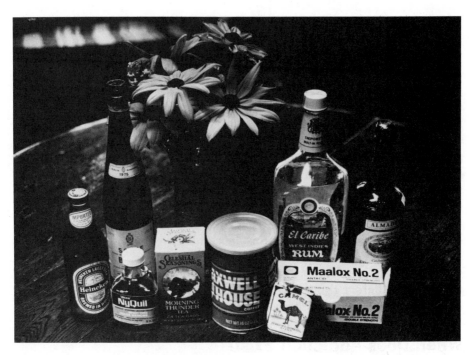

Commonly abused substances found in the home.

from a variety of sources, none of which need include an addictive substance.

A good example of addiction involves something that we all have to do — eat. While everyone has to eat, some people eat to the point of severely limiting (and even shortening) their lives. The relationship of excess weight to heart attack, strokes, and other physical ailments, and the pain that comes from obesity, professionally and personally, clearly indicate that there are people who are well aware of how much they are hurting themselves and yet who are powerless to control their compulsive eating. A person who is rewarded as a child for cleaning up his plate may become obese due to overeating; when he is shunned by social contacts, excluded from physical activities, and snubbed professionally, he has one refuge to which he can turn — eating.

But eating — and all other activities, including drug use — does not have to lead to addiction. Addiction can occur as a result of any involvement with any activity, but it is critical to realize that *no* activity is necessarily addictive.

What makes a substance or activity nonaddictive? The key is being able to control use and to fit the substance or activity, in its proper perspective, into the rest of your life. You must be able to stop doing something (taking drugs, eating, gambling) when it becomes harmful. It means having a well-balanced life with a variety of activities so that stopping that one harmful activity (taking drugs, eating compulsively, gambling) does not leave you "high and dry." Nonaddiction is characterized by a person who has other meaningful relationships and substances in his life. He is a person who likes himself and respects himself enough not to want to hurt himself. He has enough pride that he does not want to be out of control — both for his own benefit and for the benefit of others. He accepts himself, combatting the guilt and anxiety that are at the center of any addiction cycle, no matter what the substance. And, perhaps most critical, he can acknowledge and confront his problems before they become life-threatening or defeating, requiring an addiction to suppress the conflict.

When Does Addiction Exist?

In developing a model of addiction, Stanton Peele, a member of Harvard University's organizational behavior faculty, identified four major characteristics of all addiction.[5]

1. **Addiction is a continuum.** Addiction is not an "all-or-nothing" phenomenon. There is no distinct psychological or physiological mechanism that triggers addiction — no one point at which addiction occurs. As with all other aspects of life, it is indefinite, on a continuum that may progress in one direction or regress in another. An individual may be addicted only in one area of his or her life — an area in which he or she feels particularly unable to cope — or the addiction may spread to various areas of a person's life and may include complex overlapping.
2. **Addiction detracts from all other activities and involvements.** To be addictive, an activity must be harmful. Obviously, some things are balantly harmful: overeating, alcoholism, excessive tobacco smoking, and drug-taking can harm a person's health and can even cause death. Other activities are not so obviously harmful. But with

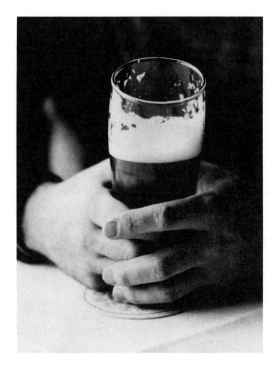

The path of abuse leads from amusement to addiction.

addiction, no matter what the substance, the same process occurs: the involvement with the substance grows stronger and stronger until the person's overall scope diminishes, and there is only one point of focus left for the person — the object of the addiction. A full-blown addiction exists when the individual can gain satisfaction and gratification from *nothing* except the addictive substance or activity.

Obviously, only the individual involved can determine when something is harmful to the point that it becomes the primary source of gratification and all other meaning in life is lost. For this reason, technicians and medical professionals cannot always accurately define an addiction. Only the individual can tell when the addictive point has been reached and surpassed.

3. **Addiction is not a pleasurable experience.** During the cycle in which addiction develops, the user turns to the involvement or substance as a release from pain, anxiety, tension, fear, guilt, or discomfort. At first, the user *does* receive such relief from use of the substance. As

the addiction increases and deepens, the euphoria that at first occurs is lost. True, chemical substances in drugs and alcohol still serve to deaden pain and provide anxiety relief, but they no longer provide pleasure in and of themselves. Thus, we see another major criterion for addiction: addiction is present when a substance is used not for its pleasurable aspects, but only for its ability to combat anxiety, guilt, fear, tension, and pain. In other words, the substance is not used for its own merit, but only for what it can do.

4. **Addiction is the inability to choose not to do something.** Obviously, an addict cannot choose to stop using a substance even though he is well aware that the use is hurting him. He cannot stop using something even when it ceases to be pleasurable for him. If a person has no choice concerning involvement with the substance, an addiction has developed. Here, then, is the final criterion of addiction: the addicted individual cannot stop. He has no choice.

DRUG TAKING AND STRESS

Continual recourse to alcoholic beverages or drugs to substitute for any unmet human need can result in serious problems. Repeated use of alcohol or drugs as a way of dealing with stress is an ineffective and harmful way to try to cope with tension. It does not resolve the stress, and it can create new problems that did not previously exist. This practice can be called "flight behavior." It does not deal constructively with stress, but instead brings other problems in its train.

What about drinking or drug taking when conflict or stress makes you want to hide, run away, or become aggressive about a problem? Is drug taking for these reasons always ill-advised?

Escape is generally presented as a totally negative response to frustration, stress, and anxiety. However, there is another side to it. In some circumstances, getting away may be the only sensible thing to do. It is possible to wax eloquent about the creative and restorative qualities of escape. Many problems can be successfully confronted and resolved if you learn to cope — if you modify the way in which you respond to difficulties. Other problems cannot be dealt with by changing your usual approach. A destitute person cannot be taught to cope with hunger but must be helped to learn how to get food. If you are well fed, safe,

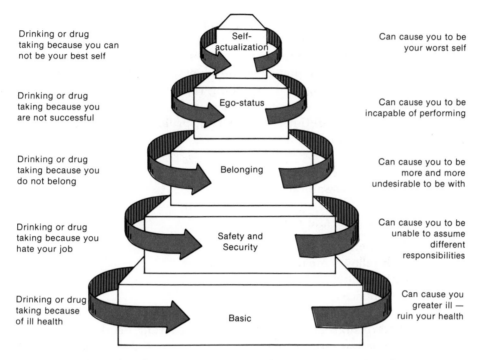

Drinking or drug taking because you can not be your best self

Self-actualization

Can cause you to be your worst self

Drinking or drug taking because you are not successful

Ego-status

Can cause you to be incapable of performing

Drinking or drug taking because you do not belong

Belonging

Can cause you to be more and more undesirable to be with

Drinking or drug taking because you hate your job

Safety and Security

Can cause you to be unable to assume different responsibilities

Drinking or drug taking because of ill health

Basic

Can cause you greater ill — ruin your health

Figure 5-8. Recurrent drinking or drug taking to compensate for unfulfilled ego and human needs can make it more difficult to ever fulfill these needs.

respected, and loved, you should be able to explore undeveloped capacities. Some problems require a change in people; others require a change in the environment that people inhabit.

It is not uncommon to hear people who have no apparent drinking problem say that they occasionally "drink to cope" with no apparent ill effects. Should you allow for that possibility when it is rather clear that such behavior is potentially dangerous? When you continually use alcoholic beverages or drugs to compensate for the frustration of human needs and aspirations, a red flare should go up.

Although there is little consensus on how to define and measure drinking and drug-related problems, one useful way is in terms of the consequences to self or others. A drinking or drug-related problem is one occasioned by the use of alcoholic beverages or drugs that results in harm to yourself or others. Under this definition, any problem closely associated with drinking or drugs can be considered a problem.

Drinking and drug problems can be more or less serious, depending on the severity and/or frequency of the adverse consequences associated with the drugs. Drinking or drug-taking repeatedly in ways that cause harm to self or others is obviously a matter of more concern than doing so once or twice in a lifetime. Most lists of problems include categories that are familiar to all of us:

Interpersonal problems
    with spouse and family
    with relatives
    with friends and neighbors

Social problems
    with fellow employees and employer
    with creditors
    with police

This lists brings around full circle. Recurrent drinking or drug-taking to compensate for unfilled ego and human needs can make it more difficult to ever fulfill these needs. For example, drinking heavily and constantly because you hate your job can make you incapable of performing in a more desirable job. Drinking because of marital problems makes the problems worse. Drinking because you consider yourself a failure makes it less likely that you will ever be a success. In short, drinking or drug-taking to substitute for frustrated human needs makes it harder to achieve the real thing.

PREVENTION

Of course, the best method of coping with substance abuse is prevention of the problems and situations that cause the abuse itself.

Teresa Kurzman-Seppala has indicated several helpful means of prevention of substance abuse. First, prevention can be partially accomplished by enhancing your social competencies — competencies that promote healthy personal functioning. The following have been cited as elements of social competencies that can be capitalized upon: trust (reliance upon the affection of other people), self-confidence (confidence in your capabilities and capacities to effect change in the environment), directionality (a sense of purpose and direction in life), identity (an integrated and coherent self-identity), perspective-taking (the ability to empathize with others), and interpersonal skills (those skills used to build and maintain productive and fulfilling relationships so that you are socially effective).

In addition, prevention can be effected by providing information on drug use. It is hoped that through informing people about the consequences of substance use and abuse, educating them about responsible use of substances, and through an indication of how to deal with behavioral problems, substance abuse will become less attractive.

Lastly, prevention may be achieved by promoting alternative ways of feeling good and of coping with problems.

ALTERNATIVES TO SUBSTANCE ABUSE

Treatment efforts aimed at substance abuse need to center on the behavioral aspects of substance abuse — *why* people resort to using drugs, alcohol, and tobacco — and they need to center on providing alternatives to satisfy the needs that drugs, alcohol, or tobacco fulfill in the mind of the user.

Those who use drugs, alcohol, or tobacco for physical relaxation or for increased physical energy should be trained in relaxation exercises (including yoga, dance movement, and others) and should participate in physical recreation that includes competitive athletics, individual physical conditioning (jogging or exercise), hiking, or training in the martial arts. They should become attuned to the positive sensations provided by a healthy body in motion.

Those who use drugs, alcohol, or tobacco to relieve the anxiety of possible illness should receive training in good dietary habits, positive health habits, and preventive health care. Those who seek an intensification of sensory input (such as sight and sound) should undergo sensory awareness training, should learn massage, and should participate in regular visual exploration of nature using the principles learned in sensory awareness training. In these ways, the senses can become trained to transcend some mundane aspects of the environment.

Those who use alcohol, tobacco, or drugs to fulfill emotional needs such as reduction of anxiety and tension, avoidance of decisionmaking, desire for aloneness and privacy, rebellion, or increase in self-esteem should be provided with careful, competent, empathic counseling designed to center on those needs — not on the particular substance abuse. Such counseling should be professional in nature and should also concentrate on helping the individual identify needs.

Those who use alcohol, tobacco, or drugs to gain a sense of "community" and belonging should engage in positive, goal-directed activities such as those provided by professional organizations, church organizations, community clubs, scouting programs, and 4-H programs. Counseling and family therapy should be provided, as should marriage counseling and individual counseling if it is needed.

Those who use substances to relieve boredom should develop mental/intellectual hobbies and games or should strive for intellectual stimulation through reading, discussion groups, or student caucuses. Those trying for an increase in creative ability can gain training and experience in artistic, communication, or theatric skills and may consider joining other students in forming a community center for the arts.

The above are loosely structured ideas for specific needs that cause people to turn to substance abuse. The main idea is to identify what made you turn to drugs or alcohol or tobacco, and then to find an alternative way of satisfying the need or desire that the substance now satisfies. You may require professional counseling, training in alternative behaviors, or the simple suggestions of others to come up with your own alternatives.

Meeting your full range of needs — physical, mental, emotional, spiritual, social, and intellectual — can start you on the path away from addiction and habit. Good principles of physical and mental health can enable you to maintain control and avoid the traps of addiction.

Notes

1. Second Annual Report on Drug Abuse, Prevention, Treatment, and Rehabilitation, Department of Health, Education, and Welfare, 1979.
2. Mark Keller, "Alcoholism. Nature and Extent of the Problem," *Annals of Political and Social Science,* 315:1-11.
3. This and parts of the following discussion taken from Stanton Peele, "The Addiction Experience, Part II," *Addictions* (Ontario, Canada: Addiction Research Foundation of Ontario, Fall 1977), p. 37.
4. This and parts of the following discussion taken from Stanton Peele, "The Addiction Experience, *Addictions* (Ontario, Canada: Addiction Research Foundation of Ontario, Summer 1977), p. 3.
5. Peele, "The Addiction Experience," Part II, pp. 42-44.

Much of this chapter is adapted from Second Annual Report on Drug Abuse Prevention, Treatment, and Rehabilitation, Department of Health & Human Services.

Self-Evaluation

Why do you smoke?

Here are some statements made by people to describe what they get out of smoking cigarettes. How *often* do you feel this way when smoking them? Circle one number for each statement.

Important: Answer every question.

	Always	Frequently	Occasionally	Seldom	Never
A. I smoke cigarettes in order to keep myself from slowing down.	5	4	3	2	1
B. Handling a cigarette is part of the enjoyment of smoking it.	5	4	3	2	1
C. Smoking cigarettes is pleasant and relaxing.	5	4	3	2	1
D. I light up a cigarette when I feel angry about something.	5	4	3	2	1
E. When I have run out of cigarettes I find it almost unbearable until I can get them.	5	4	3	2	1
F. I smoke cigarettes automatically without even being aware of it.	5	4	3	2	1
G. I smoke cigarettes to stimulate me, to perk myself up.	5	4	3	2	1
H. Part of the enjoyment of smoking a cigarette comes from the steps I take to light up.	5	4	3	2	1
I. I find cigarettes pleasurable.	5	4	3	2	1
J. When I feel uncomfortable or upset about something, I light up a cigarette.	5	4	3	2	1
K. I am very much aware of the fact when I am not smoking a cigarette.	5	4	3	2	1
L. I light up a cigarette without realizing I still have one burning in the ashtray.	5	4	3	2	1
M. I smoke cigarettes to give me a "lift."	5	4	3	2	1
N. When I smoke a cigarette, part of the enjoyment is watching the smoke as I exhale it.	5	4	3	2	1

DRUGS AND PARAPHERNALIA

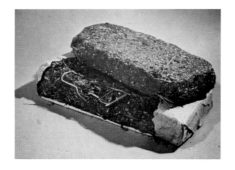

Kilo Bricks of Marijuana

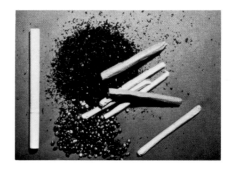

Manicured Marijuana

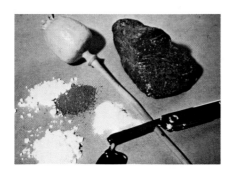

Opium, Poppy, and Derivatives

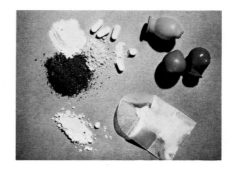

Forms of Heroin

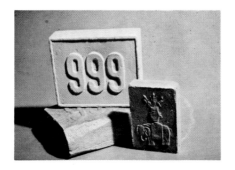

Morphine Base

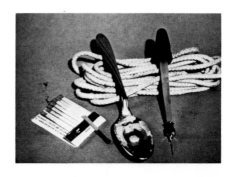

Addict's Equipment

DRUG SOURCES

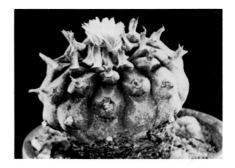

Marijuana Plant

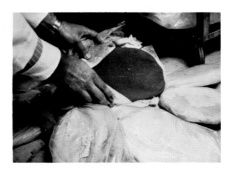

Peyote Cactus

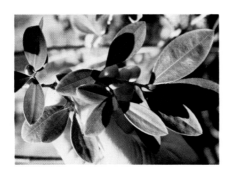

Coca Plant

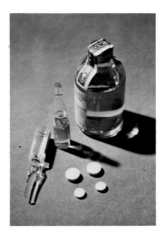

Hashish

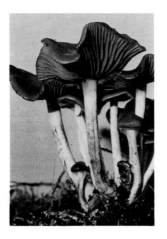

Psilocybin Mushroom

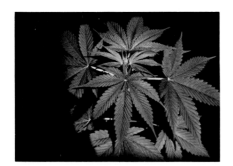

Synthetic Narcotics

ALCOHOL & DRUG ABUSE DISORDERS

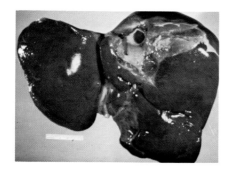

Normal Liver

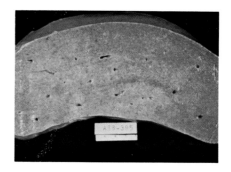

Alcoholic Cirrohsis

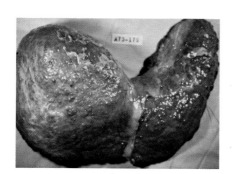

Fatty Liver (Alcohol)

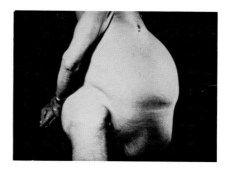

Advanced Alcoholic Cirrhosis

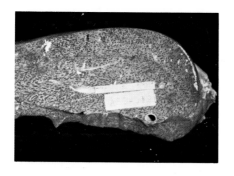

Liver Damage - Drug Overdose

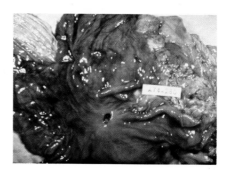

Chronic Gastric Ulcer

DRUG & ALCOHOL RELATED DISORDERS

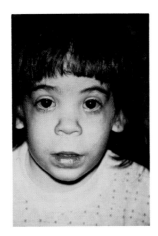

Fetal Alcohol Syndrome

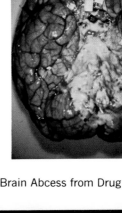

Brain Abcess from Drug Injection

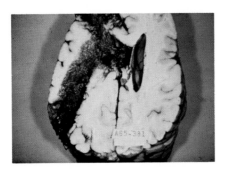

Fetal Alcohol Brain Damage

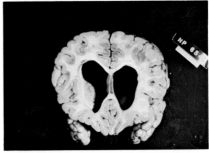

Bullet Wound to Brain Alcohol Related

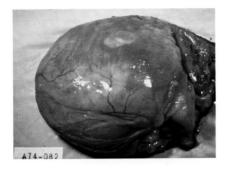

Alcohol Induced Cardiomyopathy

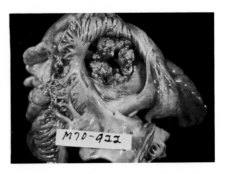

Fungal Damaged Heart from Drug Injection

CHRONIC & DEGENERATIVE DISORDERS

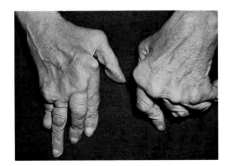

Rheumatoid Arthritis

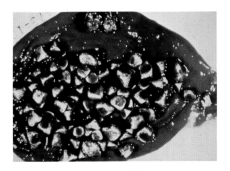

Gallstones

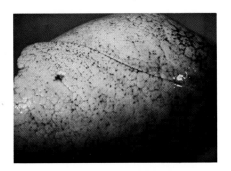

Normal Lung City Dweller

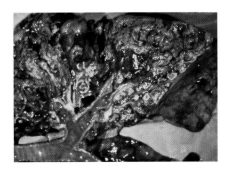

Lung Cancer and Emphysema

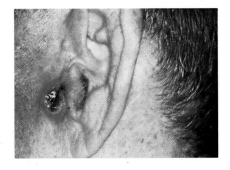

Advanced Skin Cancer

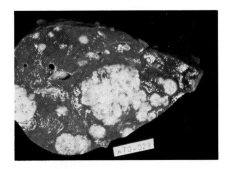

Liver Cancer

VENEREAL DISEASE

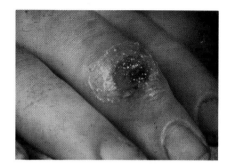

Syphilitic Chancre of Hand

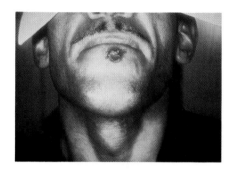

Syphilitic Chancre of Lip

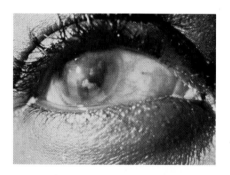

Syphilitic Involvement of Eye

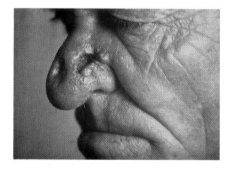

Late Stage Syphilis

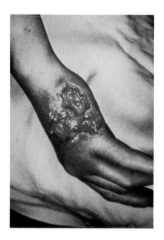

Syphilitic Gumma (Late Stage)

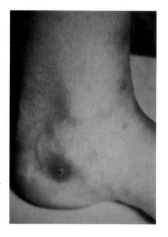

Gonorrhea Skin Lesion

VENEREAL DISEASE

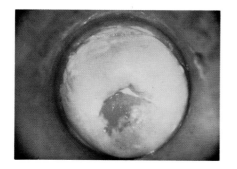

Cervical Gonorrhea

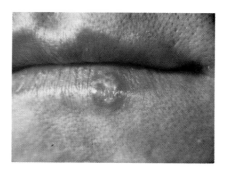

Herpes

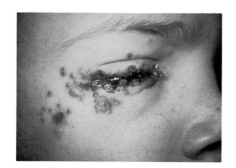

Herpes

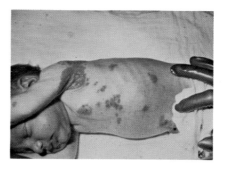

Neonatal Herpes

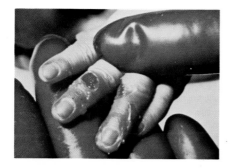

Neonatal Herpes

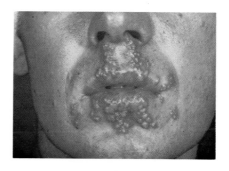

Herpes

COMMON EMERGENCIES

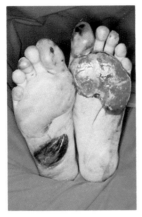

Frostbite

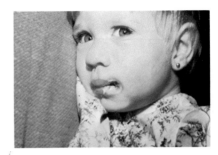

Electrical Burn
Chewing on Electrical Cord

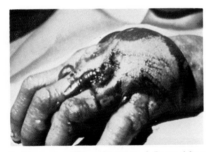

Rattlesnake Bite - Approx. 4 Days After

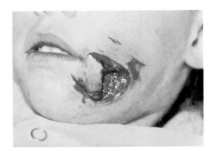

Dog Bite

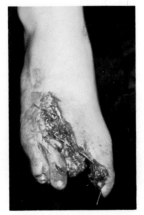

Rotary Lawn-Mower Injury

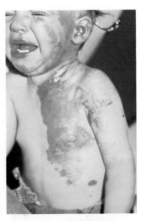

Third Degree Scald Burn

O. I want a cigarette most when I am comfortable and relaxed.   5   4   3   2   1

P. When I feel "blue" or want to take my mind off cares and worries, I smoke cigarettes.   5   4   3   2   1

Q. I get a real gnawing hunger for a cigarette when I haven't smoked for a while.   5   4   3   2   1

R. I've found a cigarette in my mouth and didn't remember putting it there.   5   4   3   2   1

How to score:

1. Enter the numbers you have circled to the Test questions in the spaces below, putting the number you have circled to question A over line A, to question B over line B, and so on.

2. Total the three scores across on each line to get your totals. For example, the sum of your scores over lines A, G, and M gives you your score on *Stimulation* —lines B, H, and N give the score on *Handling*, etc.

Totals

_____ + _____ + _____ = _____   11 or above suggests you are
  A   G   M   Stimulation   stimulated by the cigarette to get going and keep going. To stop smoking, try a brisk walk or exercise when the smoking urge is present.

_____ + _____ + _____ = _____   11 or above suggests
  B   H   N   Handling   satisfaction from handling the cigarette. Substituting a pencil or paper clip, or doodling may aid in breaking the habit.

_____ + _____ + _____ = _____   11 or above suggests you
  C   I   O   Pleasurable relaxation   receive pleasure from smoking. For this type of smoker, substitution of other pleasant habits (eating, drinking, social activities, exercise) may aid in eliminating smoking.

____ + ____ + ____ = _____
  D   J   P   Crutch: tension
                   reduction

11 or above suggests you use cigarettes to handle moments of stress or discomfort. Substitution of social activities, eating, drinking, or handling other objects may aid in stopping.

____ + ____ + ____ = _____
  E   K   Q   Craving: psychological
                   addiction

11 or above suggests an almost continuous psychological craving for a cigarette. "Cold turkey" may be your best method of breaking the smoking habit.

____ + ____ + ____ = _____
  F   L   R   Habit

11 or above suggests you smoke out of mere habit and may acquire little satisfaction from the process. Gradually reducing the number of cigarettes smoked may be effective in helping you stop.

Scores can vary from 3 to 15. Any score 11 or above is *high;* any score 7 and below is *low.*

What do you think the effects of smoking are?

For each statement, circle the number that shows how you feel about it. Do you strongly agree, mildly agree, mildly disagree, or strongly disagree?

Important: Answer every question.

	Strongly agree	Mildly agree	Mildly disagree	Strongly disagree
A. Cigarette smoking is not nearly as dangerous as many other health hazards.	1	2	3	4
B. I don't smoke enough to get any of the diseases that cigarette smoking is supposed to cause.	1	2	3	4
C. If a person has already smoked for many years, it probably won't do him much good to stop.	1	2	3	4

D. It would be hard for me to give up
smoking cigarettes.   1   2   3   4

E. Cigarette smoking is enough of a
health hazard for something to be
done about it.   4   3   2   1

F. The kind of cigarette I smoke is much
less likely than other kinds to give me
any of the diseases that smoking is
supposed to cause.   1   2   3   4

G. As soon as a person quits smoking
cigarettes he begins to recover from
much of the damage that smoking
has caused.   4   3   2   1

H. It would be hard for me to cut down
to half the number of cigarettes I now
smoke.   1   2   3   4

I. The whole problem of cigarette
smoking and health is a very minor
one.   1   2   3   4

J. I haven't smoked long enough to
worry about the diseases that cigarette
smoking is supposed to cause.   1   2   3   4

K. Quitting smoking helps a person to
live longer.   4   3   2   1

L. It would be difficult for me to make
any substantial change in my smoking
habits.   1   2   3   4

How to score:

1. Enter the numbers you have circled to the Test questions in the spaces below,
putting the number you have circled to question A over line A, to question B
over line B, and so on.
2. Total the three scores across on each line to get your totals. For example, the
sum of your scores over lines A, E, and I gives you your score on *Importance*
—lines B, F, and J give the score on *Personal Relevance,* and so on.

Totals

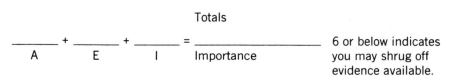

_____ + _____ + _____ = _____   6 or below indicates
  A   E   I   Importance   you may shrug off
                                                     evidence available.

_____ + _____ + _____ = _____   6 or below may
   B   F   J   Personal relevance   indicate the
                                                     "it-can't-happen-to-
                                                     me" attitude.

_____ + _____ + _____ = _____   6 or below suggests
   C   G   K   Value of stopping   an unawareness of
                                                     health benefits
                                                     occurring when you
                                                     quit.

_____ + _____ + _____ = _____   6 or below suggests
   D   H   L   Capability for stopping   you feel stopping
                                                     would be difficult.

Scores can vary from 3 to 12. Any score 9 and above is _high;_ any score 6 and below is _low._

National Clearinghouse for Smoking and Health

Could You Be In Danger of Alcoholism?

Directions: Respond to the following questions by answering "yes" or "no."

Yes   No

_____ _____ 1. Do you occasionally drink heavily after a disappointment, a quarrel, or when the boss gives you a hard time?

_____ _____ 2. When you have trouble or feel under pressure, do you always drink more heavily than usual?

_____ _____ 3. Have you noticed that you are able to handle more liquor than you did when you were first drinking?

_____ _____ 4. Did you ever wake up on the "morning after" and discover that you could not remember part of the evening before, even though your friends tell you that you did not "pass out?"

_____ _____ 5. When drinking with other people, do you try to have a few extra drinks when others will not know it?

_____ _____ 6. Are there certain occasions when you feel uncomfortable if alcohol is not available?

188

		7.	Have you recently noticed that when you begin drinking you are in more of a hurry to get the first drink than you used to be?
_____	_____	8.	Do you sometimes feel a little guilty about your drinking?
_____	_____	9.	Are you secretly irritated when your family or friends discuss your drinking?
_____	_____	10.	Have you recently noticed an increase in the frequency of your memory "blackouts?"
_____	_____	11.	Do you often find that you wish to continue drinking after your friends say that they have had enough?
_____	_____	12.	Do you have a reason for the occasions when you drink heavily?
_____	_____	13.	When you are sober, do you often regret things that you have done or said while drinking?
_____	_____	14.	Have you tried switching brands or following different plans for controlling your drinking?
_____	_____	15.	Have you often failed to keep the promises that you have made to yourself about controlling or cutting down your drinking?
_____	_____	16.	Have you ever tried to control your drinking by making a change in jobs, or moving to a new location?
_____	_____	17.	Do you try to avoid family or close friends while you are drinking?
_____	_____	18.	Are you having an increasing number of financial and work problems?
_____	_____	19.	Do more people seem to be treating you unfairly without good reason?
_____	_____	20.	Do you eat very little or irregularly when you are drinking?
_____	_____	21.	Do you sometimes have the "shakes" in the morning and find that it helps to have a little drink?
_____	_____	22.	Have you recently noticed that you cannot drink as much as you once did?
_____	_____	23.	Do you sometimes stay drunk for several days at a time?
_____	_____	24.	Do you sometimes feel very depressed and wonder whether life is worth living?

_____ _____ 25. Sometimes after periods of drinking, do you see or hear things that are not there?

_____ _____ 26. Do you get terribly frightened after you have been drinking heavily?

Scoring: Those who answer **yes** to **any** of these questions may have some symptoms of alcoholism and should seek help. **Yes** answers to **several** of the questions indicate these stages of alcoholism:

Questions 1-8:   early stage
Questions 9-21:   middle stage
Questions 22-26: beginning of the final stage.

_____

Source: From the brochure, *What are the Signs of Alcoholism?* published by the National Council of Alcoholism.

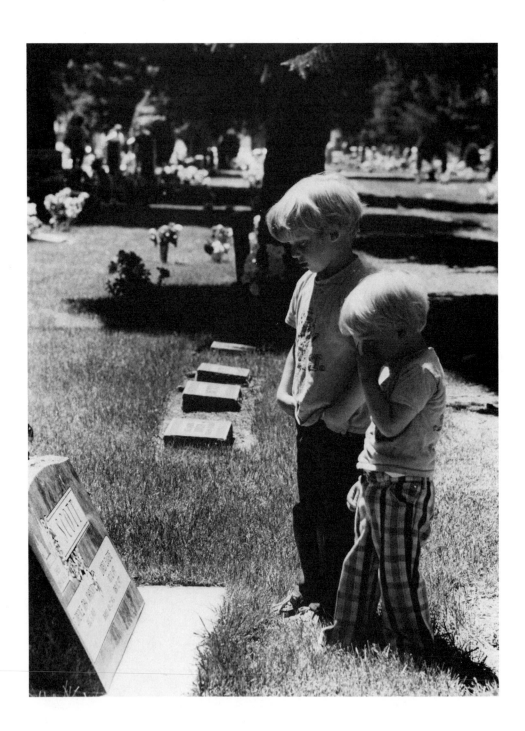

6
Life Crises: From the Beginning to the End

CHILD ABUSE

One of the most devastating and tragic crises of childhood is child abuse and neglect, a problem that affects an estimated million children every year in the United States. Approximately six a day — one every four hours — die from the ravages of child abuse and neglect.[1] Every segment of society is affected by child abuse; race, socioeconomic level, education, and size of community have no relation to the frequency or occurrence of child abuse and neglect.

Child abuse and neglect can result in death or permanent injury: they can also cause serious irreversible damage to the child's personality. In short, child abuse or neglect can make it impossible for a child to grow up and develop into a healthy human being.

And it is a vicious cycle: most people who mistreat children were abused themselves when they were children. In other words, the abused

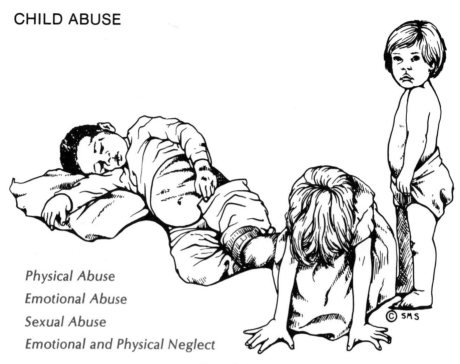

Physical Abuse

Emotional Abuse

Sexual Abuse

Emotional and Physical Neglect

Figure 6-1.

grow up to become abusing adults themselves, and the cycle continues.

There are four basic kinds of abuse and neglect: physical abuse, physical or emotional neglect, emotional abuse, and sexual abuse.

Physical Abuse

A child who is physically abused will have unusual bruises, welts, burns, or fractures. Sometimes he will have bite marks. He will seem to suffer from many injuries, but his parents will always be able to explain them as "accidents." The child's behavior is vastly affected. He may tell you that his parents have hurt him. Many are unpleasant, hard to get along with, demanding, and disobedient. Many abused children frequently cause trouble or break and damage things. Others are unusually shy; they avoid people, and they seem too eager to please. Such a child will not often protest.

A school child who is abused at home is usually late to school much of the time; he often is absent. An abused child may either arrive at school too early or loiter around after school has been dismissed, reluctant to go home. In some cases, the abusing parent will seem unconcerned about the child; in others, the parent will perceive the child as a bad, evil monster and will exercise discipline that seems excessively harsh or inappropriate for the child's age.

Emotional or Physical Neglect

The victim of emotional or physical neglect is characteristically tired, lacking in energy, and usually is not clean; his clothes are generally dirty or inappropriate for the weather conditions (a child who wears no coat in a snowstorm), and many neglect victims are badly in need of dental care, eyeglasses, or other medical attention.

A neglected child will often come to school without having eaten any breakfast, and many will not bring a lunch and will have no money to buy lunch. He usually has not completed homework assignments, and he seems to be alone often, isolated from the other children for long periods of time.

Misbehavior is common among victims of neglect. Such a child will frequently cause trouble in school, will participate in vandalism or destruction of property, will beg for or steal food, or will use alcohol and/or drugs. A common problem with neglected children is their tendency to sexual misconduct. They are frequently absent from school.

The parent or caretaker who neglects a child emotionally or physically usually has a history of neglect as a child and lives a life that is very isolated from neighbors, friends, and even other relatives; he or she often lacks the skills of socializing.

The parent often seems to have an apathetic attitude; he or she does not seem to care what happens (to the child or anyone else) and often gives the impression that he or she is powerless to do anything to solve current problems or resolve the situation.

Emotional Abuse

It is difficult to tell whether a child is being emotionally abused because there are few physical signs. Behavioral indicators include being behind for his age in emotional, intellectual, or physical development;

Physical and Behavioral Indicators of Child Abuse and Neglect

TYPE OF CA/N	PHYSICAL INDICATORS	BEHAVIORAL INDICATORS
PHYSICAL ABUSE	Unexplained Bruises and Welts: - on face, lips, mouth - on torso, back, buttocks, thighs - in various stages of healing - clustered, forming regular patterns - reflecting shape of article used to inflict (electric cord, belt buckle) - on several different surface areas - regularly appear after absence, weekend or vacation Unexplained Burns: - cigar, cigarette burns, especially on soles, palms, back or buttocks - immersion burns (sock-like, glove-like, doughnut shaped on buttocks or genitalia) - patterned like electric burner, iron, etc. - rope burns on arms, legs, neck or torso Unexplained Fractures: - to skull, nose, facial structure - in various stages of healing - multiple or spiral fractures Unexplained Lacerations or Abrasions: - to mouth, lips, gums, eyes - to external genitalia	Wary of Adult Contacts Apprehensive When Other Children Cry Behavioral Extremes: - aggressiveness, or - withdrawal Frightened of Parents Afraid to go Home Reports Injury by Parents
PHYSICAL NEGLECT	Consistent Hunger, Poor Hygiene, Inappropriate Dress Consistent Lack of Supervision, Especially in Dangerous Activities or Long Periods Unattended Physical Problems or Medical Needs Abandonment States There Is No Caretaker	Begging, Stealing Food Extended Stays at School (early arrival and late departure) Constant Fatigue, Listlessness or Falling Asleep in Class Alcohol or Drug Abuse Delinquency (e.g. thefts)

(continued)

Physical and Behavioral Indicators of Child Abuse and Neglect (continued)

TYPE OF CA/N	PHYSICAL INDICATORS	BEHAVIORAL INDICATORS
SEXUAL ABUSE	Difficulty in Walking or Sitting Torn, Stained or Bloody Underclothing Pain or Itching in Genital Area Bruises or Bleeding in External Genitalia, Vaginal or Anal Areas Venereal Disease, Especially in Pre-teens Pregnancy	Unwilling to Change for Gym or Participate in Physical Education Class Withdrawal, Fantasy or Infantile Behavior Bizarre, Sophisticated, or Unusual Sexual Behavior or Knowledge Poor Peer Relationships Delinquent or Run Away Reports Sexual Assault by Caretaker
EMOTIONAL MALTREATMENT	Speech Disorders Lags in Physical Development Failure-to-thrive	Habit Disorders (sucking, biting, rocking, etc.) Conduct Disorders (antisocial, destructive, etc.) Neurotic Traits (sleep disorders, inhibition of play) Psychoneurotic Reactions hysteria, obsession, compulsion, phobias, hypochondria) Behavior Extremes: - compliant, passive - aggressive, demanding Overly Adaptive Behavior: - inappropriately adult - inappropriately infant Developmental Lags (mental, emotional) Attempted Suicide

being either unusually mature or immature (may suck his thumb or rock constantly); or being unusually shy and avoiding others. A child who is emotionally abused is often too anxious to please others and will not protest even in situations that are unpleasant. Some children are unpleasant, hard to get along with, and demanding; many will not leave others (children or adults) alone, and may cause trouble.

A parent or caretaker who emotionally neglects a child usually does so by withholding love, blaming or belittling the child constantly, and treating the children in the family unequally. The parent is often cold and rejecting and usually does not seem to care much about the child's problems.

Sexual Abuse

The child who is the victim of overt sexual abuse will often have torn, stained, or bloody underwear and may experience pain or itching in the genital area. Some have venereal disease.

The child generally has poor relationships with other children and is unwilling to participate in physical activities with others — even innocuous activities like tetherball, volleyball, or hopscotch. Often, the child appears to be withdrawn into a fantasy world and may exhibit babylike behavior; some will tell a teacher or other adult that they have been sexually assaulted by a parent. Many run away from home or engage in delinquent behavior at school or in the community.

The parent who abuses a child sexually is usually very protective or jealous of the child. Such a parent is frequently absent from the home and often misuses drugs or alcohol. Some will even openly encourage a child to participate in sexual acts or prostitution in the presence of other adults.

Causes of Child Abuse and Neglect

No one knows for sure what causes child abuse and neglect, because there is no simple "cause." The situation that results in abuse or neglect is usually a composite of a number of factors. These include:

1. **Characteristics of society,** including violence portrayed on television and in movies, lack of willingness to get involved, discrimination

because of color or class, and society's encouragement of physical methods of disciplining children.

2. **Social and institutional factors,** such as competition among professionals, gaps in service for families that are in trouble, and the kinds and quality of services that society is willing to provide.

3. **Immediate life circumstances,** such as unemployment, poor housing, financial problems, or marital problems.

4. **Personal factors,** including everything that has combined to make up the individual: personality, intelligence, previous experiences, and so on. Of special impact is the parent's own experiences as a child and his or her relationships to parents.

5. **Absence of bonding.** Several investigators have discovered that premature infants who spend a long period of time away from their mothers following birth frequently wind up back in the hospital battered and abused even though they had been sent home intact and thriving. When postnatal separation does not occur, the relationship between the mother and infant is much closer. This enhanced closeness is called "bonding." It would be interesting to learn whether bonding might also occur with the father and, further, whether it might influence relationships between children and their aging and dependent parents.

Identifying the Potential Abuser

A potential abuser can be identified in many cases before the child is even born or shortly after the child is born by the way in which the parents act during pregnancy, childbirth, and immediate postnatal periods.

Before the Child is Born

Those who are prone to abuse or neglect will express great concern over the sex of the child; one or both parents may seem preoccupied with the child's future performance, concerned that he will not "measure up" in some way. The mother may continue to deny her pregnancy into the second trimester and may refuse to talk about the baby or make plans that involve the baby. One or both of the parents may feel great depression over the pregnancy and may comment that the child was an "accident" or is unwanted. Either one may have considered an abortion

Indicators of Emotional Maltreatment

PARENT BEHAVIOR	CHILD BEHAVIOR	
CONSISTENT/GROSS FAILURE TO PROVIDE:	TOO LITTLE MAY RESULT IN:	TOO MUCH MAY RESULT IN:
Love (empathy) (praise, acceptance, self-worth)	Psycho-social dwarfism, poor self-esteem, self-destructive behavior, apathy, depression, withdrawn	Passive, sheltered, naive, "over self-esteem"
Stimulation (emotional/cognitive) (talking-feeling-touching)	Academic failure, pseudo-mental retardation, developmental delays, withdrawn	Hyperactivity, driven
Individuation	Symbiotic, stranger and separation anxiety	Pseudo-maturity
Stability/permanence/continuity of care	Lack of integrative ability, disorganization, lack of trust	Rigid-compulsive
Opportunities and rewards for learning and mastering	Feelings of inadequacy, passive-dependent, poor self-esteem	Pseudo-maturity, role reversal
Adequate standard of reality	Autistic, delusional, excessive fantasy, primary process, private (unshared) reality, paranoia	Lack of fantasy, play
Limits, (moral) guidance, consequences for behavior (socialization)	Tantrums, impulsivity, testing behavior, defiance, antisocial behavior, conduct disorder	Fearful, hyperalert, passive, lack of creativity and exploration
Control for/of aggression	Impulsivity, inappropriate aggressive behavior, defiance, sadomasochistic behavior	Passive-aggressive, lack of awareness of anger in self/others

Indicators of Emotional Maltreatment (continued)

PARENT BEHAVIOR	CHILD BEHAVIOR	
CONSISTENT/GROSS FAILURE TO PROVIDE:	TOO LITTLE MAY RESULT IN:	TOO MUCH MAY RESULT IN:
Opportunity for extrafamilial experience	Interpersonal difficulty (peer/adults), developmental lags, stranger anxiety	Lack of familial attachment, excessive peer dependence
Appropriate (behavior) model	Poor peer relations, role diffusion (deviant behavior, depending on behavior modeled)	Stereotyping, rigidity, lack of creativity
Gender (sexual) identity model	Gender confusion, poor peer relations, poor self-esteem	Rigid, stereotyping
(Sense of) (Provision of) security/safety	Night terrors, anxiety, excessive fears	Oblivious to hazards and risks, naive
Scape-goating, ridicule, denigration		Poor self-esteem, depression
Ambivalence	Rigidity	Lack of purpose, determination, disorganization
Inappropriate expectation for behavior/performance	Poor self-esteem, passivity	Pseudo-maturity
Substance abuse	(Depends on behavior while intoxicated)	
Psychosis	(Depends on behavior/type/frequency)	
Threats to safety/health		Night terrors, anxiety, excessive fears

*Ira S. Lourie M.D. and Lorraine Stefano. On Defining Emotional Abuse: Results of an NIMH/NCCAN Workshop. *Proceedings of the Second National Conference on Child Abuse and Neglect,* Volume 1.

WHY SHOULD YOU GET INVOLVED?

The best reason is to help someone . . . you help the child; you help the parent(s); you help the family as a whole.

If someone — like you — doesn't get involved, the abuse or neglect is very likely to continue. If it does, it may get worse. If it gets worse, a child could die or suffer permanent injury. If that happens, the abusing parent may well go to jail and the family will be broken up. (Also, no parent is likely to get much help in jail).

None of this needs to happen. It rarely does happen if someone gets involved because when you care enough to do something about it, the family can get help.

Some parents — or even older children — seek it on their own. Most do not. They need an outsider to get the help process started.

Most of us don't realize it, but there is a lot of help available for children and parents with child abuse or neglect problems.

There are, for example:

- hospitals (if injuries are severe enough);
- public and private organizations offering a wide range of services, like:

  - protective services
  - emergency shelter for children
  - day care
  - self-help groups
  - help or "hot" lines
  - counseling for parents, children, families

  - homemaker service
  - transportation
  - financial help
  - employment help
  - courses in education for parenthood
  - mental health services

You can put a stop to the abuse or neglect and get help for the family by getting involved!

How? If you are a friend or relative, talk to the parent(s); offer your friendship and help; offer to baby-sit or take care of the child for a few days if you can; tell them about the various kinds of help available; urge them to seek it; offer to make an appointment for them; offer to go with them on their first visit; offer, if you can, to take care of the child for a day or two till things calm down.

If efforts of this kind do not succeed . . . or if the child is hurt, you have no choice but to report it to the proper authority.

but changed his or her mind, or simply waited too long. The woman may be single, may lack the support of her husband, or may lack the support of family members and others who are important to her.

During Birth

The father may refuse to be with his wife during childbirth. Either the mother or father may appear to be apathetic, uninterested, or hostile during the birth process; after birth, they may not express interest in seeing the baby, holding it, or talking about it. They may not establish eye contact with the baby even if they do hold it. Either may become upset or hostile if the baby starts to cry and cannot be quieted. They may express great disappointment over the sex of the baby.

Following Birth

Parents may remain upset over the sex of the child. The mother may find feeding or caring for the baby unpleasant; either parent may become hostile or upset when the baby cries. The parents may name the baby after someone whom they dislike; the father may refuse to participate in child care. The parents may wait an abnormal length of time before naming the baby and may proceed with necessary tasks reluctantly and slowly — including medical checkups, immunizations, purchase of shoes when they are needed, and so on. The mother may be repulsed by the baby's messiness and may find it so difficult to change diapers that the baby develops a severe diaper rash. Trouble is in the offing if the husband is excessively jealous of the infant and resents the amount of time that his wife spends in child care and attention. Parents are in serious trouble if they do not have fun with the baby, if they strike out — verbally or physically — at an infant, or if they seem hostile instead of comforting when the child cries.

DIVORCE

Marital failure, a common life crisis in this country, is a phenomenon that occurs in several degrees. Some people never realize complete

- The recent rapid rise in the American divorce rate, to heretofore unprecedented levels, must be counted among the major demographic changes occurring in the United States since World War II.
- Immediately following World War II, there was a sudden surge of divorce reaching a rate of 4.3 divorces per 1,000 population, more than double the rate occurring before 1940. This sudden surge ended as promptly as it began and rates declined rapidly, returning to pre-war levels.
- More recently, the formal dissolution of marriage through divorce has once again climbed rapidly. Between 1966 and 1976, the annual American divorce rate doubled, rising from 2.5 to 5.0 divorces per 1,000 population. Although the 1977 rate was the same as in 1976, provisional rates showed a slight movement upward in 1978, 1979, and 1980.
- Marriage is less likely to end in divorce as the duration of the marriage increases. For example, 49.6% of newly contracted marriage will end in divorce. Of marriages reaching the 10th anniversary, 26.8% will end in divorce, while only 6.6% of couples reaching their 25th anniversary will divorce.

fulfillment or even find a comfortable degree of companionate love, but nevertheless establish a workable relationship, a kind of corporate coexistence under the same roof. Other couples stay together because of their commitment to the idea of permanence in the marriage relationship but waste their lives in quiet desperation, making no attempts to resolve their conflicts. Many more each year, however, are finding a quick solution to their frustrations, or so they suppose, in the divorce courts. The whole concept of marriage and family is beleaguered. In fact, the divorce rate in the United States leads all other nations in the world.[2]

Although internal conflicts still play the major role in marital failure, external forces also contribute:

1. The change from an agrarian life-style took fathers out of the home to work in the city, thus fracturing cooperative leadership in the home.
2. The fracturing of extended family relationships produced by job relocation has disrupted continuity and traditional ties supportive of

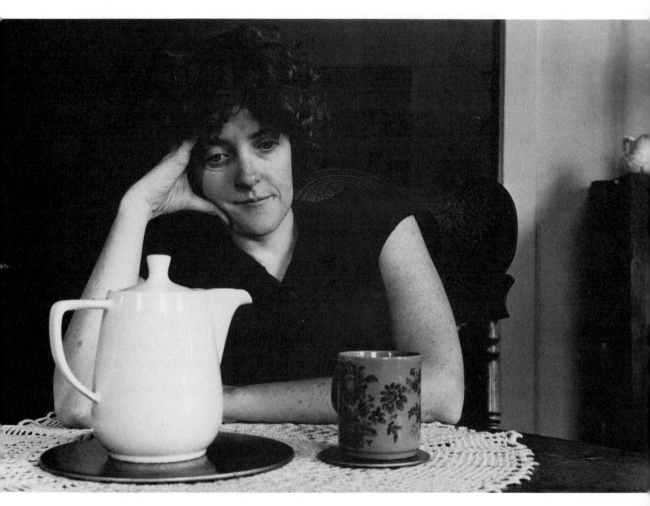

Presently, 50 percent of those married experience the crisis of a divorce.

family relationships. Children too rarely relate to their grandparents, a peculiar benefit in these times of extended life expectancy.

3. The "liberation" of women has encouraged greater independence from or her dependence on the marriage relationship for material and psychological support.

4. The move away from religious tenants, which circumscribed behaviors related to fidelity and commitment, has prompted a more casual orientation to marriage covenants.

5. Various states have instituted laws that provide contraceptive and other services to minors without parental consent. Such legislation suggests a lack of public confidence in the parenting function of the home.

6. Media tends to glamorize the unattached adult or the promiscuous spouse, at the same time ignoring the gratifications of family life. Television in particular is a negative influence, glorifying inhumanity and usurping valuable time that might otherwise be spent in family involvement.

7. Somehow the notion has developed that the activities of a woman caring for her family are not work, while the paid profession of the husband, no matter what he is doing, is the only activity that qualifies.

8. The contractural nature of society has prompted parents to relegate care and training of children to outside agencies. Some parents spend less involved time with their children than the babysitter.

9. Erroneous expectation of the marriage relationship as portrayed in the media and as interpreted from sexology texts leads to disillusionment and frustration.

Whatever the external pressures, there are as many or more problems from within that erode the relationship. The detection of early warning signs that trouble is brewing might allow the couple to ward off the separation and/or divorce if corrective steps are taken. Such signs usually fall into the following categories:[3]

1. **Denial** — lack of honesty and integrity with yourself.
2. **Avoidance** — not talking over with your partner concerns about the relationship.
3. **Repetition** — attempting to discuss problems but achieving no lasting solution.

4. **Detachment** — lack of true commitment to the quality of the relationship.

If these problems are not attacked early, deterioration is likely to continue with the development of further emotional separation from each other. This leads to:

1. **Self-incrimination** — the individual feels negative toward self, fearful that he or she is to blame for the failure in the relationship.
2. **Divided effort** — trying to solve the problem without involving the spouse, a procedure that frequently leads to:

   a. Alienation — ignoring the spouse and divulging private matters to people outside the relationship who are frequently biased, untrained, and emotionally involved. With few exceptions, these forays aggravate rather than alleviate the problem.
   b. Apathy — developing a feeling or attitude of unconcern about which way the marriage goes — giving up on the spouse and the relationship.
   c. Fault-finding — denigrating the spouse in your own mind, to his or her face, and to others.

When relationships have progressed to this point, redemption is more difficult, requiring not only changes in behavior, but changes in attitudes and feelings about each other.

The Trauma of Divorce

Part of the reason why divorce is so common is the perception by troubled couples that it is the most painless solution to their problem. Few fully realize the trauma associated with dissolution of the family, particularly when children are involved:

1. The finances required to run one family rarely support two families at the same level of affluence.
2. Dividing the family does not solve the emotional and personality problems that may have led to the split and that the children continue to endure.

3. Adjustment to single living is frequently prolonged and difficult.
4. When the divorce is not sought mutually, considerable resentment and bitterness remain in the offended spouse.
5. The pressures of working out of the home frequently disrupt the family orderliness previously enjoyed in the home.
6. There is an aloneness resulting from the necessity of assuming the jobs and decision-making responsibilities of the other spouse.
7. The absence of another adult being brings its onmipresent feelings of loneliness, particularly for the woman who elects to devote herself to the care of her children.
8. There are frequently feelings of failure and guilt, the combined effect of "I couldn't make a go of it" from within and "You couldn't make it" from without.
9. For a woman, there is the spectre of the "divorcee," right or wrong, a label that she encounters with great discomfort in many males, both married and single.
10. A divorced individual, whose self-image includes continence outside of marriage, is under considerable emotional strain after several years of regular sexual involvement.
11. The ramifications of a divorce very often plague the new relationship of those who remarry, particularly when children are involved.

These constitute a miniscule listing of the general problems facing the divorced and include none of the trivial day-to-day experiences that are so often magnified into mountains. Regarded as a significant source of stress, the trauma of marital failure should be approached in a fashion similar to other health problems:

Prevention

It is generally easier to stay out of trouble than to get out of trouble. Many second marriages work simply because the couple has learned through the trauma of the first marriage those things that they should have learned before they were married in the first place.

1. Children should be raised to become responsible, loving individuals, able to empathize, finding greatest joy and satisfaction in the happiness of others.

2. Dating couples should carefully determine the strengths and weaknesses of their relationships early, before the involvement evolves into commitment and becomes difficult to terminate.
3. Parents should help children look realistically at the marriage relationship — at its responsibilities, challenges, rewards, and operations.

Treatment

Once in trouble, it is frequently possible to resolve the problems by attacking their causes.

1. Seek help from outside sources, such as books written by professionals who deal with marital difficulties, and the professionals themselves (for example, counselors, clergy).
2. Try to correct those personal and interpersonal defects in attitudes, communication, and behavior that impede the development of a good, charitable, and compassionate relationship.
3. Spend time assessing your personal and joint orientations to life and each other:

    a. Value priorities — what things are important, and how important are they?
    b. Feelings — what hurts, what helps in the relationship?
    c. Goals — what should be coming out of the relationship? Family? Growth?
    d. Options — consequences of various alternatives — what happens if we do this? Where does this discussion lead? What are the risks?
    e. Discussions — what commitments need to be made? What principles need to be held inviolate?

4. Avoid isolation — loneliness is one of the greatest problems that follows divorce. Hold on to the friends that you and your spouse shared; they will still like you, even if your spouse is not there anymore. You will probably feel more comfortable interacting on a one-to-one basis with another couple or hosting a party where both single people and couples are invited. It will help to avoid strictly "couple" situations. Do not feel stupid about going to parties or other

social activities without an escort: the host likes *you,* or he would not have invited you. Or try going out with members of your own sex — there is nothing wrong with enjoying dinner at a restaurant with a group of women whom you have always liked and admired.

5. Listen to the advice of others, but do not be pressured into an uncomfortable situation just because well-meaning friends or relatives are pressuring you. Make your own decisions; you need the support of being in control of your own life.

6. Do not be afraid or embarrassed to ask for help. There are agencies, physicians, and psychologists who specialize in helping separated or divorced individuals.

DEATH AND DYING

All of us as members of the human race suffer differences in the color of our skin, the language that we speak, the foods that we eat, and the very personal ways in which we worship. But there are two things that each of us shares: each of us is born, and each of us dies.

Birth signifies new beginnings — the miraculous unfolding of a human soul, the embryo of countless dreams, the vision of hope in a

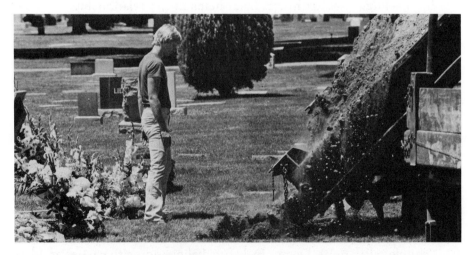

Death represents an ending, a finality, a cessation of all that is good.

bright future. Birth makes us reverent and peaceful. We are eager for birth.

But we dread death. Too often it represents an ending, a finality, a cessation of all that is good. We fear death; we envision blackness, sorrow, cobwebbed tombstones marching across the dying grass of a weed-choked cemetery. We cling tenaciously to life, even when life's melody has struck its final chord and we need to experience that other universal part of living: dying.

We can learn to appreciate death, to dread its coming less, if we understand what happens during the dying process, and if we come to terms with the ways in which our bodies, our minds, and our spirits are affected as we experience death. And because death is common to the human race, the effort to understand death is an effort to understand the human experience a little better.

What Is Death?

To understand death, we must first examine the clinical aspects of dying — that is, we must understand completely what happens to the body and how others determine that death has occurred.

We die in orderly stages; the rate at which we move from one state to another may be very slow (as in those with terminal disease) or very rapid (this rapid progression usually occurs in people who die of a heart attack, stroke, or some kind of an accident that takes life very quickly). The stages of death are clinical death (the body's vital functions cease), brain death (because of lack of blood and oxygen, the brain ceases functioning), biological death (the complete lack of function of all body organs), and cellular death (failure of individual body cells to sustain any kind of life).[4] The first two stages of death — clinical and brain — are especially important to understand.

It appears that some people are able to tell that they are going to die, that during the last days of life some inner kind of premonition allows the individual to begin to expect death (this phenomenon has been observed even when there was absolutely no sign that the person might die — no sign of physical illness or impending accident).

What actual physical changes occur as a person dies? Visible physical changes occur in the body during the last hour of life. The circulatory system slows down, and the lips, fingernails, and toenails turn slightly blue. The skin usually starts to look mottled and blotchy.

As the circulatory system slows down, the person's pulse weakens, and his blood pressure drops; body temperature becomes abnormal, either rising or lowering significantly. The sensation of touch and reflex action are lost in first the legs and then the arms; the person is unable first to move his legs, then his arms. But just because he cannot move does not mean that he is insensitive to pressure such as that exhibited by a squeeze of the hand. Unless he is in deep coma, he is aware that his loved ones are nearby, and he is comforted by their presence. Immediately before death, respiration becomes increasingly difficult.

After clinical death has occurred — that is, after respiration and heartbeat have stopped — brain death occurs. The brain, like the rest of the body, dies in stages. The outer layer of the brain — the cortex — is first; the midbrain follows, and the brainstem is last. Because the outer layer of the brain, which controls thought processes and memory, dies before the brainstem, which controls basic life functions, it is possible for a person to completely lose consciousness on a permanent basis and yet remain "alive"; for weeks or months (a condition referred to as *coma*); in this condition, it is even possible for the body to survive without the aid of respirators or other life-sustaining machinery. Even when the brainstem is dead, it is possible for technicians to keep the heart beating for a limited amount of time (a factor that makes it possible for dying persons to donate organs, since cellular death does not begin as long as blood is circulating).[5]

According to the Harvard definition, brain death has occurred when:[6]

1. The person is completely unresponsive to stimulus and completely unaware of his own internal needs.
2. The person does not respond at all to pain, touch, sound, or light, and the person does not breathe on his own or move his muscles by himself.
3. The person completely loses muscle tone and reflexes.
4. The person exhibits a flat electroencephalogram (test to detect the presence of brain waves), even when the test is conducted under ideal conditions.
5. There is no change in any of the above conditions twenty-four hours later.

Emotional Stages of Dying

How do the person's emotions and feelings enter in? Of course, people who die suddenly do not have time to think about their death situation, to compose their thoughts, to become emotionally involved with this ultimate in growth experiences. But those people who learn that they will die sometime soon have the marvelous opportunity of preparing for death in many ways, chief among them being the emotional preparation.

There are five stages that a dying person goes through, and they are much like the stages that grieving people experience.[7]

When a person is first told that he is going to die, he reacts with **shock** and **disbelief.** He denies that this is happening to him. In a very real sense, he refuses to believe the news that he will die. Some people maintain such a denial for only a few seconds; in the most extreme cases, the denial period may last as long as several months. Eventually, however, people accept the truth of the news regarding their illness and death.

Once a person accepts the fact that he is going to die, he enters the second stage of reaction: **anger.** "Why me?" is a normal question. This stage is characterized by bitterness: the person becomes difficult, nasty, and demanding. He often criticizes viciously the ones who are trying the most to help him. This stage is extremely difficult for both the dying person and those who surround him — loved ones, family members, and doctors and nurses. Relief of this anger is essential, and it eventually comes. One person may need to finally take a drive in the car and scream until she is exhausted; another may simply need to discuss the problem with someone who understands.

Then the person enters the third stage of **bargaining.** Whether it is subconscious or overt, the person promises something in exchange for an extension of life: he might promise to donate his kidneys or eyes, might start going to church every Sunday, or might patch up an old quarrel that had been causing unhappiness for years. But in this bargaining stage, promises are rarely kept — for instance, a woman who begs to be kept alive just until her daughter finishes high school then wants to see her through college, see her son-in-law, hold her grandchild. This stage is earmarked by a frantic, desperate attempt to work something out — to make things better. But eventually the realization comes. The individual does not have control over death.

Enter stage four: **depression.** This can be another period of difficulty for those who surround the dying person. In some patients who are terminally ill, the stage of depression can last for months. The dying person must grieve over impending loss, and it might help us to understand (and tolerate) him better if we realize the magnitude of that loss. Imagine the prospect facing the dying person: he is going to lose not one, but *all* of the people who are dear to him — he is losing everyone he has ever loved. As people who support and care for those who are dying, we need to understand and respect that kind of loss and the courage that it takes to face it.

As the dying person eventually learns to cope with this depression and sense of loss, he finally begins to separate himself from those he knows he will lose. He asks to see people — his cousin, a friend at work, a favorite aunt — for the last time. And then he chooses one special person with whom he wants to spend a great deal of time (this is usually a spouse or, in the case of a child, a parent). He will choose a person whose companionship offers him comfort, peace, and warmth — someone who will sit and hold his hand and be near.

At this point, the dying person has entered the final stage of emotional adjustment: **acceptance.** This is *not* resignation. Resignation means giving up, losing hope. Rather, the dying person comes to terms with himself. He accepts his condition, but he is not defeated. His time is near, and he is all right. People who have come to this point have a great deal to teach us all about living and dying; their experience is one of growth for them and one of progression for those who are lucky enough to share in it. There is no more fear and anger; there is peace and hope for what is to come

Unfortunately, death is usually a time of fear — fear of loneliness, fear of pain, and fear of meaninglessness. A dying person has a vast network of needs, most of which can be fulfilled by concerned and loving family members in the home:

1. **The need to feel secure, to feel that those who are caring for him are competent.**
2. **The need to feel that others are concerned about him.**
3. **The need to be comfortable.**
4. **The need to communicate.** Be a good listener; try to really understand what he is trying to say.
5. **The need to be with his children.**
6. **The need for family cohesion.** It is critical that the dying person feel the support and concern of loved ones.
7. **The need for cheerfulness.** A dying person is not dead yet — he still

possesses the same wit and sense of humor he always has. Help him have fun.

8. **The need for consistency and perseverance.** A great fear of the dying is isolation — do all you can to alleviate that concern.

In addition to the things listed above, there are a number of things you can do to meet the needs of a dying person:

1. **Help him maintain his dignity until the end.**
2. **Offer him hope.**
3. **Help him know that he is still valuable and worthy of self-esteem.** Even in the most outrageous stages of disease, let him do things for himself if it is at all possible.
4. **Let him participate in giving and receiving.**
5. **Let him act out his frustrations and angers without censure or ridicule.**
6. **Allow the dying person to have privacy when he needs it.**
7. **Touch and hold the dying person.**
8. **Help the dying person work out matters of concern to him.**
9. **Give the person permission to die.**

Euthanasia

Euthanasia — the voluntary ending of life — is a complex and highly volatile subject. Such emotionally filled incidences as the Karen Quinlan episode adequately testify to the controversy and stress evoked by the issue of euthanasia. Proponents of the right to die — or dying with dignity, or euthanasia (both passive and active) — tell us that death is often less cruel than a life filled with pain and misery, that death to a suffering person is a blessing and a relief, that every person has the right to die a dignified death, not a death marked by excruciating pain and mindless vegetation. Opponents warn us sternly that none of us has the right to play God — that the right to give life and the right to take away life rest with a higher power than the human family, that we are bound by duty and honor to do everything possible to sustain life. In answer, proponents tell us that "life" is not valuable or real if it is simply a battered existence of pain and agony and tubes and resuscitators. Opponents answer back that "life" is life if the heart is beating and the lungs are expanding with air — no matter what the condition of the mind.

There is even more controversy within the proponents and opponents themselves. For instance, is there a difference between failing to start life-saving treatment and stopping life-saving treatment once it has been initiated? Is there a moral and ethical difference between "letting" someone die (by withholding treatment) and "killing" someone (by offering a painless termination of life)? And then comes the ultimate distinction — that between *life-sustaining* procedures (giving a patient food and oxygen) and *extraordinary* procedures (giving a patient a blood transfusion, heart massage, respirators). Doctors continue to argue, to avoid making a stand, to beg for a legal decision.

Some states have already made that decision. California was the first state to legally recognize a "living will" — a document signed by a person stating his wish that he be allowed to die and not be kept alive by artificial means. Arkansas, Idaho, and New Mexico followed suit. Similar legislation was defeated in Maryland and Utah by legislators on the floor of state assemblies; it was withdrawn or failed in the committees of assemblies in Illinois, Indiana, Massachusetts, Mississippi, Montana, New Hampshire, New York, Vermont, Virginia, and West Virginia. Legislation to recognize a living will and allow death with dignity has been passed by both the assembly and the senate in Nevada; it was postponed in Colorado, Connecticut, Georgia, Hawaii, Kansas, Nebraska, and Oregon. Legislation is still active in the states not listed above.[8]

What about the American Medical Association? Statements released are purposefully vague, but one sentiment rings through with stunning clarity: the doctor must never kill a patient. So far, there has not been a ruling about "letting" a patient die as a result of neglecting to offer treatment — only the definite ruling that a doctor should never *kill* a patient (administer a lethal dose of medication, disconnect life-saving machinery, give a patient opportunity and instruction on killing himself).[9]

Exactly what makes the issue so difficult for physicians to deal with? There are nine major areas of ethical uncertainty connected with the issue of euthanasia, or "mercy killing":[10]

1. **Death usually is not instantaneous.** There are several stages of death — clinical, in which the heart stops beating and the person stops breathing; brain, in which brain activity ceases and brain cells die from lack of oxygen; and cellular, in which the cells of various

216

body organs die. These organs die at different rates (making possible the modern miracle of donating organs for transplantation), and even when part of an organ has died, the entire organ has not undergone total destruction. So when is a person *dead?* His heart may have stopped beating, but his brain may still be active and his other organs alive. On the other hand, a person may be breathing and experiencing a heartbeat as a result of a machine, but his brain may have ceased all activity and function. His blood is still circulating — so he is alive, or is he dead because he cannot think? Can a physician pull the plug on a patient whose brain has stopped functioning, even though blood is circulating? Or can he stop trying to resuscitate someone whose heart has stopped beating, even though his brain is very much alive?

2. **There is no solid definition of professional etiquette and professional ethics.** Professional etiquette and ethics demand that a physician exercise courtesy and concern for his patients and colleagues. What happens when his concern for a patient clouds his ability to judge a course of action? Or what happens when the patient is another doctor, and he demands to be left alone? Where does respect enter in here?

3. **The physician's own interests and idealism inevitably enter the picture.** And often these come into conflict, such as when an elderly patient has no ability to pay for expensive, long-term medical treatment. Should a doctor burden the patient and his family (and possibly not receive pay), or should the doctor allow the elderly person to die?

4. **Medical truth is not absolute.** There is the truth as it relates to the patient, and the truth as seen through the eyes of the physician. So many factors affect the "truth" — every patient poses a unique, individual case in which the truth may be entirely different than that which applies to a patient a week later in a different hospital. For a stable, alert patient, a detailed and complete diagnosis might constitute the "truth"; for a patient who might not be able to accept news of his impending death, partial report of his condition may be the "truth."

5. **Medical mores change and respond to cultural changes.** A good example of this is abortion — a medical practice that was unheard of in this country even fifty years ago (except in the most extreme cases) and that is now legal in several states and is performed in

many others as a result of intense pressure on the part of women's groups. But cultural pressures are an inadequate reason for medical mores to be changed. And before such changes can be recognized widely in the medical community, legislation needs to be enacted to define exact boundaries.

6. **The welfare of the many sometimes conflicts with the welfare of the few.** Of course, a physician's primary concern is with the patient. But he must of necessity also be concerned with that patient's family. It may seem kind to shorten the life of a terminally ill patient who is suffering, but his family may have very valid reasons for wanting him kept alive. The family has the responsibility for disposition of the patient's body after death finally works its course, so they must be able to exercise an opinion about the patient's final stages of medical care. On the other hand, a patient who is terminally ill may be placing a severe financial drain on a family, a hardship from which they may never recover.

7. **Physicians are expected to regulate themselves.** That is, physicians are expected every day to make moral decisions — some minor, such as *how* to treat a patient, and some major, such as whether to allow a patient to die — and, as such, they are generally protected from prosecution and are generally free from restricting supervision. This freedom is cherished by most physicians; yet, it becomes somewhat of a difficult burden when the physician is confronted with a painful, confusing situation concerning the life and death of an individual patient.

8. **Technology has perhaps advanced beyond wisdom.** New technology is being developed at such a rapid pace that it is difficult (and sometimes impossible) for physicians to keep up a current and workable understanding of how to put that new technology to use in their individual practices. And there is an even deeper complication when it comes to the terminally ill: many of them are elderly, and many more are so weakened and devastated by their conditions that it is almost impossible for the physician to judge how they will react to a treatment involving new technology. There is a second problem, too: some physicians are resistant to change and are reluctant to begin using new technology that may needlessly prolong a patient's life.

9. **Problems arise from the concept of a "useful" life.** What eventually becomes a very significant question is this: Is it worth prolonging a life that is no longer "useful" — that only becomes a scenario of pain-

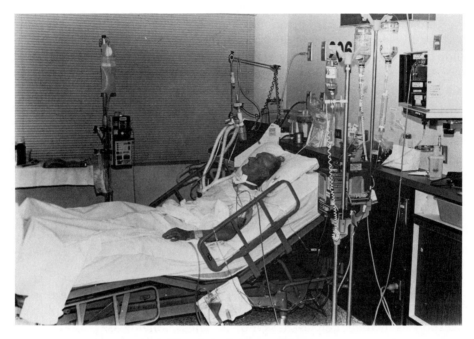

When is it all right to die?

ful hospital residence? Is it worth prolonging the life of an individual who has become a mindless vegetable, a man or woman who can only lie in bed, fed through tubes and breathing through a machine, who will never think or run or talk again? What, exactly, is "life"?

Among the medical profession, the stiffest critics have relied on the argument that professionally they are unable to justify euthanasia — that they spoke the Hippocratic Oath, promising to do everything in their power to sustain and save lives. Not just sometimes, or when it is convenient, or when the patient is in good condition and has a happy chance for a bright future — but always. A doctor promises to give treatment that will sustain life, and euthanasia — no matter how it is practiced — goes directly against that promise.

And there is the final argument — and one that many religious organizations support — that life is holy, sacred, and God-given; none of us has the right to take away what God has given. If we do, we, in a very real way, are "playing God."

So the controversy continues. Some believe they have the answers; others live daily with the guilt of either taking a life or of not taking it. For some, life is ended when a doctor walks quietly through a darkened corridor and secretly administers too much pain medication to a patient whom he has seen suffer for months. For others, life ends only after months of legal battles waged by family members who are unable to persuade their own doctors to walk that same darkened corridor. We sometimes think that life should never be taken or determined by a physician — until that person lying on the table, writhing in pain and violated with tubing, is our brother, our wife, our infant daughter.

GRIEF AND MOURNING

Grief is a word used to describe suffering, sorrow, and failure. It includes a series of emotional responses that follow the perception or anticipation of a loss of one or more valued or significant objects. Responses include: helplessness, hopelessness, loneliness, sadness, guilt, anger, and the like. It is an unpleasant and usually avoided emotional experience accompanying the loss of something valued.

Mourning is the psychological process that follows a loss of a significant or valued object or the realization that such a loss may occur. Mourning includes the processes necessary to overcome the subjective state of grief.

The healing power of grief and mourning is so well known that wise doctors encourage its full expression. However, many factors operate in our society to restrict or prevent the full expression of grief.

Grief and mourning are generally thought of as phenomena that follow the death of a loved one. However, many other losses are equally painful — loss of a loved person by divorce or separation; loss of a job, money, prestige, or status; loss of health through sickness, surgery, or accident; loss of body parts, such as a limb or an eye; loss of sight or hearing; and inability to walk or talk.

The degree of loss is a highly individual perception that will affect the course of grief and mourning. Those who perceive a loss as minor, temporary, or of value in a larger context ("hidden blessings") may experience grief and mourning qualitatively and quantitatively different than those who view it as a major calamity.

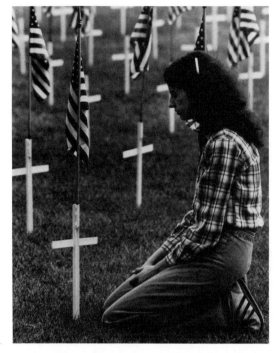

Loss of a loved one is a most difficult crisis.

It should also be noted that research into the grief and mourning experience is in its infancy. The information that follows is based on the best accumulated evidence available at present but may not fit every situation of loss.

Normal Grief Reactions

A healthy and normal reaction — one that eventually leads to healing and cessation of mourning — proceeds through five basic phases. These are denial, awareness, restitution, resolution, and idealization.

Denial

The initial normal reaction to loss is denial — shock and disbelief, stunned refusal to believe that the loss has occurred. The victim simply refuses to accept or comprehend what has happened. Sometimes a victim

NORMAL GRIEF REACTIONS

IDEALIZATION

DENIAL

AWARENESS

RESOLUTION

RESTITUTION

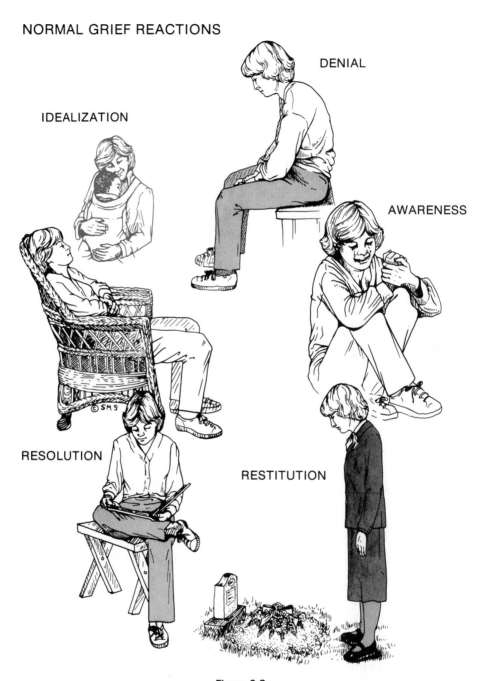

Figure 6-2.

may accept the fact intellectually, while emotionally he still denies it — such an individual will not react emotionally in any way that conveys knowledge of the loss. Some may try to carry out normal activities as though nothing has happened. Others may become dazed and may sit completely motionless, unable to move.[11]

The numbness that victims experience during this stage of grief enables them to attend to the necessary arrangements required after the loss of a loved one. For most, the period of disbelief or denial is short — lasting anywhere from a few minutes to a few days. When the period of denial lasts longer than a few days, it is a signal that something is wrong.

Awareness

Following the period of denial, the individual usually develops a sense of awareness in which he *emotionally* acknowledges the loss. At this point, the victim will begin to feel the anguish and emptiness of the loss. In essence, the loss is no longer simply a part of the surroundings; the loss is a very real part of himself.[12]

During this phase, the individual begins to experience feelings toward the loss. Anger is commonly expressed, especially if the individual feels that a person or institution was to blame for the loss. (Some individuals even strike out in anger against a nurse or doctor who treated a loved one who subsequently died.) Some may blame themselves instead and may try to harm themselves because of extreme guilt. Others may act on impulse and may harm themselves quite unintentionally — such as a victim who pounds on his chest, thrusts his fist through a window, or drives irrationally and gets in an accident.

Several specific behaviors are common during this stage: crying with tears is a typical reaction. Some may cry inwardly while not crying outwardly; others may not be able to cry at all, a problem that interferes with the normal grief process.

It is during this stage that the most anguish is felt; that anguish is often a result of the culture, and the expression of the anguish depends on what is expected of the individual. Emotions and reactions expressed during this stage may be triggered by a number of incidents, such as a friend's comment or a place associated with the loss. Expressions of grief during this stage tend to be especially tense and painful during the night, when the activities and distractions of the daytime are not present. In the case of loss of a loved one, there is often preoccupation with the memory of the individual; some victims even experience visual images of the dead person.

During this stage, it is important that the grieving individual feel free to express his emotions; too often, well-meaning friends and relatives encourage the individual not to cry, not to concentrate on the death or loss. On the contrary, the bereaved needs to vent full expression to the emotions so that he can heal and move on to other, more constructive emotions.

Somatic manifestations often appear during the second stage of mourning, including digestive difficulties, poor appetite, weight loss, insomnia, and loss of libido. Women often manifest menstrual difficulties, and the elderly usually show less overt grief but suffer more physical complaints. Many victims display irritability, restlessness, and the inability to concentrate on ordinary tasks.

The most important and effective treatment during this phase is the support and understanding of loved ones. The victim should be encouraged to express his emotions and should be told that those emotions are normal. The victim should be aided in making cultural and religious adjustments if those are indicated.

This stage usually peaks between two and four weeks after the death or loss and begins to subside after three months (but may last up to one year).

Restitution

During this phase, the individual is helped more clearly to see the reality of the loss — in the death of a loved one, for instance, the victim has a chance to view the body, participate in a funeral, and see the casket lowered into the grave. Far from being a disturbing sequence of events, these often take place while the victim is in the company of friends and loved ones, who can help him to cope better with the loss.

Resolution

It is during this, the fourth stage of grief, that the individual accepts the loss or the death and begins to pick up the threads of his life. He begins to visualize, for the first time, the possibility of functioning well without the spouse, job, money, or whatever it is he has lost. This stage

— resolving the loss and reorganizing life to accommodate the changes —
should be completed within one year after the loss.

The individual first begins to deal with the emptiness within. He
progressively regains interest in the ordinary activities of his life; at first,
memories of the loss or of the dead person will be painful and will evoke
emotional reactions. Eventually, the individual will be able to remember
the dead person with pleasure and interest and will be able to accept a
new love object.

The individual commonly suffers various physical sensations, sometimes identical to a symptom suffered by the deceased person (especially
common when a loved one dies of a long terminal illness). These
symptoms, a way for the mourner to suffer on behalf of the deceased
person and thereby ease his guilt toward the deceased person, usually
last a brief time.

For a long time during this phase, the mourner will seem completely
preoccupied with thoughts of the deceased person — he will place a great
deal of emphasis on the person who died and will want to bring up, talk
about, and think over memories. At times this becomes a long and painful
process and continues until the mourner has developed an image of the
deceased that is almost devoid of negative or undesirable traits.

The mourner's religious beliefs — particularly regarding his beliefs
about whether he will meet the deceased person after this life — will play
a big role in how he is able to resolve the loss.

Idealization

The fifth and final stage of mourning involves repression of all negative and hostile feelings toward the deceased. There is a disadvantage to
this repression: the victim often experiences fluctuating guilt feelings
that may lead to fear and that often involve regret for past acts or fan-
tasies of inconsiderateness, unkindness, or hostility toward the deceased.

But two important things are achieved by idealization. First, the recurring thoughts and memories help the individual to create a vivid image
of the deceased — the person then does not seem quite so lost. Second,
the individual is able to remember — and eventually to concentrate on —
the more positive aspects of the relationship with the deceased.

The successful process of mourning usually requires a year or
longer. Those who are able to comfortably and realistically remember

both the pleasures and the disappointments of the relationship have healed most successfully. The healing process requires a great deal of support and comfort during the first stages and relatively little assistance or support during the final stages. During even the final stage, however, it is not uncommon for the individual to experience brief recurrences of his grief and feelings of loss; as in the earlier stages, the victim should be encouraged to express his feelings openly.

The success of the grief process depends on a number of factors — the major determinant of the outcome is the degree to which the loss was a source of support. The more dependent the relationship, the more difficult will be the task of resolving its loss. Some believe that the loss of a child — usually an adolescent or young adult — causes a grief that never completely heals.

OLD AGE

There has always been a tendency to ignore the elderly — those quiet, gray-haired folks who slipped unnoticed between decades and remembered the years gone by. But we cannot afford to ignore them: approximately one in 35,000 Americans now reaches 100 years of age; more than two million are over eight-five years of age. Approximately every ninth American is over sixty-five. It is projected that in the near future, one in every six Americans will be sixty-five or older.[13]

Growing old will happen to everyone — and we each need to learn how it happens and what we can do to make old age a healthy, happy time of life.

The Process of Aging

As we grow older, a number of physical, emotional, and mental changes take place simply as a by-product of the natural wear and tear on the body.

Physical Changes

The wearing out of body parts is not well understood, but we do

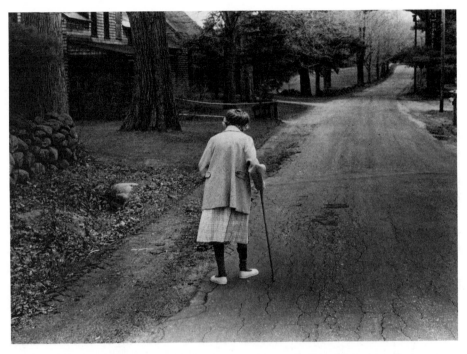

For too many, old age is seen as a dreary path of failing health and loneliness.

know that it occurs at different rates for different body systems. The skeletal system is among the first to be affected by aging — the bones lose calcium and become brittle and fragile. The bones break more easily, and it is more difficult for them to heal. The muscular structures supporting the skeleton and body organs begin to lose their tone, flexibility, and strength, eventually becoming weak. The amount of body fat generally increases.

The heart and respiratory systems deteriorate, affecting the body's ability to get enough oxygen and use it most efficiently in the blood. The ability to ventilate the lungs fully, diffuse the oxygen into the bloodstream, and utilize the oxygen in the tissues is sharply reduced, as are the strength of the heartbeat and its rate. Some organs actually change size — the brain gets smaller and the prostate gland gets larger, for example.

Almost 20 percent of all elderly suffer from chronic brain syndrome, a physical disorder that has often been labeled *senility*. While the effects of senility seem to be intellectual — including personality changes and a change in the ability to think clearly, with memory loss becoming worse with time — senility is a physical disorder, with physical causes. While the exact cause is unknown, researchers know that metabolism, heredity, and atherosclerosis (accumulation of fatty tissue in the arteries of the brain) all play a significant role.

Some physical changes are actually beneficial. The elderly seem to be less affected by poor nutrition and are less susceptible to a number of illnesses (including the common cold).

Probably the most noticeable changes that accompany old age are those that affect the reflexes and the senses. The elderly are slower on their feet, a little more clumsy, and are slower to respond. All fives senses are dulled, affecting their ability to hear, see, smell, taste, and perceive skin sensations. Poor eyesight and hearing have almost become the trademarks of old age.

Emotional Changes

The most marked emotional change of old age is depression — but there are plenty of reasons for it. An elderly person is often lonely, having lost his or her spouse and many friends. It is obvious that the person's days are numbered — we can only live so long — and the individual has to cope with the increasing disabilities that earmark old age. For many, depression is a by-product of lack of activity — though such lack of activity may be a cultural or social product than a physical one (in a number of foreign countries, people work well into their old age and often live longer than they do in the United States). Depression can also be due to personal financial conditions — people who had plenty of money when they were younger are forced to live on dwindling savings, meager pensions, or small social security checks while coping with the ever-increasing cost of living.

Some emotional changes are results of medication given to relieve physical and medical conditions.

Social Changes

Sociologists have found that many — not all — elderly people gradually withdraw from society, and society gradually withdraws from them. There are five basic steps that make the final disengagement (death) easier for the elderly person to handle:[14]

1. The aging person comes to a realization of his own mortality.
2. The aging person, realizing his own mortality, comes to terms with the fact that some of his dreams and goals will never be achieved. To compensate, he resets his priorities, bringing his dreams and goals more in line with what is now possible to achieve.
3. Earlier in his life, he was able to replace most of what was lost. Now, the losses far outnumber the gains — he cannot replace what is lost so easily. He loses his spouse; his children move away; his friends die. He is no longer employed. He may lose his own health and abilities.
4. As his life changes, he sets new rewards. These rewards often have much less status than the rewards that he once established. Where he once sought fame and wealth, he may now seek companionship and health.
5. As a final step, the aging person seeks freedom from his obilgations. As he perceives death to draw nearer, he wants to take care of his financial obligations as well as his obligations to other people. He wants to die in peace, knowing that he has taken care of the things for which he was responsible.

While not all elderly people undergo these changes, they are common and can occur at any period during old age.

Intellectual/Mental Changes

While many old people suffer some degree of senility, research has shown that for most, intellectual capacity remains unchanged until shortly before death.[15] Most retain their mental and intellectual abilities, with thinking processes sharp. There *does* seem to be a decrease in mental or intellectual abilities if the individual suffers from chronic disease, such as diabetes, high blood pressure, or kidney disease.

Factors Contributing to Deterioration

Four major factors contribute primarily to physical deterioration in the aging:

1. The cross-sectional area of the blood vessels decreases in size, with

FACTORS CONTRIBUTING TO PHYSICAL DETERIORATION IN AGING

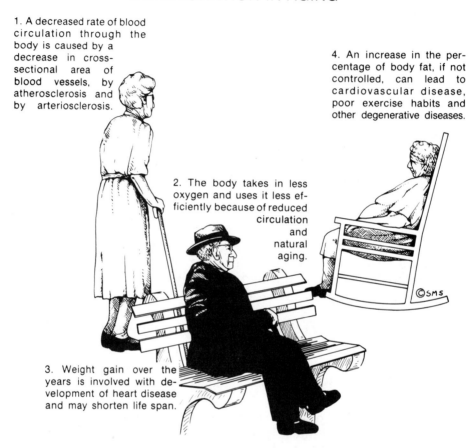

1. A decreased rate of blood circulation through the body is caused by a decrease in cross-sectional area of blood vessels, by atherosclerosis and by arteriosclerosis.

4. An increase in the percentage of body fat, if not controlled, can lead to cardiovascular disease, poor exercise habits and other degenerative diseases.

2. The body takes in less oxygen and uses it less efficiently because of reduced circulation and natural aging.

3. Weight gain over the years is involved with development of heart disease and may shorten life span.

©SMS

Figure 6-3.

the important result that less blood can circulate through the body in equivalent amounts of time. By the time a person is fifty, the area that he has open to blood flow is about 35 percent less than it was when he was thirty — and the area keeps diminishing. Add atherosclerosis (fatty deposits on the linings of the vessels), and circulation is further jeopardized; arteriosclerosis (hardening of the arteries) can cause even further damage.

2. Partly as a result of reduced circulation and partly as a result of natural aging, the body is able to take in less oxygen and is not able to

utilize the oxygen that it does take in as efficiently as it once did.

3. As elderly people gain weight slowly over the years, they develop heart disease; if the weight gain is substantial, their life may be shortened due to the excess weight.

4. There is a steady rise in the percentage of body fat — the ratio of muscle mass to body fat — as we grow older. This steady rise can be controlled but often is not, leading to cardiovascular disease, poor exercise habits due to impaired ability, and development of certain other chronic and/or degenerative diseases.

While aging is a certainty and nothing can be done to avoid it, certain good health practices — good nutrition, proper weight, and continuous exercise — can slow down some of the deterioration as aging progresses.

Myths About the Aged

Perhaps one of the reasons why the elderly are so misunderstood is because you cannot really know what it is like to be old until you *are* old. A number of common myths and misconceptions have added to the tendency of people to misunderstand the elderly and to hold fast to incorrect perceptions about old age.

Myth: Old people cannot learn anything new.

Fact: Anyone who puts himself in a stimulating atmosphere will continue to learn as long as his health permits it. Some changes do occur with aging — reaction time and maximum work capacity are usually reduced — but verbal intelligence, the ability to retain information, vocabulary, and comprehension are generally unchanged. People who do stop learning usually do so because they specialized in one narrow career and stopped getting exposed to new ideas while they were still young. As long as health is generally good, most elderly people stay acutely sharp intellectually up until death — and anyone who wants to learn and stay active mentally usually can (and does).

Myth: Old people are too feeble to get around by themselves — certainly too feeble to enjoy normal activities.

Nothing could be farther from the truth! Of course, some elderly people are plagued by disease that disables them and makes them incapable of functioning independently — but there are also younger people who have disabling diseases. But the vast majority of the elderly — more than 80 percent of them — get around without help, and only about 5 percent require institutionalization. It is best for older people to participate as much as they can in all kinds of activities — including physical, mental, and social ones. It is inactivity that causes a withering of the will to live — not old age

Myth: Aging is an inescapable process — so most disabilities associated with old age cannot be avoided or prevented.

Of course, everyone grows old — that cannot be prevented. But many of the major diseases and disabilities that affect the aged *can* be prevented. The major killer of people over sixty-five — cardiovascular disease — can be lessened enormously by proper diet, reduction of cholesterol intake, and regular exercise. In fact, if all people followed a sensible course of prevention while they were younger, the average lifespan would be extended by at least ten years![16]

Many of the other disabilities that have become an accepted part of old age could be reduced in severity by seriously practicing good health habits during youth and young adulthood. Remember: the seeds of good health in old age must be carefully planted in youth and nurtured throughout an entire lifetime.

Myth: The menopause causes women to lose interest in sex.

Some women — about 20 percent — do find a reduction in their sex drive after menopause. But about 60 percent experience no change, and the other 20 percent actually find their sex drive increased after menopause! The menopause is strictly a hormonal change in the body (men undergo a similar hormonal change, too), and there is no need for it to alter a woman's abilities, interests, and activities.

Problems of the Aged

The elderly, as all people, have unique problems individual to each person. One man may suffer poor health, another loneliness from losing his wife. But certain problems are common to the elderly as a group.

Imbalance of the Male/Female Ratio

A man who reaches the age of sixty-five usually lives about ten more years; a woman, almost twenty. Around the age of seventy, 143 men die for every 100 women who die.[17] So there are many more widows and older women than there are widowers and older men. This statistic alone dictates one of the reasons why many elderly women abandon satisfactory sexual expression — they no longer have a partner.

Lack of Quality Medical Care

Health programs available to help the elderly in the United States, including Medicare and Medicaid, pay only a percentage of the cost of medical care for those over the age of sixty-five; the patients must pay the rest out of their own pockets. In a day when the cost of health care is on a seemingly endless upward spiral, the amount left for the elderly person to pay grows more and more each year. When an elderly person lacks financial resources, he often neglects routine medical and preventive care, waiting until a problem is critical before he seeks help.

Retirement

When this country was younger, elderly people worked long past the age of sixty-five; even though they sometimes worked at a slower pace, they worked until their vigor no longer permitted it — sometimes well into their eighties. Today, it is almost impossible for a person over the age of sixty-five to find a job. In most industry and government corporations, retirement is mandatory at the age of sixty-five — the employee has no choice. It is as though all the years of experience and expertise are for nothing. Even when the person finds a job, he is penalized. His social security benefits are cut if he earns too much. On the job, many elderly are passed over for promotions and raises.

The inactivity associated with retirement can sometimes have devastating effects, including depression and a sense of uselessness. In reality, those over sixty-five are often good job risks: they have fewer accidents, they lose less time from work than younger workers, and they have greater job stability. When these workers are forced to quit, and when they lose interest and become inactive, poor health results. In fact, some researchers have found a direct link between forced inactivity (as in retirement) and a sharp increase in the number of chronic complaints and illnesses.[18]

Since the number of elderly is growing, their voice is also growing, and their votes at the polls are having increased impact. Part of this influence caused the 1978 Congress to up the retirement age from sixty-five to seventy in some industries; perhaps changes will occur that will allow the elderly to gradually retire — to work shorter work weeks as they grow older, retaining them in the work force as their health permits.

Financial Problems and Poverty

An elderly person is twice as likely to be poor as a young person; while the elderly make up 10 percent of the nation's population, they constitute 20 percent of the nation's poor. With social security and retirement benefits failing to keep pace with inflation, more than 15 percent of the nation's elderly lived below the national poverty level at the end of the 1970s. Even those who do not qualify for the poverty classification usually suffer — some with extreme hardships. Many, too proud to seek help, abandon first the luxuries (movies and vacation trips) and then some of the necessities (nourishing food, warmth, good clothing).

Health Status of the Elderly

Elderly people were asked in a Harris poll to rate their own health. The results were surprising: 22 percent said that they were in fair health, while only 9 percent said that their health was poor. Of those polled, 68 percent said that they enjoyed excellent health — dispelling the myth of the infirmed aged.[19] In the survey, the aged ranked as their most frequent medical problems arthritis, hearing impairments, digestive disturbances, chronic sinusitis, mental and nervous conditions, genito-urinary problems, and circulatory problems.[20]

234

While disease attacks people of all ages, the elderly have a higher incidence of chronic disease — disease that is long-term and that tends to incapacitate the victim for a long period of time. About 72 percent of those between the ages of forty-five and sixty-five suffer from chronic disease conditions; of those over the age of sixty-five, the percentage climbs to 86.[21]

Certain health problems are more common for the elderly and can be anticipated and, to a certain extent, prevented earlier in life.

Hospitalization

The aged are more likely than other groups to require short-term hospitalization; about 18 percent of older people are hospitalized each year as compared to about 10 percent of the general population. The conditions for which the elderly are most frequently hospitalized include diseases of the circulatory system, digestive system, tumors, diseases of the respiratory system, accidents, poisonings, and injuries resulting from violence.[22]

Lack of Exercise

Many people become sedentary with advancing age, but exercise throughout life can improve health and can reduce some of the problems normally experienced by the elderly. People in Pakistan, the Soviet Union, and Ecuador often live to be 100 or 120 years of age — and they all work hard, expending intense physical activity.[23]

It is best to exercise throughout life, but a comeback after years of inactivity can even have benefits. In one instance, a seventy-seven-year-old man who started jogging ten years earlier was found to have the physiology of a much younger man.[24]

The benefits of exercise to the elderly (as to all people) include improved health, improved circulation, reduction in the risk of heart attack, lowering of the blood pressure, higher survival rates following illness or heart attack, improved posture and gait, improved sleeping patterns, reduction in stress, greater joint mobility, improved feeling of self-worth, and increased muscular strength.[25]

Poor Nutrition

Undernutrition and starvation always reduce the lifespan sharply; of all the factors affecting quality of life, nutrition is probably the most important. Yet, a ten-state study conducted in the United States between 1968 and 1970 found that iron and vitamin C deficiencies were pronounced among the elderly, and obesity was found to be a significant problem, especially among elderly women.[26]

Since the taste buds remain receptive to sweet tastes longer than to other tastes, the consumption of sweets among the elderly is often extreme and is a major contributing factor to obesity — considered by some to be the major nutritional problem of the elderly.[27] The caloric needs of the body decrease with age, but many people do not adjust their eating habits accordingly. Overweight in the elderly is serious, since it compounds the problems of diseases such as arthritis, diabetes, arteriosclerosis, varicose veins, hernias, cardiovascular disease, ulcers, and high blood pressure. The obese elderly are also much more prone to accidents than those of normal weight.

Reducing the Effects of Aging

You can start early in life — in your late teens and early twenties — to take measures that will prolong your life and reduce the effects of aging. All of the following can extend your life and can make your older years less troubled by disease:

1. **Reduce stress.** Stress causes all kinds of physical reactions. Continued for long periods, stress simply wears out the body. You can do plenty to reduce your own stress levels. Identify which situations in your life cause stress — your job, your education, your life-style. Do what you can to make things better. Avoid the urge to be competitive, driving, and ambitious to a fault. Try to relax and be more tolerant of your own failings.
2. **Eat a balanced diet.** A balanced diet can promote longevity and good

health; a poor diet, high in fatty and processed foods, can lead to disease and deterioration of the body tissues (especially disorders of the circulatory system). Keep your fat content low; increase your fiber content. Eat foods from all the basic food groups (fruits, vegetables, cereals/grains, milk/dairy, meat/protein) each day.

3. **Exercise.** Exercise strengthens all the body tissues and improves the performance of all the body functions — especially the circulatory and respiratory systems, which are most vulnerable to disease in the elderly. Exercise also keeps you limber, helping to combat the tendencies toward arthritis, rheumatism, and other effects of inactivity. You can exercise all your life — and can continue mild exercise well into old age. Best are the exercises that are rhythmic, controlled, and mild — bicycling, walking, and swimming are good lifelong activities.

4. **Keep your weight down.** Eating a balanced diet and getting the proper amount of exercise is almost certain to keep your weight where it should be. Fat people are more likely to die at any age, but with old age, the risks are even greater. Controlling weight is not easy, since as age increases the caloric needs of the body decrease — and you have to eat less and move around more to maintain the same body weight. But controlling your weight pays dividends in avoidance of serious disease and sharply reduced lifespan.

5. **Use alcohol in moderation.** It is best if you do not drink — but if you do drink, do not drink too much. Alcohol leads to liver and kidney impairment, plus heavy drinkers jeopardize normal brain function.

6. **Do not smoke.** Cigarette smoking has now been identified as the leading cause of preventable death and illness in the United States. We know now that cigarette smoking leads to early death, cancer, cardiovascular disease, emphysema, general illness, and premature aging. Smoking even results in early wrinkling; a fifty-year-old smoker has the wrinkles of a sixty-year-old nonsmoker! Heavy smokers cut from five to twenty years off their lives due to the toxins contained in cigarettes.

7. **Have regular medical checkups.** Even if you do not think that you are sick, you can detect serious diseases in their early stages with regular medical checkups — and many serious diseases can be cured or controlled when detected early enough. Many forms of breast and cervical cancer are considered curable if caught early enough; early detection of high blood pressure, diabetes, and other conditions can lead to control before the disease wreaks havoc on the body. Good

medical care throughout life can add years and can mean a better-quality life, especially during old age.

8. **Stay active.** Even while you are young, look ahead to old age: what will you do when you cannot work anymore? How will you spend your time when your employer puts you out to pasture at the age of sixty-five, when you still have plenty of energy left? Establish interests and hobbies now that will occupy and interest you then. Make sure that you find some hobbies that you can do indoors, sitting down — just in case your health does dwindle. Stay involved with those around you now, and your involvement will continue to your old age. Studies have established the fact that those who are involved and active suffer fewer physical complaints and live longer, happier lives.

Notes

1. Head Start Bureau and the National Center on Child Abuse and Neglect, *New Light on an Old Problem* (Washington, D.C.: U.S. Department of Health, Education, and Welfare, 1978), DHEW Publication No. (OHDS) 79-31108.
2. "What Future for the American Family?" *Changing Times*, December 1976, p. 7.
3. William V. Arnold, et al., *Divorce: Prevention or Survival* (Philadelphia: Westminster Press, 1977), p. 18.
4. Frank J. Ayd, Jr., "What Is Death?" *Medical Counterpoint*, March 1974, p. 26.
5. Ibid.
6. Ibid., p. 27.
7. Summarized from Elisabeth Kubler-Ross, *On Death and Dying* (New York: Macmillan Publishing Company, 1969).
8. Karen Waugh Zucker, "Legislatures Provide for Death with Dignity," *The Journal of Legal Medicine*, August 1977, pp. 21-23.
9. "Mercy Killing," *The Encyclopedia of Health Sciences*, vol. 13 (Stanford, Calif.: Medical Readings, Inc., 1974), p. 1263.
10. Barbara Littlewood, "Interpreting Death," source unknown, p. 110.
11. Annette Edwards, Pamela Hay, and Lois Thompson, "Grief and Mourning," unpublished manuscript in the possession of Brent Q. Hafen, p. 269.
12. Information adapted from Edwards et. al., "Grief and Mourning," and Hafen, "Grief and Mourning."
13. *Fact Book on Aging* (The National Council of Aging, Inc., 1821 L Street NW, Washington, D.C. 20036, 1978).
14. Elaine Cumming, "Further Thoughts on the Theory of Disengagement," *International Social Science Journal*, vol. 15, pp. 377-393.

15. Lissy F. Jarvik, "Thoughts on the Psychobiology of Aging," *American Psychology* 30 (no. 5): 576-585.

16. Harry A. Brotman, "The Fastest Growing Minority: The Aging," *American Journal of Public Health* 64 (March 1964): 250.

17. *Monthly Vital Statistics Report*, Provisional Statistics, Annual Summary for the United States, 1977, DHEW Publication Number (PHS) 79-1120, Volume 26 (December 7 1978), p. 25.

18. Jack Ossofsky, Statement of the National Council of the Aging to the Subcommittee on Equal Opportunity, Committee on Education and Labor, United States House of Representatives, September 14, 1976.

19. Charles S. Harris, *Fact Book on Aging: A Profile of America's Older Population* (Washington, D.C.: The National Council on Aging, 1978).

20. Ibid.

21. Ibid.

22. Ibid.

23. Ibid.

24. Ibid.

25. Ibid.

26. Ibid.

27. Ibid.

Self-Evaluation

Could You Become a Child Abuser?

Child abuse is a very common occurrence in the modern family. Have you ever wondered how you might treat your own children after you bring them into this world? Read each of the following questions below, and answer each either "yes" or "no," depending on which *best* describes your thoughts or behavior. If you fall somewhere in between, circle the response that comes closest to describing you.

AS A CHILD . . .

Yes No 1. Did you become extremely apprehensive when other children cried?

Yes No 2. Did you frequently cause trouble or break and damage things?

Yes No 3. Were you extremely shy to the point of avoiding people?

Yes No 4. Were you overly anxious to please others, even in unpleasant situations?

Yes No 5. Were you reluctant to go home?

Yes No 6. Were you frequently absent from school?

Yes No 7. Were your clothes frequently dirty or inappropriate for the weather conditions?

Yes No 8. Did you frequently fail to eat breakfast and/or lunch during your school years?

Yes No 9. Did you feel that your parents treated your brothers and sisters better than you?

Yes No 10. Did your parents fail to show they cared when you had a problem?

Yes No 11. Did either or both of your parents beat you to the point of severe bruises, burns, lacerations, or broken bones?

Yes No 12. Were you afraid of either of your parents?

Yes No 13. Did your parents leave you alone during "dangerous" activities or for long periods of time?

Yes No 14. Did you abuse alcohol or drugs?

Yes No 15. Were you sexually abused by either of your parents?

Yes   No   16. Did you suck your thumb or exhibit any other infantile be-
                  haviors longer than your peers?

Yes   No   17. Did you feel like your parents had overly high expectations
                  for you?

Yes   No   18. Were you unable to depend on your parents for love and
                  nurturance?

Yes   No   19. Were you neurotic? (i.e., exhibited sleep disorders, obses-
                  sions, compulsions, phobias, etc.)

Yes   No   20. Did you ever attempt suicide?

DO YOU FEEL THAT . . .

Yes   No   21. You are an extremely poor socializer?

Yes   No   22. You are powerless to solve personal problems or resolve
                  situations?

Yes   No   23. Children are "bad", "evil", or "monsters"?

Yes   No   24. You have many unmet emotional needs?

Yes   No   25. A child would fill an emotional void in you?

Yes   No   26. You have poor impulse control?

Yes   No   27. You have very low self-esteem?

Yes   No   28. You are unable to cope with many situations?

Yes   No   29. You abuse alcohol?

Yes   No   30. The sex of your future child is extremely important?

Scoring: In each instance, the "yes" response reflects the thoughts or behavior often associated with child abusers. Obviously, a random yes answer here or there does not mean you will become a child abuser. A preponderence of "yes" responses in questions 1-20 and/or questions 21-30 *may* indicate that you have a tendency towards child abuse. In that case, if you are planning to have children in the future, it may be a good idea to discuss this subject with a professional counselor.

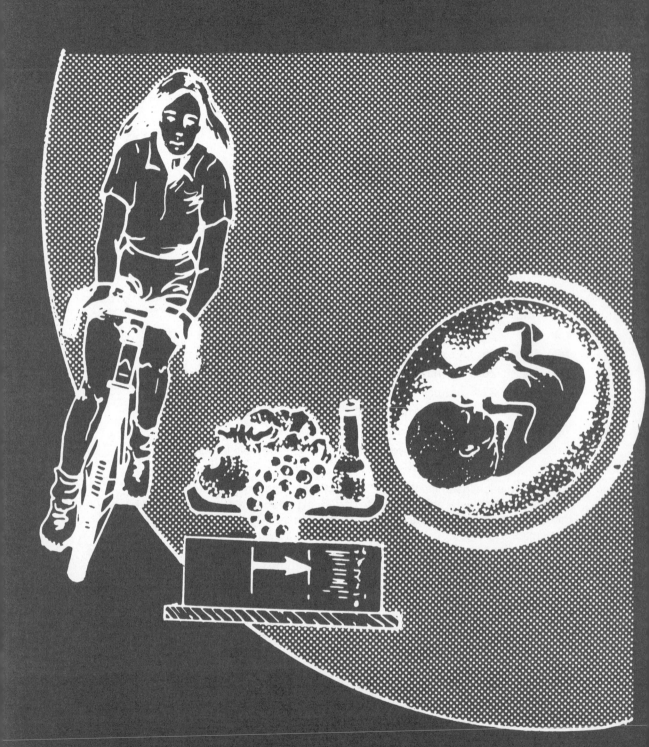

Part III
Health Maintenance

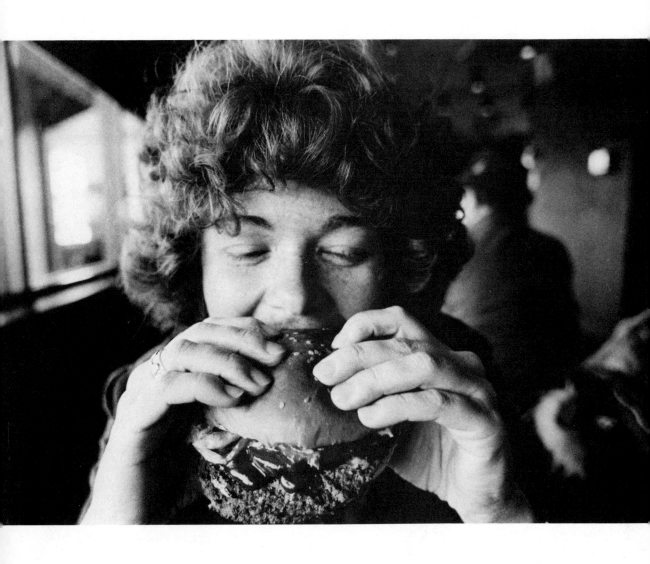

7
Nutrition: Basic Life Support

You probably do it at least three times a day — probably up to about 100,000 times in your life. It affects the way you feel and function on a day-to-day basis. It determines in part how long you will live. It can cause — or prevent — disease. It influences how well you can deal with stress, either emotional or physical. It influences your health and the health of your children.

It is eating. And the decisions that you make about eating are some of the most important of your life. Good nutrition can improve your health, expand your capabilities, keep you from developing a host of diseases, and increase your life span.

BASIC NUTRIENTS

Each important nutrient found in food is essential to the function of the body and the maintenance of proper health. In the United States today, an abundance of good foods is available everywhere and within the economic reach of most people. A variety of different types of foods will provide all of the nutrients that most of us need. No one food does everything, and all foods have something to offer.

245

LIFE SPAN OF AMERICANS ⟹

HOW IT HAS LENGTHENED

	Males			Females		
	Years of Life Remaining			Years of Life Remaining		
	75 Years Ago	Today	Increase (in years)	75 Years Ago	Today	Increase (in years)
At birth	48.23	69.4	21.17	51.08	77.2	26.12
Age 20	42.19	51.4	9.21	43.77	58.6	14.83
Age 25	38.52	46.9	8.38	40.05	53.8	13.75
Age 30	34.88	42.2	7.32	36.42	49.0	12.58
Age 35	31.29	37.6	6.31	32.82	44.2	11.38
Age 40	27.74	33.0	5.26	29.17	39.4	10.23
Age 45	24.21	28.5	4.29	25.51	34.8	9.29
Age 50	20.76	24.3	3.54	21.89	30.3	8.41
Age 55	17.42	20.4	2.98	18.43	26.0	7.57
Age 60	14.35	16.8	2.45	15.23	21.9	6.67
Age 65	11.51	13.7	2.19	12.23	18.1	5.87
Age 70	9.03	10.9	1.87	9.59	14.4	4.81
Age 75	6.84	8.5	1.66	7.33	11.2	3.87
Age 80	5.10	6.7	1.60	5.50	8.6	3.10
Age 85	3.81	5.2	1.39	4.10	6.5	2.40

Figure 7-1. The biggest gains in this century have come from the sharp reduction in deaths during infancy and childhood. In recent years, however, life expectancy for older persons has begun to lengthen faster than in the past because of medical advances, especially in the treatment of heart disease. Good nutrition, too, is a factor influencing lifespan. Source: U.S. Department of Health, Education, and Welfare.

Recommended Dietary Allowances

The Recommended Dietary Allowances (RDA) are generally accepted in the United States as typical dietary standards. The RDA are the levels of intake of essential nutrients considered to be adequate to meet the known nutritional needs of practically all healthy persons. The allowances are intended to provide for variations among most normal persons as they live in the United States under usual environmental stresses.

Diets should be based on a variety of common foods in order to provide other nutrients for which human requirements have been less well defined.

In addition to being guides to human needs for nutrients, the RDA have become guides for regulatory agencies that are responsible for nutrition labeling, for regulations designed to ensure nutritional quality of foods, and for development of new food products.[1]

Proteins

Protein, the chief tissue builder, is the basic substance of every cell in the body, including muscle, blood, and bone; protein supports growth and maintains healthy body cells. Antibodies that assist the body in resisting infection are protein, as are enzymes.

All protein is made up of smaller units called amino acids; during the process of digestion, proteins are broken down into the most simple amino acids. After absorption into the body, the amino acids are rearranged in the cells to form the many special and distinct proteins in the body. The proteins in food are usually composed of eighteen or more amino acids. The body can manufacture its own supply of more than half of them, but the others — essential amino acids — must be supplied through the intake of food.

The amino acid makeup of a food protein determines its nutritive value. Those proteins that supply all of the essential amino acids in about the same proportions as they are needed by the body are considered highest in value; most are foods of animal origin, and they include eggs, fish, poultry, meat, and milk.

While they do not supply as good an assortment of amino acids as animal proteins do, the proteins from cereal and grains, vegetables, and fruits still supply valuable amounts of many amino acids. Proteins from legumes — especially soybeans and chickpeas — are almost as good as the proteins derived from animal sources.

To improve the percentage of essential amino acids that you receive from your food, you should combine foods that do not provide optimum amino acids with those that do — for instance, have milk with cereal or macaroni with cheese. Foods of vegetable origin can also be combined to improve protein quality. Try combining beans and corn, beans and rice, and wheat bread with peanut butter. If meat is not included in a meal,

FOOD AND NUTRITION BOARD, NATIONAL ACADEMY OF SCIENCES-NATIONAL RESEARCH COUNCIL

"Recommended Daily Dietary Allowances,"[a] Revised 1979

Designed for the maintenance of good nutrition of practically all healthy people in the USA

	Age (years)	Weight (kg)	Weight (lbs)	Height (cm)	Height (in)	Protein (g)	Fat-Soluble Vitamins Vitamin A (μg R.E.)[b]	Vitamin D (μg)[c]	Vitamin E (mg α T.E.)[d]	Water-Soluble Vitamins Vitamin C (mg)	Thiamin (mg)	Riboflavin (mg)	Niacin (mg N.E.)[e]	Vitamin B6 (mg)	Folacin[f] (μg)	Vitamin B12 (μg)	Minerals Calcium (mg)	Phosphorus (mg)	Magnesium (mg)	Iron (mg)	Zinc (mg)	Iodine (μg)
Infants	0.0-0.5	6	13	60	24	kg × 2.2	420	10	3	35	0.3	0.4	6	0.3	30	0.5[g]	360	240	50	10	3	40
	0.5-1.0	9	20	71	28	kg × 2.0	400	10	4	35	0.5	0.6	8	0.6	45	1.5	540	360	70	15	5	50
Children	1-3	13	29	90	35	23	400	10	5	45	0.7	0.8	9	0.9	100	2.0	800	800	150	15	10	70
	4-6	20	44	112	44	30	500	10	6	45	0.9	1.0	11	1.3	200	2.5	800	800	200	10	10	90
	7-10	28	62	132	52	34	700	10	7	45	1.2	1.4	16	1.6	300	3.0	800	800	250	10	10	120
Males	11-14	45	99	157	62	45	1000	10	8	50	1.4	1.6	18	1.8	400	3.0	1200	1200	350	18	15	150
	15-18	66	145	176	69	56	1000	10	10	60	1.4	1.7	18	2.0	400	3.0	1200	1200	400	18	15	150
	19-22	70	154	177	70	56	1000	7.5	10	60	1.5	1.7	19	2.2	400	3.0	800	800	350	10	15	150
	23-50	70	154	178	70	56	1000	5	10	60	1.4	1.6	18	2.2	400	3.0	800	800	350	10	15	150
	51+	70	154	178	70	56	1000	5	10	60	1.2	1.4	16	2.2	400	3.0	800	800	350	10	15	150
Females	11-14	46	101	157	62	46	800	10	8	50	1.1	1.3	15	1.8	400	3.0	1200	1200	300	18	15	150
	15-18	55	120	163	64	46	800	10	8	60	1.1	1.3	14	2.0	400	3.0	1200	1200	300	18	15	150
	19-22	55	120	163	64	44	800	7.5	8	60	1.1	1.3	14	2.0	400	3.0	800	800	300	18	15	150
	23-50	55	120	163	64	44	800	5	8	60	1.0	1.2	13	2.0	400	3.0	800	800	300	18	15	150
	51+	55	120	163	64	44	800	5	8	60	1.0	1.2	13	2.0	400	3.0	800	800	300	10	15	150
Pregnant						+30	+200	+5	+2	+20	+0.4	+0.3	+2	+0.6	+400	+1.0	+400	+400	+150	[h]	+5	+25
Lactating						+20	+400	+5	+3	+40	+0.5	+0.5	+5	+0.5	+100	+1.0	+400	+400	+150	[h]	+10	+50

a The allowances are intended to provide for individual variations among most normal persons as they live in the United States under usual environmental stresses. Diets should be based on a variety of common foods in order to provide other nutrients for which human requirements have been less well defined. See text for detailed discussion of allowances and of nutrients not tabulated.

b Retinol equivalents. 1 Retinol equivalent = 1 μg retinol or 6 μg β carotene. See text for calculation of vitamin A activity of diets as retinol equivalents.

c As cholecalciferol. 10 μg cholecalciferol = 400 I.U. vitamin D.

d α tocopherol equivalents. 1 mg d-α tocopherol = 1 α T.E. See text for variation in allowances and calculation of vitamin E activity of the diet as α-tocopherol equivalents.

e 1 NE (niacin equivalent) is equal to 1 mg of niacin or 60 mg of dietary tryptophan.

f The folacin allowances refer to dietary sources as determined by Lactobacillus casei assay after treatment with enzymes ("conjugases") to make polyglutamyl forms of the vitamin available to the test organism.

g The RDA for vitamin B12 in infants is based on average concentration of the vitamin in human milk. The allowances after weaning are based on energy intake (as recommended by the American Academy of Pediatrics) and consideration of other factors such as intestinal absorption. see text

h The increased requirement during pregnancy cannot be met by the iron content of habitual American diets nor by the existing iron stores of many women; therefore the use of 30-60 mg of supplemental iron is recommended. Iron needs during lactation are not substantially different from those of nonpregnant women, but continued supplementation of the mother for 2-3 months after parturition is advisable in order to replenish stores depleted by pregnancy.

REPRODUCED FROM RECOMMENDED DIETARY ALLOWANCES, NINTH EDITION (1980) with the permission of The National Academy of Sciences, Washington, D.C.

you should try to eat a variety of vegetable proteins. Beans, peas, soybeans, grains, and nuts are good choices.

Carbohydrates

Foods supply carbohydrates chiefly in three forms — starch, sugar, and cellulose (fibrous material). Cellulose furnishes bulk in the diet, and starches and sugars are the major sources of energy.[2]

Glucose, commonly called blood sugar, is the form in which starches and sugars are used by cells to furnish energy for body processes. The energy cells derived from glucose (carbohydrates) allow protein to be used for building and rebuilding. Carbohydrates also assist the body in utilizing fat and in achieving normal and regular elimination.

Good sources of starches include grains (such as wheat, oats, corn, and rice), products made from grains (such as macaroni, flour, spaghetti, noodles, grits, breads, and breakfast cereals), potatoes, sweet potatoes, and dry beans and peas. Most vegetables contain some starch; most fruits contain some sugar. Cane and beet sugars, jellies, jams, candy and other sweets, honey, molasses, and syrups contain carbohydrates that are highly concentrated sugars.

Fruits, vegetables, and whole-grain cereals provide the most effective bulk for normal functioning and health of the digestive tract; you should eat some fruits and vegetables raw and avoid peeling as many as possible.

Fats

Concentrated sources of energy, fats give more than twice as much energy, weight for weight, as do either carbohydrates or protein. Fats make up part of the structure of every cell, they form a protective cushion around vital internal organs, they supply an essential fatty acid (linoleic acid), and they carry fat-soluble vitamins such as A, D, E, and K. Because the body does not manufacture its own linoleic acid, this substance must be provided by food. The best sources include oils that come from plants — particularly corn, cottonseed, safflower, sesame, soybean, and wheat germ. Many margarines, salad dressings, mayonnaise, and cooking oils are manufactured from plant oils and are referred to as polyunsaturated. Nuts contain less linoleic acid than do most vegetable oils; walnuts rank quite high among the nuts. Poultry and fish oils have more linoleic

CALORIES

A calorie is a unit of measurement that tells you how much energy you get from food. The body needs energy for activity and even at rest. Eating foods day after day that have fewer total calories than you use up will help you lose weight. If you eat foods that have more total calories than you need, the extra energy is stored as fat and you can gain weight. All foods provide calories.

On labels, the calorie content is shown to the nearest 2 calories (2, 4, 6 etc.) up to 20 calories; to the nearest 5 calories (20, 25, 30, etc. up to 50 calories; and to the nearest 10 calories (50, 60, 70 etc.) above 50 calories.

PROTEIN

Protein is the basic part of every cell in your body. The kind of protein that best meets the body's needs comes from animal foods — meat, fish, poultry, eggs, and milk. Protein from legumes, especially soybeans and chickpeas, is almost as good. Protein from cereals and vegetables performs best when these foods are used with a little meat, egg, milk, or cheese in the meal.

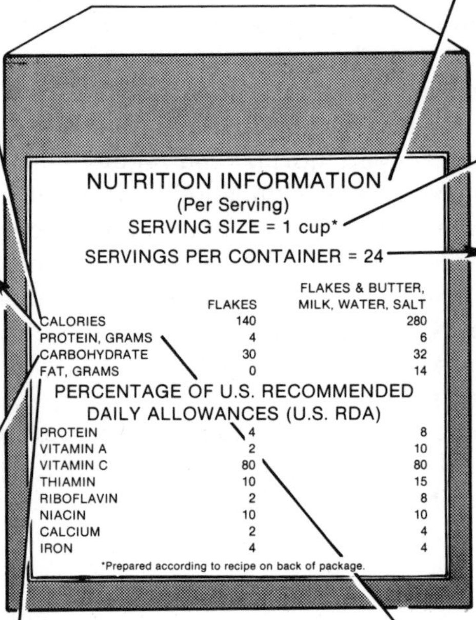

CARBOHYDRATE

Foods contain three types of carbohydrate — starch, sugar, and cellulose. Starch and sugar give energy. You get starch from grain products (cereal, flour, breads, pastas), potatoes, and dry beans and peas. Concentrated sugar comes from such sources as cane and beet sugar, jellies, candy, honey, molasses, and syrup. Cellulose, important for bulk or roughage in the diet, is found in fruit, vegetables, and whole grain cereals.

NUTRITION INFORMATION

Information must be given for a specified serving of the product as found in the container. This label shows information for a serving of potato flakes. Additional information may be listed for the product in combination with other ingredients — flakes prepared with butter, milk, salt, and water, for example.

SERVING (portion) SIZE

The amount of food for which nutrition information is given. It might not be the same as the amount you eat.

SERVINGS PER CONTAINER

The number of servings of the size shown that are in the container. This number may help you visualize the size of the serving. For example, if there are four servings in the container, you know that one serving is equal to one-fourth of the amount in the container.

To find the cost of a serving, divide the price for the container by the number of servings per container.

NUTRITION INFORMATION
(Per Serving)
SERVING SIZE = 1 cup*
SERVINGS PER CONTAINER = 24

	FLAKES	FLAKES & BUTTER, MILK, WATER, SALT
CALORIES	140	280
PROTEIN, GRAMS	4	6
CARBOHYDRATE	30	32
FAT, GRAMS	0	14

PERCENTAGE OF U.S. RECOMMENDED DAILY ALLOWANCES (U.S. RDA)

PROTEIN	4	8
VITAMIN A	2	10
VITAMIN C	80	80
THIAMIN	10	15
RIBOFLAVIN	2	8
NIACIN	10	10
CALCIUM	2	4
IRON	4	4

*Prepared according to recipe on back of package.

FAT

Fat is a concentrated source of energy. (A gram of fat provides roughly twice as much energy as a gram of protein or carbohydrates.) Fat in food digests slowly and helps keep you from feeling hungry. Fat carries the fat-soluble vitamins A, D, E, and K.

Some foods are high in fat, for example, butter, margarine, shortening, cooking and salad oils, cream, nuts, and bacon. Meat, whole milk, and eggs also have some fat. Many popular snacks, baked goods, pastries, and desserts contain substantial amounts of fat.

GRAMS

Grams are units of weight. They are used on the label to express amounts of protein, fat, and carbohydrate. A gram is a much smaller unit of weight than an ounce (1 ounce = 28 grams). A paper clip weighs about an ounce.

Figure 7-2. Nutrition information. From *Nutrition Labeling,* U.S. Department of Agriculture Information Bulletin No. 382, pp. 2-5.

acid than other animal fats, which rank fairly low as sources of linoleic acid.

Because fats digest slowly, they delay feelings of hunger after a meal; used in cooking, they add flavor and variety to many foods. In planning meals, you should keep the total amount of fat at a moderate level, and you should include some foods that contain polyunsaturated fats.

Fats and Health

Of late, the cholesterol question has come to the forefront in relationship to heart disease. It has been found that saturated fats (or those found in animal fats) produce larger concentrations of cholesterol in the blood than unsaturated and polyunsaturated fats (or those found in vegetable fats). Cholesterol is used beneficially in the body to form sex and adrenal hormones, produce bile acids, form cell membranes, and provide Vitamin D. However, when cholesterol from dietary sources (such as animal fats) combines with already existing sources of cholesterol in the body, a high cholesterol blood level is produced in some people. Increased blood cholesterol can be deposited in blood vessel walls so that placques are formed. These placques may in turn contribute to heart and vessel problems by the formation of clots or the closure of vessels.

Certain foods are high in animal fats and raise blood cholesterol levels in the body. Some of these foods are as follows: red meats (especially those that are marbled with fat), butter, egg yolk, cheese, chocolate, whole milk, and ice cream. It has been found that to protect the body from too much cholesterol in the blood, less than 10 percent of the fats found in the diet should be saturated. That means that you should eat less high-fat meats (and more low-fat meats such as fish and poultry). It also means that you should cut off all fat on meat before cooking, and you should bake, broil, roast, and stew your meat rather than fry it. You should substitute skim or low-fat milk for whole milk. You should consider using margarine rather than butter and eating fewer eggs. You should use polyunsaturated fats in cooking, such as vegetable oils (remember, polyunsaturated fats may in fact lower blood cholesterol levels). You should, lastly, achieve and maintain an ideal body weight by eating more fruit, vegetables, and whole grains and less sugar-sweetened foods and foods that contain saturated fats.[3]

Cholesterol and Lipoproteins

As we know, fat and water do not mix, so the body needs a system for carrying fats through the bloodstream (the major component of which is water). The combination of fat, cholesterol, and the blood protein that serves as the medium of transport is called a lipoprotein.

Scientists have classified two protein-cholesterol combinations that may be vital to the health of your heart and circulatory system: high-density lipoproteins (HDL) and low-density lipoproteins (LDL). LDLs seem to pick up cholesterol and deposit it in cells (and on the walls of blood vessels), while HDLs seem to collect excess cholesterol and perhaps even remove it from cells. HDLs may also prevent LDLs from entering into cells to form fatty-cholesterol deposits, and they may help clear the blood of triglycerides that are also instrumental in cholesterol formation.

What does this mean for you? It has been known for over twenty-five years that men with coronary heart disease also have high LDL levels in the blood. Conversely, it is now thought that high HDL levels are associated with low cholesterol levels. Thus, HDL and LDL levels give us a major clue in predicting heart disease.[4]

Minerals

A number of minerals are required by the body to give strength and rigidity to body tissues and to maintain basic body functions. Some are major minerals that are required by the body in large amounts, and others are metals that are required only in traces.

Vitamins

"Vitamins are chemical substances essential in the diet for the growth and maintenance of body tissue."[5] Typically, vitamins are said to be used in conjunction with enzymes to promote growth, maintenance, repair, and coordination of cell and tissue functions.

Most nutritionists agree that individuals can get all of the vitamins that they need to fulfill the RDA from the foods that they eat — provided they get the right kinds of foods. Eating the proper foods in the proper amounts from the basic four food groups (meat, milk and dairy products, fruits and vegetables, and breads and cereals) can insure adequate intake of the vitamins that can help you maintain a healthy body. It must be remembered, though, that even if you are taking in the right foods in the proper amounts, you may not be getting all of the vitamins that your body needs. Certain vitamins can be easily destroyed by several means. Exposure to air, light, heat, and multiple handling can destroy the vitamin value of many of our foods. To insure that you get the most from your food in the way of vitamins, you should use fresh foods, use a minimum of water in cooking, and cook foods for the least possible time.

Although there are very few full-blown, clinical cases of vitamin deficiencies in the United States, nutritionists feel that there are many subclinical deficiencies where individuals do not manifest gross abnormalities or symptoms of the deficiency. If you notice abnormalities in body tissues, it could mean a vitamin deficiency. Check with your doctor to be sure.

The "Natural" Craze

This is a generation of nature lovers, and everything is geared to "getting back to nature," even vitamins. A vitamin that would cost one dollar in its "synthetic" form costs five dollars "natural."

Two fallacies are behind this "natural" vitamin craze: (1) natural vitamins are superior to those synthesized by man, (2) vitamin products sold as "natural" do not contain synthetic ingredients.

Chemists tell us that each vitamin, in order to be called such, must have a particular molecular structure. This remains the same whether the vitamin is synthesized in a laboratory or extracted from an animal or plant. For example, to be called vitamin A, a substance, no matter what its source, has to have a specific molecular arrangement. The body cannot tell the difference between a vitamin from an animal or plant and the same vitamin from a laboratory.

An investigator discovered some interesting things while visiting two manufacturers of "natural" vitamins: Their Rose Hips Vitamin C Tablets are made from natural rose hips combined with chemical ascorbic acid, the same vitamin C used in standard pharmaceutical tablets. Natural rose hips contain only about 2 percent vitamin C, and if no vitamin C were added, the tablet "would have to be as big as a golf ball."[6]

In any case, all vitamins, "natural" or synthetic, must contain a certain number of binding additives, such as ethyl cellulose, polysorbate 80 (a synthetic emulsifier), gum acacia, etc. It comes back to the same old story — if you want natural vitamin C, go buy an orange. Your pocketbook will appreciate it.

Water

Water is essential for life. If you are not drinking enough, you may tire easily and find it hard to concentrate. Many people drink less water than is optimum for the best functioning of the body. The shipwrecked sailor who goes without water for much more than forty-eight hours will die.

Your need for liquids depends on your size and weight. As a general guide, adults should drink between one and one-half and two quarts of fluid a day. Children, of course, need proportionately less. Water, which makes up more than half your body weight, is constantly being lost and must be replaced. Not all of this water is lost through urination. It is also lost through perspiration and unseen and unfelt evaporation through the skin. Some water comes from your lungs; you can see this moisture by breathing on a mirror.

It is very important that you drink enough. If you drink too little, the salts and minerals excreted by your kidneys may not be flushed completely from your system. These minerals are the building blocks for kidney stones. Also, many doctors believe that bacteria, which cause infections, can grow more easily when urine flow is low. However, very large amounts of urine may weaken certain protective mechanisms that suppress the growth of bacteria.

NUTRITION LABELING

To decide what kind of nutrients that you are getting when you take a chicken pot pie out of the box or when you open a can of tomato soup, you should learn what nutrition labels are and what they can tell you about your food. All labels — on cans, boxes, bags, and cartons — have to list certain basic information:[7]

- The name of the product.
- The net contents or the net weight. Net weight of canned food includes the weight of the liquid in which the food is canned.
- The name and place of business of the manufacturer, packer, or distributor.

In the case of most foods, the ingredients must be listed on the label; the only foods not required to list ingredients are foods that qualify under the Food and Drug Administration as standardized foods: all foods by that particular name (catsup or mayonnaise, for example) contain certain mandatory ingredients. Under law, those mandatory ingredients do not need to be listed, but if the manufacturer adds any optional ingredients, those must be listed on the label.

For those foods that list ingredients, the ingredient that is listed first is the one that is present in the food in the largest amount, by weight. Others are listed in descending order, by weight. You can learn a lot about what you are getting by reading the list of ingredients. For example, the primary ingredient in Jello Banana Cream Instant Pudding and Pie Filling is sugar; in Campbell's Cream of Mushroom Soup, it is water. Hunt's Fruit Cocktail lists peaches first, but they are followed by water; Kraft's Macaroni and Cheese Dinner has enriched macaroni as its primary ingredient — and the side of the box lists the enriching agents as thiamin, niacin, and riboflavin, among others. Lipton's Lite-Lunch Oriental Style lists enriched wheat flour first; soy sauce is fourth. Instant Quaker Oatmeal with Apples and Cinnamon lists specially processed rolled oats as the primary ingredient, followed by sugar; dehydrated apple flakes are third.

━━━ VITAMIN AND MINERAL SUPPLEMENTS

What if you think that you are not getting all of the nutrients that you need? Is it time to turn to vitamin and mineral supplements? The National Dairy Council has come up with what it considers to be the ten

255

leading nutrients — those most important to health: protein, carbo-hydrates, fat, vitamin A, vitamin C, thiamin, riboflavin, niacin, calcium, and iron. About fifty nutrients are needed to maintain optimum health; according to National Dairy Council officials, if you eat foods that will supply you with the ten leading nutrients, you will almost certainly get the other forty nutrients in the same food.

If you are eating a relatively well-balanced diet, then, you probably do not need vitamin or mineral supplements. In fact, vitamin and mineral supplements that you do not need can cause toxic effects if you take too many of them in too short of a time.[8] Especially dangerous are the fat-soluble vitamins (A, D, E, and K). While water-soluble vitamins are eliminated in the urine if you take any excess, fat-soluble vitamins are stored in the body, where they may lead to a toxic condition serious enough to cause severe illness or death.

Certain life-style patterns or events can lead to destruction of vita-mins in the body. If you drink alcohol, coffee, or tea; smoke tobacco or

SITUATIONS WHERE SUPPLEMENTS ARE USEFUL

The following are common conditions in which vitamin supplements are valuable — or an increased consumption of vitamin-rich foods.
1. **Pregnancy and breast-feeding** boost a woman's vitamin requirements. A multi-formula tablet with iron guarantees meeting these clearly-defined needs. In fact, *every* woman of child-bearing age needs extra iron, whether from foods or supplements.
2. **Oral contraceptives** lower bloodstream vitamin levels by disrupting the body's ability to utilize B vitamins (particularly niacin and B_6). Some physicians recommend a B-complex tablet to counter this.
3. **Smoking** cuts vitamin C supplies by as much as 30 percent, which can be harmful, depending upon dietary habits. A small supplement (100 mg.) will be enough to compensate.
4. **Dieting** reduces overall vitamin intake, at times dangerously, especially among the fad diets. Unless the diet is nutritionally balanced (an example is Weight Watchers), multivitamin tablets are needed.
5. **Alcohol** can disrupt diet. Multi-tablets (especially those high in B-complex vitamins, which absorb alcohol) may prevent serious physical damage.
6. **Caffeine,** taken in large quantities from coffee, tea, or cola drinks, causes the body to flush out the water-soluble vitamins more rapidly. Small daily supple-ments of the B-complex and C vitamins will replenish supplies.

Reprinted with permission from Consumer's Digest, July/August 1981, p. 47.

marijuana; take birth control pills, iron pills, sleeping pills, or aspirin; undergo excessive mental or physical stress or surgery; eat an excess of sugar or if you eat egg whites or raw clams; if you ingest rancid oil or fat; or if you are exposed to chlorine or radiation, you may want to ask your doctor about vitamin supplements. You should be cautious about self-prescribing supplements of either vitamins or minerals.

NEEDLESS VITAMIN SUPPLEMENTS

The following are heavily-advertised vitamins you should never need to take.

Vitamin	General Sources
A	Dairy products, meat and vegetables; excessive dosage causes health damage, particularly to children
D	Potentially lethal in large doses; the body manufactures sufficient quantities from sunlight
K	Is produced internally as needed by the body
Pantothenic Acid	Present in almost all foods and cannot be destroyed by cooking — adequate supply is guaranteed by almost all people
Biotin	Useful in only small amounts, otherwise eliminated by the body, survives cooking and processing so is present in many foods

Reprinted with permission from: Consumers Digest, July/August 1981, p. 48.

PLANNING MEALS

At Each Meal

1. **One serving of a protein.** You could try eggs, meat, fish, poultry,

257

cheese, seafood, or lentils. Peanut butter counts as a protein. So do certain combinations, such as whole-grain cereal with milk or macaroni with cheese.

2. **At least one grain food.** Depending on your protein, you can try bread, rice, noodles, macaroni, or cereal. If you choose rice, cereal, macaroni, noodles, or similar products, they should be enriched. If you can, eat whole-grain cereals. Whole-grain or whole-wheat bread is best, but make sure that you eat it enriched if you choose white bread.

3. **At least one fruit or vegetable.** Raw is best; frozen is second best. The canning process sometimes removes nutrients, so cook your vegetables as little as possible if you are using canned items out of season. Use fresh fruit if it is in season. Once a day you should have a deep yellow or a dark green vegetable; once each day you should have a citrus fruit (or its juice).

4. **A beverage.** You need eight to twelve cups of fluid a day; you can drink juice or water. If you want to use a milk serving here, you could have a glass of milk. You should try to drink at least one cup of beverage so that you can begin to fulfill your daily requirement. If you do not drink milk, you need to plan cheese, cottage cheese, or yogurt into two of your meals for the day, or you need to have two milk group snacks during the day.

At One Meal

At one meal, or with a snack sometime during the day, you need to include the following:

1. A food high in fiber (try bran muffins, whole-grain bread, raw carrots, sunflower seeds, and so on).
2. Iodized salt (this may be contraindicated for those with severe acne or for those who are on salt-free diets).
3. A food high in vitamin C (try tomato juice if you are tired of citrus fruit juice).
4. An unsaturated oil (you can get it in cooking, in salad dressings, and in margarines).

FAST FOODS AND NUTRITION

If you are an average American, you eat out from four to seven times a week at one of the nation's close to 50,000 fast food restaurants, and you contribute to the multibillion-dollar industry that has made Kentucky Fried Chicken a household word.[9] There is good news and bad news nutritionally when it comes to fast foods. If you learn the benefits and the drawbacks, you can control the nutritional aspects of fast-food eating. A number of general conclusions can be drawn in relation to the basic nutrients and fast foods:[10]

Fats and Carbohydrates

Most fast foods are high in both fats and carbohydrates; while these nutrients are essential to energy, too much of them can lead to overweight. Two points bear mention. The ground beef used in most fast-food chains to prepare hamburgers is, in most cases, lower in fat content than the ground beef purchased in the grocery store by the average consumer. In addition, most thick shakes are made with a nonfat powdered milk base and vegetable fats; the thick shakes have more nutritional value than regular milkshakes.

Protein

The amount of chicken, fish, and hamburger served at the average fast-food establishment and the amount of meat on an average pizza do qualify for servings of protein — although not very abundant servings. To boost the amount of protein in the meal, you can order a thick shake — low in fat and a good source of protein.

Minerals

The only fast food that is a good source of minerals is pizza, with its cheese topping providing a serving of calcium. Hamburgers are the only fast food that supply a significant amount of iron, and adolescent and adult women who need more iron than men of the same age may be prone to pick chicken, fish, or pizza, which contain no significant iron.

Among the drinks, the thick shake also provides a significant amount of calcium.

Protein and Calories at Fast Food Chains

RESTAURANTS (In alphabetical order)	MENU ITEMS (Main dish, side dish and beverage)	PROTEIN	CALORIES (in grams)
A&W	Super Papa Burger	19	448
	Small fries	3	249
	Root Beer Float	3	200
	TOTAL	25	897
BURGER CHEF	Super Chef	23	423
	Small fries	4	285
	Large Chocolate Shake	9	361
	TOTAL	36	1069
BURGER KING	Whopper	29	563
	Small fries	2	218
	Large Chocolate Shake	7	407
	TOTAL	38	1188
DAIRY QUEEN	Super Brazier	43	732
	Small fries	3	239
	Large Chocolate Shake	10	376
	TOTAL	56	1347
HARDEE'S	Deluxe Huskee	32	635
	Small fries	4	283
	Large Chocolate Shake	10	328
	TOTAL	46	1246
JACK-IN-THE-BOX	Jumbo Jack	28	558
	Small fries	2	226
	Large Chocolate Shake	13	540
	TOTAL	43	1324

(All data compiled by Jacobs-Winston Laboratories Inc., New York, N.Y.)

Vitamins

Most fast-food meals are low in vitamin A, vitamin C, and most B vitamins, but most contain sufficient amounts of thiamin, niacin, and riboflavin. To boost your intake of vitamins A and C, try ordering orange juice, taking a trip to the salad bar (and stocking up on lettuce and fresh vegetables), ordering a lemonade, or getting tomatoes on your hamburger.

Calories

Almost all fast-food meals are high in calories, easily providing many people — especially children — with well over half of their daily caloric requirements. You are getting 1,000 calories with the average fast-food meal consisting of a quarter-pound hamburger, french fries, and a chocolate shake. Half of a thirteen-inch pizza is 900 calories, and an average two-piece fried fish dinner is almost 1,000.

Even if you are not overweight now, frequent trips to the fast-food restaurants can add on extra unwanted pounds unless you increase your physical exercise to balance your caloric intake.

Sugar Versus Fiber

Most fast foods are extremely high in refined sugars.[11] Commercial chicken batters and barbecue sauces are usually more than 50 percent refined sugar. Aside from meat, sugar is unnecessarily added to almost every item on a fast-food menu — including the mustard, catsup, "secret" sauce, pickles, relish, and processed cheese that you put on your hamburger. Even the bun that you put around your hamburger has sugar added, as do sodas, frozen desserts, milkshakes, and pizza fillings. Even hot dogs have sugar added at many fast-food restaurants. The sugar content in simple catsup is, on the average, about 30 percent, and the coffee creamers used in most fast-food restaurants are about 65 percent sugar.

Just as there is sugar in almost everything, there is fiber in almost nothing. The typical quarter-pound hamburger, french fries, and shake have no dietary fiber at all.

High Salt Content

Almost all fast foods are high in sodium content; one Big Mac, for example, supplies almost the full day's allotment for someone on a low-sodium diet. Add a dill pickle, and you have doubled it.

Improving the Picture

If you frequently eat at fast-food restaurants, there are things that you can do to improve the picture nutritionally. Add condiments to your hamburger: raw onions, cheese, and tomatoes all help provide vitamins and minerals. If you can, get lettuce, too. On the other hand, limit catsup, relish, mustard, and special sauces that are high in salt and sugar.

If you are concerned about calories, drink milk or fruit juice instead of a carbonated beverage or a milkshake. Choose a regular hamburger or cheeseburger instead of a quarter-pounder. If there is a salad bar, take advantage of it, but go light on dressing.

Opt for extra ingredients on your pizza that will add some nutrition. In addition to cheese topping, choose meats, green peppers, onions, tomatoes, shrimp, pineapple, or other vegetables.

Finally, and most important, choose your foods for the rest of the day carefully. Make sure that you include fruits and vegetables in your other meals — especially a citrus fruit and some dark green and deep yellow vegetables. Because the caloric content of most fast foods is high, choose broiled fish or baked poultry for the proteins in your other meals; meat is also a good choice if it is a lean cut and is roasted or broiled. Make sure to include milk or milk products and some foods that will provide fiber (it is a good idea if you can eat fresh fruits and vegetables raw; whole-grain cereals and nuts will also help). You need to pay special attention to your other meals to guarantee that you have chosen foods from all four basic food groups in their proper proportion.

FOOD ADDITIVES

The Food and Drug Administration defines additives as "substances added directly to food, or substances which may be reasonably expected to become components of food" as a result of processing or packaging or "substances that may affect the food without becoming part of it."[12]

Food additives have become so common in the foods that we purchase and eat that it would be difficult to serve a complete meal that did not include them. A typical lunch, for instance, might consist of a sandwich, a bowl of instant soup, a gelatin dessert, and a cola drink. The additives in that simple lunch include:

1. **Sandwich.** The bread contains an additive to keep it fresh, and it has been fortified with vitamins. The margarine has been colored a pale yellow; the mayonnaise contains emulsifiers that keep it from separating. The luncheon meat on the sandwich contains nitrite, added during the curing process to keep the meat from spoiling.
2. **Soup.** The soup contains an additive that prevents it from becoming rancid.
3. **Gelatin.** The dessert's red color is a result of an additive designed to make it more appealing.
4. **Cola drink.** This drink is stocked with artificial flavoring, artificial coloring, sweetners, and artificial carbonation; without them all, it is just plain water.

Additives are intentionally used in foods for one or more of several reasons:

1. **To maintain freshness.** Without additives, foods on the shelf or in the refrigerator would spoil, lose their color and flavor, or turn rancid. Vitamin C is added to peaches to keep them from turning brown. Nitrite is added to meats during the curing process to protect them from contamination by the bacteria that causes botulism. Antioxidants help prevent changes in flavor, color, and texture that occur when foods are exposed to air.
2. **To maintain or improve nutrition.** A number of foods are fortified or enriched with vitamins and minerals that have otherwise been lost or destroyed during processing. Common additives include vitamins A, B, C, and D and iodine (in table salt).
3. **To make food more appealing.** The most widely used additives are the ones designed to make food more appealing — to add color and flavor. By far, the most common are sugar, salt, and corn syrup.
4. **To aid in processing or preparation.** A number of additives are used during preparation or processing of food to prevent caking or

DIETARY GUIDELINES FOR AMERICANS

The U.S. Department of Agriculture has given the American public seven dietary guidelines that are based on the assumption that food alone cannot make you healthy, but good eating habits based on moderation and variety can help keep you healthy and even improve your health.

1. Eat a variety of foods. To assure yourself an adequate diet, eat a variety of foods daily, including selections of:
   - Fruits
   - Vegetables
   - Whole grains and enriched breads, cereals, and grain products
   - Milk, cheese, and yogurt
   - Meats, poultry, fish, and eggs
   - Legumes (dry peas and beans)

2. Maintain an ideal weight. To improve your eating habits that may contribute to weight:
   - Eat slowly
   - Prepare smaller portions
   - Avoid "seconds"
   To lose weight:
   - Increase physical activity
   - Eat less fat and fatty foods
   - Eat less sugar and sweets
   ° Avoid too much alcohol

3. Avoid too much fat, saturated fat, and cholesterol. To accomplish this:
   - Choose lean meat, fish, poultry, dry beans and peas as your protein source
   - Moderate your use of eggs and organ meats (such as liver)
   - Limit your intake of butter, cream, hydrogenated margarines, shortenings and coconut oils, and foods made from such products
   - Trim excess fat off meats
   - Broil, bake or boil rather than fry
   - Read labels carefully to determine both amounts and types of fat contained in foods

4. Eat foods with adequate starch and fiber. To eat more complex carbohydrates daily:
   - Substitute starches for fats and sugars
   - Select foods which are good sources of fiber and starch, such as whole grain breads and cereals, fruits and vegetables, beans, peas, and nuts

5. Avoid too much sugar. To avoid excessive sugars:
   - Use less of all sugars including white sugar, brown sugar, raw sugar, honey, and syrups
   - Eat less of foods containing these sugars, such as candy, soft drinks, ice cream, cakes, and cookies
   - Select fresh fruits or fruits canned without sugar or light syrup rather than heavy syrup
   - Read food labels for clues on sugar content — if the names sucrose, glucose, maltose, dextrose, lactose, fructose, or syrups appear first, then there is a large amount of sugar
   - Remember, how often you eat sugar is as important as how much sugar you eat.

6. Avoid too much sodium. To accomplish this:
   - Learn to enjoy the unsalted flavors of foods
   - Cook with only small amounts of added salt
   - Add little or no salt to food at the table
   - Limit your intake of salty foods, such as potato chips, pretzels, salted nuts and popcorn, condiments (soy sauce, steak sauce, garlic salt, etc.), cheese, pickled foods, and cured meats
   - Read food labels carefully to determine the amounts of sodium in processed foods and snack items

7. If you drink alcohol, do so in moderation.

---

lumping, to control acidity or alkalinity, to retain moisture, to affect cooking or baking results, to give body and texture to foods, or to evenly distribute particles in liquid. Others prevent crystals from forming in ice cream, preserve the moisture in shredded coconut, and prevent the oils in mayonnaise and peanut butter from separating.

Additives are listed on ingredient labels: exercise your right to choose which additives you want to include in your food. For example, you might decide to continue buying bread that contains sodium propionate to inhibit growth of mold, but you might decide to stop buying cookies that contain artificial coloring.

Scientists will never be able to guarantee that anything added to food is completely safe; most of the time, additives perform important functions (such as preventing spoilage), but in some cases, they are not really needed. Since the long-term effects of many chemical additives are still a question of debate and concern, you should limit what you reasonably can.

FIBER

The controversy has raged for years as to the role of fiber in the diet and its relationship to various disease conditions. The major advocate of high-fiber intake as a disease-prevention technique is Dr. Denis P. Burkitt. Dr. Burkitt indicated recently that the most common cause of death in North America is coronary heart disease; the most common intestinal disease is diverticular disease; the most common emergency abdominal surgery is the appendectomy; the most common venous disorders are hemorrhoids and varicose veins; the second most common cause of death is cancer of the colon and rectum; the most common nutritional disorder is obesity; and the most common endocrine disorder is diabetes.[13] Dr. Burkitt maintains that these disease conditions could be decreased among the general population by increasing the fiber content of the diet.

What is fiber? It consists of cell walls of plants that resist the digestive enzymes in the gastrointestinal tract. Certain food types contain varying degrees of fiber. Some foods that are high in fiber are whole grains and cereals, fresh fruits (don't forget that the peelings are a good source of fiber!), berries, legumes and nuts, tuberous root vegetables (such as potatoes, carrots, turnips, and parsnips), and other fresh vegetables (such as cabbage).

So how does this all relate to disease conditions? Fiber affects the intestinal tract in several ways. Fiber collects and holds water as it passes through the intestinal tract, which makes for softer, bulkier stools. These bulkier stools pass through the intestinal tract much more rapidly than harder, smaller stools, which are characteristic of low-fiber diets. As these larger, softer stools pass more rapidly from the body, they decrease the internal pressure in the large intestine. High fiber in the diet also influences the bacterial environment of the intestinal tract. In addition, bile salts (which emulsify fats and oils so that they are absorbed from the intestinal tract into the bloodstream) and bile acids are not reabsorbed from the intestinal tract. So, more bile salts and bile acids are excreted from the body with the fats and oils that are bound to them.

Advocates of high fiber in the diet point to the fact that fiber promotes a lower blood level of cholesterol which in turn decreases coronary heart disease. Because less bile salts and acids are reabsorbed into the body, and because these salts and acids carry bound fats and oils with them as they leave the body, there is less cholesterol formation in the body. Also, because the stools produced from a high-fiber diet pass more rapidly from the body, more cholesterol is likely to be excreted from the body. Simply stated, with less cholesterol in the bloodstream, atherosclerosis, arteriosclerosis, and in turn, heart disease are all less likely. The decreased reabsorption of bile acids and salts also plays a role in decreased gallstone formation.

Scientists have not yet determined how much fiber anyone should eat. There are no Recommended Daily Allowances (U.S. RDA) for fiber. The source of the fiber is also important. Bran, for example, has a laxative effect, but some fruits and vegetables do not. Bran should never be eaten dry, because it can clog the digestive system.

Eating a high-fiber diet can have some distressing side effects, such as a feeling of being stuffed or bloated. Stomach rumblings, usually frowned on in polite society, are caused by changes in the material passing through the intestines.

Large amounts of fiber can impair the body's ability to absorb certain important minerals such as iron, copper, and calcium. Eaten over a long period of time, large amounts of indigestible material such as fiber can lead to a condition called volvulus of the sigmoid colon, which requires surgery.

Experts in nutrition point out that fiber is just one part of a properly balanced diet. Adding fiber to a poor diet probably will cause more problems than it will solve. Much more research is needed before anyone can say with certainty what the full role of fiber is in the human diet.[14]

SUGAR IN THE RAW

Another nutritional controversy centers around one of the least understood foods of all time — sugar. From one group you hear, "Sugar is a must for energy." Yet from another group, "Sugar is poison." Where is the average consumer to turn for the correct answers? Actually, neither is completely correct, but both contain some sweet truths.

Western civilization has not always had sugar. We knew very little about this sweet substance until the fifteenth century, when the Portuguese introduced sugar cane into Africa. Not until they brought it from Brazil in the sixteenth century did it become a normal commodity among Europeans.[15]

Time was when sugar was a great luxury, rather than a staple. In

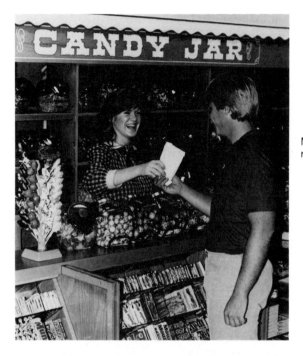

Most Americans need to
reduce their sugar intake.

1830, England, which has to import most of its sugar, consumed five pounds per person per year. Today the average Englishperson devours 125 pounds per year. In the United States, the rate of consumption has gone from nothing, when the Pilgrims first landed at Plymouth Rock, to a high of 128 pounds per person per year.[16]

The greatest factor in increased sugar use has come from the addition of refined sugar to processed foods.

Page and Friend report:

Use in processed food products and beverages has increased more than threefold from nearly 20 to 70 pounds, while household purchase has dropped one-half from a little more than 50 to about 25 pounds. Currently, food products and beverages account for more than two-thirds of the refined sugar consumed — 70 pounds out of a little over 100 pounds. Moreover, beverages now comprise the largest single industry use of refined sugar in the United States diet, or nearly 23 pounds. Futhermore, the amount used in beverages has increased nearly sevenfold since early in the century when 3½ pounds per person per year was used in these products. Use of refined sugar in beverages is now second only to household use.[17]

Does the Body Require Sugar?

Contrary to popular belief, the body does not require table sugar (sucrose). It does require carbohydrates, which can be found as either sugar or starches. Although both supply energy, only starches provide other essential nutrients. Sugar is an integral part of all living substances. It is produced in plants through photosynthesis. Animals eating the plants also contain sugar in their makeup. Therefore, we cannot escape it. However, only lactose (milk sugar) fructose (sugar found in fruits), and glucose (blood sugar) are essential to life. Sucrose (table sugar) can be eliminated from the diet almost completely, and, at least in the case of many diabetics, probably should be.

The impact on health of increasing sugar use is not well understood. The relationship of sugar to coronary artery disease and cancer is a controversial issue with little pertinent data. The most immediate problem is the danger of displacing complex carbohydrates, which are high in micronutrients, with sugar, which is essentially an energy source offering little other nutritional value. This not only increases the potential for depriving the body of essential micronutrients, but may actually increase the body's needs for certain vitamins.

What Part Does Sugar Play in Dental Decay?

Authorities all agree that sugar can promote tooth decay and gum disease. Although tooth decay is not by any means deadly, it can be painful and is expensive. Americans today spend about 2 billion dollars a year treating it.

Progressively, tooth decay has become more common as we use grain rather than meat and fruit as our main sources of food, as we make refined flours and sucrose abundantly available, and, most recently, as we vastly increase use of the packaged, ready-to-eat sweetened snacks and candies that flood the modern market. The important matter is not the amount of sugar eaten, but the kind. Sweets such as sticky candies tend to adhere to teeth more than others.

The decay process begins with colonies of bacteria (called dental plaque) that stick to your teeth. When you eat, the bacteria break down your food and change the sugar to acid. The sticky bacterial plaque then holds the acid to the tooth surface, allowing it to attack the enamel on your teeth, resulting in tooth decay.[18]

Another causative factor in dental caries is frequency of intake. Dr. Abraham Nizel explains:

> Each time the dental plaque on the tooth surface is exposed to sweets, twenty to thirty minutes of acid is produced. So, if five lozenges or cough drops are eaten, one after another, within a space of fifteen minutes, they might produce thirty-five minutes of acid. On the other hand, if they are eaten twenty minutes apart, they will produce one hundred minutes of acid.[19]

Is It Healthier To Use Honey Instead of Sugar?

Honey is formed by an enzyme from nectar gathered by bees. Depending on where the nectar comes from, honey can differ in composition and flavor. But all honey is a blend of a number of different sugars, largely fructose and glucose. Like brown sugar, honey has a few nutrients — mainly potassium, calcium, and phosphorus. But, again, they are scant. You would have to eat 91 tablespoons of honey each day to get your recommended daily requirement of potassium, 200 for calcium, and 267 for phosphorus. The only nutrient of any significant value found in honey is iron. And still you would need to eat over five tablespoons of honey (310 calories) to obtain 0.9 mg of iron — the amount found in one medium egg yolk.[20] There is no evidence that honey is easier to digest than other sugars. When you eat table sugar, your body breaks the sucrose down into fructose and glucose, the two leading ingredients of honey.

The idea that honey is natural and, therefore, nutritionally wiser than sugar is a great hoax. In fact, the late Dr. Adelle Davis admits:

> Despite the fact that honey is a natural sweet, it contains only traces of nutrients and appears to cause tooth decay as quickly as does refined sugar. Persons who are convinced that honey is "good for them" often eat large amounts, gain unwanted pounds, and spoil their appetite for more nutritious foods.[21]

Is Fructose a Sugar Substitute?

Fructose is a type of sugar that has been touted as a "natural" replacement for table sugar, as the "newest, most effective diet aid," as a sugar substitute for diabetics, and as a hunger appeaser. Major sources of fructose are honey and fruits.

Although the scientific and medical community is by no means unanimous over the merits of fructose as an "ideal substitute" for table sugar (sucrose), this is how most health professionals respond to such claims:

The prevailing medical opinion, according to a report prepared for FDA, is that there are no "clinical advantages" in substituting fructose where diabetics are concerned.

The available scientific data, according to a recent report to the FDA, is regarded as insufficient "to determine if fructose or any other carbohydrate has beneficial properites for the long-term dietary management of diabetes."

The claim that fructose is a natural replacement for ordinary sugar can be misleading. Commercially sold fructose is produced from sucrose (table sugar).

Fructose provides the same number of calories as table sugar, so health experts say there is little if any advantage in using fructose for weight reduction.[22]

VEGETARIANISM

Vegetarianism (in which meat or animal products are not eaten) is becoming more widespread in this country. People give various reasons for not eating meat, such as expense, desire not to exploit animals, religious reasons, and personal taste, but whatever the reason, the question always exists as to whether vegetarian diets are indeed adequate nutritionally.

To assess the adequacy of vegetarian diets, we must consider the fact that there are various degrees and types of vegetarians. Total vegetarians, or vegans, are persons who consume no animal foods, including meat, poultry, fish, eggs, and dairy products. Strict vegans also refuse to wear or use products that have come from animals, such as fur, leather, or wool. Lacto-vegetarians are persons who do not eat meat, poultry, fish, or eggs, but who do consume milk or milk products. Lacto-ovo-vegetarians do not eat meat, poultry, fish or seafood, but do include dairy products and eggs in their diets. Semi or partial vegetarians consume some groups of animal foods but not all of them. For example, they may not eat red meat, but may eat poultry or fish.

Strict vegetarians who exclude all animal products including milk and eggs risk the danger of vitamin B12 deficiency. The Vegans, a popular dietary group, prescribe such a diet which frequently causes a degeneration of the spinal cord (now known as Vegan back) which is usually not detected until the condition is irreversible. Vitamin B12 is essential for blood cell formation and normal functioning of the nerves. No known vegetable source can supply this much-needed vitamin; consequently, a supplement is mandatory when animal products are eliminated from the diet.

Vegetarian women must also consider the fact that they chance a loss of iron in their systems if they are of childbearing age. The needed iron may be obtained through the eating of eggs if they have not been eliminated from the diet.

The American Dietetic Association has stated that well-planned vegetarian diets can be sources of good nutrition and can ensure good nutritional status. However, poorly planned or unplanned diets should be avoided, because they can produce diet-related nutritional disorders. Vegetarians should also be aware that there are special health conditions for which careful and meticulous diet planning must be achieved to ensure health. These conditions include pregnancy, lactation, adolescence (or other growth periods), and diabetes.

"The most important safeguard for average [vegetarian] consumers," said a Committee of the National Academy of Sciences — National Research Council, "is a great variety in the diet."[23] This is, indeed, sound advice for anyone — whether he eats meat or not.

ORGANIC AND NATURAL FOODS

One of the most heated controversies in nutrition and health centers around organic and natural foods and nutrients. *Organic* refers to carbon-

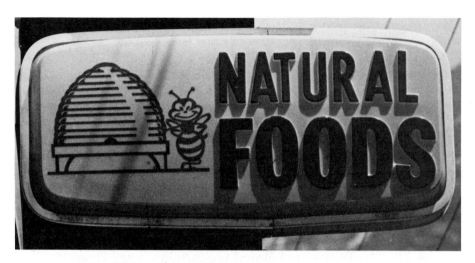

The term "natural food" is an advertising gimmick.

based molecules, which also contain oxygen and hydrogen, that are characteristic of living protoplasm. Proponents of organic foods believe that foodstuffs grown in soil should be fertilized with decomposed plant material (called *humus)* rather than inorganic, chemically produced fertilizers, which contain materials such as potash, nitrates, and phosphates. Those advocating this type of nutrition feel that the active organic substances used in soil fertilization and the organic foods resulting from this fertilization are more in harmony with the components of our bodies.

This concept is interesting, but many refute it by saying that organically grown foods are not necessarily superior to synthetically fertilized foods. The reason: plants cannot tell the difference between inorganic and organic fertilizers; they use the available chemicals regardless of the source. One other consideration is that organically grown foods cost more. This, and the fact that plants cannot differentiate between organic and inorganic fertilizers, may help you to be a wiser consumer in the area of organic foods.

Natural foods are those derived from plant or animal sources, including foods that do not contain artificial colors, flavors, or synthetic ingredients such as chemical additives. Advocates of natural foods and of other nutrient materials consider the following concepts important:

- Whole foods are more nourishing than processed foods, because they contain more vitamins and minerals and less chemical additives.
- Americans eat too much sugar.
- Survival depends on the intake of complete proteins, which supply all the essential amino acids for growth, repair, and maintenance of body tissues.
- Individuals should take into account seasonal dietary changes and occasional cleansing (fasting) regimes to ensure health.
- There is no need to eat when hunger is not present; eating three meals a day is merely a cultural habit.
- Specific foods are medicines for specific conditions.[24]

Considering the characterisitcs of natural foods, however, finding foods that do not contain additives or artificial colors or flavors of some type is difficult. Today, agricultural productivity is enhanced by fertilizers, pesticides, and other substances. These substances are in turn taken into the plants that grow in the area and into the animals that ingest the plants. So chemicals such as DDT, DES (diethylstilbesterol — a hormonelike substance), Dieldrin, Aldrin, and PCBs (polychlorinated biphenyls) get into our food sources. Then, other foreign substances are added when foods undergo chemical processing. Of the 10,000 items in your local grocery store, it has been established that 8,000 have undergone some type of major chemical processing.[25] Each year, 140 pounds of additives are consumed by every man, woman, and child in this country.[26] Our meats contain drugs, antibiotics, pesticides, and environmental pollutants. Our fruits and vegetables contain fumigants, retardants, preservatives, drugs, and antisprouting chemicals.

Although it is frightening to know that we are taking in so many harmful substances each time we eat, there is another side to the story. Most of our natural foods also contain these same harmful chemicals as a natural part of their makeup. For example, cranberry juice naturally contains sodium benzoate, a chemical preservative added to many foods. Nitrates and nitrites, the additives that help preserve cured meats, occur naturally in many green, leafy vegetables.

Summary of Vitamins & Minerals

Essential Nutrients	Function in the Body	Good Food Sources	Comments
Vitamin A	Important for skeletal growth and normal tooth structure; necessary for health mucous membranes in mouth, nose, throat, digestive and urinary tracts; and essential for night vision.	Fish-liver oils, liver, butter, cream, milk, cheese, egg yolk, dark green and yellow vegetables, yellow fruits, and fortified margarine.	Fat soluble; destroyed by oxidation and very high temperatures.
Vitamin B_1 (Thiamine)	Necessary to help convert sugar and starches into energy.	Pork, liver, heart, kidney, milk, yeast, whole-grain and enriched cereals and breads, soybeans, legumes, peanuts, and wheat germ.	Quickly destroyed by heat in neutral or alkaline solutions.
Vitamin B_2 (Riboflavin)	Essential link in the body's use of protein, carbohydrates, and fats for energy.	Milk, powdered whey, liver, kidney, heart, meats, eggs, green leafy vegetables, dried yeast.	Decomposes quickly in light or in alkaline solutions.
Vitamin B_6 (Pyridoxine, pyridoxal, pyridoxamine)	Important for the body's use of protein, carbohydrates, and fat; aids in formation of hemoglobin.	Wheat germ, meat, liver, kidney, whole-grain cereals, soybeans, peanuts, corn; some in milk and green vegetables.	Water soluble; destroyed by ultra-violet light and heat.
Vitamin B_{12} (Cobalamin)	Essential for forming red blood cells; helps in forming all cells in body and in functioning of nervous system.	Milk, eggs, cheese, liver, kidney, muscle meats contain small amounts needed for normal body functioning.	Inactivated by air or light; water soluble.
Folic acid	Needed for use of protein in body and for regeneration of blood cells.	Green leafy vegetables, liver, kidney, yeast, and — in lesser quantities — many foods.	Easily inactivated in sunlight and acid solutions.

Summary of Vitamins & Minerals (continued)

Essential Nutrients	Function in the Body	Good Food Sources	Comments
Pantothenic acid	Necessary for the body's use of carbohydrates, fats, and protein in conjunction with other substances.	Almost universally present in plant and animal tissue. Loss of fifty percent in milling of flour; thirty-three percent lost in cooking meat.	Water soluble; destroyed easily by dry heat and alkaline.
Niacin	Active in normal functioning of tissues, particularly of the skin, gastrointestinal tract, and nervous system; with other vitamins, used in converting carbohydrates to energy.	Lean meat, liver, kidney, whole-grain and enriched cereals and breads, green vegetables, peanuts, yeast.	Water soluble; stable to heat, air, light.
Biotin	Essential for the functioning of many body systems and use of food for energy.	Liver, kidney, molasses, milk, yeast, egg yolk, and green vegetables.	Water soluble; quite stable in heat, air, and light.
Vitamin C (Ascorbic acid)	Essential for the formation of collagen, a protein which supports the body structures; needed for the absorption of iron, some proteins, and folic acid.	Citrus fruits, strawberries, cantaloupe, tomatoes, cabbage, potatoes, green peppers, and broccoli.	Water soluble; destroyed by heat, air, and light, as well as by aging, drying, and copper contact.
Vitamin D	Promotes normal bone and tooth development; necessary for absorption and stabilization of calcium and phosphorus.	Fish-liver oils, fortified milk, exposure to sunlight; very small amounts in butter, liver, and egg yolks.	Fat soluble: stable to heat and air.
Vitamin E (Tocopherol)	Protects the body's store of vitamin A and the tissue fat from destructive oxidation; also prevents breakdown of red blood corpuscles.	Oils of wheat germ, cottonseed, and the germs of other seeds; green leafy vegetables, nuts, and legumes.	Fat soluble: breaks down in presence of lead and iron salts, alkalies, and ultraviolet light.

Summary of Vitamins & Minerals (continued)

Essential Nutrients	Function in the Body	Good Food Sources	Comments
Vitamin K	Essential for blood clotting.	Green leafy vegetables such as alfalfa, spinach, cabbage; liver.	Fat soluble: unstable to light.
Minerals: Calcium	Builds bones and teeth; aids in proper functioning of muscles, heart, and nerves; helps in blood coagulation.	Milk, hard cheese, and in kale, mustard, turnip, and collard greens. Also some in oysters, shrimp, salmon, clams, and in other dairy products.	Calcium is the most abundant mineral in the body.
Iron	One of the constituents of hemoglobin, which carries oxygen to the tissues by blood circulation. Iron is present in all body cells.	All kinds of liver are the best source of iron; also, meat, egg yolk, legumes, molasses, dark green leafy vegetables, peaches, prunes, apricots, raisins, and food made with enriched flour or cereal.	Iron deficiency is most common in growing children, adolescent girls, and pregnant or nursing women.
Phosphorus	Builds bones and teeth (with other minerals): important in a number of body systems involving fats, carbohydrates, salts, and enzymes.	Milk, cheese, egg yolk, meat, fish, fowl, legumes, nuts, whole-grain cereals.	Some forms of phosphorus are not utilized if the vitamin D level is inadequate in the diet.
Iodine	Required to regulate the exchange of food for energy.	Iodized salt best protection: also, salt water fish.	The need for iodine is increased in adolescence and during pregnancy.
Potassium	Needed to maintain fluid balance within the cell; regulates muscular and nervous irritability; necessary for regular heart rhythm.	Meat, fish, fowl, cereals, fruits, vegetables.	Deficiency in diet is uncommon, but may occur in connection with some diseases.

Summary of Vitamins & Minerals (continued)

Essential Nutrients	Function in the Body	Good Food Sources	Comments
Sodium	Protects body against excessive fluid loss, regulates muscle and nerve irritability, and maintains water balance.	Table salt, meat, fish, fowl, milk, eggs, and sodium compounds.	Excessive salt intake dangerous for persons subject to hypertension and kidney disorders.
Fluorine	In small quantities, protects the teeth against cavities. In larger quantities, fluorine causes mottling of the teeth.	Milk, eggs, and fish; many communities add low concentrations of fluorine to drinking water.	Prolonged high intake of fluorine may cause skeletal abnormalities.

Other minerals which are considered essential for good health are: chlorine, sulfur, magnesium, manganese, copper, zinc, cobalt, and molybdenum. In most cases, diet provides adequate intake.

Notes

1. Basics for this section adapted from Consumer and Food Economics Institute, *Nutrition: Food At Work for You* (Washington, D.C.: U.S. Department of Agriculture, 1978), revised edition, pp. 6-13.
2. Joy Gross, "Carbohydrates," *Family Health*, pp. 26, 34.
3. Edward Bauman, et al., editors, *The Holistic Health Handbook*. Berkeley, California: And/Or Press, 1978, p. 122; J. A. Scharffenberg, "Diet and Heart Disease," *Life and Health*, n.d., n.p. and Lynne Scott, et al., "The Help Your Heart Eating Plan," *Health Values: Achieving High Level Wellness*, November/December, 1978, p. 311.
4. "High-Density Lipoprotein and Heart Disease," *The Harvard Medical School Health Letter — The Medical Forum*, Vol. V, No. 1, November 1979, p. 3; "Understanding Your Cholesterol, Triglycerides and Other Blood Fats," *The Health Letter*, Vol. SV, No. 2, January 25, 1980, p. 2.
5. "Vitamins: Gear Their Intake to Your Special Needs," *Science Digest*, July 1979, p. 82.

6. Adolph Kamil, "How Natural Are Those 'Natural' Vitamins?" *Nutrition Reviews Supplement,* July 1974, p. 34.

7. Margaret Morrison, A Consumer's Guide to Food Labels, *FDA Consumer Reprint.* Washington, D.C.: United States Department of Health, Education, and Welfare, Public Health Service, Food and Drug Association, Office of Public Affairs, DHEW Publication No. (FDA) 77-2083, 1977.

8. Jean P. Darack, "Vitamin Pills You Don't Need Can Kill You," *Consumer's Digest,* July/August 1977, pp. 46-48.

9. "Fast Foods OK With Nutrition Know-How," *Medical Times,* July 1979, pp. 21-22.

10. Ibid.

11. Francis Sheridan Goulart, "The Fast Food Fantasy," *Consumer's Digest,* May/June XXXX, p. 17.

12. Information taken from Phyllis Lehmann, "More Than You Ever Thought You Would Know About Food Additives," a three-part series appearing in *FDA Consumer,* April 1979, pp. 10-12; May 1979, pp. 18-23; and June 1979, pp. 12-19; and United States Department of Health, Education and Welfare, *Some Questions and Answers About Food Additives.* Washington, D.C.: Public Health Service, DHEW Publication No. (FDA) 74-0-2056, 1974.

13. Denis P. Burkitt, "The Link Between Low Fiber Diets and Disease," p. 34.

14. Barbara Harland and Annabel Hecht, "Grandma Called It Roughage," *FDA Consumer,* July/August 1977, pp. 18-19.

15. Jean Mayer, "Scale Down Your Sugar," *Family Health,* April 1974, pp. 74-75.

16. Ibid.

17. Select Committee on Nutrition and Human Needs, U.S. Senate, *Dietary Goals for the United States.* Washington, D.C.: U.S. Government Printing Office, 1977, pp. 43, 45.

18. Excerpted from "Diet and Health," a booklet by the American Dental Association, 1975, pp. 3-4. Copyright by the American Dental Association.

19. Lou Joseph, "Foods and Drinks That Will Cause You the Fewest Cavities," *Today's Health,* October 1973, pp. 41-43.

20. American Medical Association, "Let's Talk About Food," Action, Mass.: Publishing Sciences Group, Inc., 1974.

21. Sidney Margolius, *Health Foods — Facts and Fakes.* New York: Walker and Company, 1973.

22. Chris Lecos, "Fructose: Questionable Diet Aid," *FDA Consumer,* March 1980, p. 21.

23. "Vegetarianism: Can You Get By Without Meat?" *Consumer Reports,* June 1980, p. 357.

24. Bauman, et al., p. 121.

25. Robert J. Benowicz, Vitamins and You. New York: Grosset & Dunlap, Inc., 1979, p. 18.

26. Benowicz, p. 20.

27. Elise Kay Lindvig, *Nutrition and Mental Health.* Moscow, Idaho: The University Press of Idaho, 1979, p. 3.

Self-Evaluation
WEEKLY DIETARY INDEX

Scoring the Diet Index

This instrument has not been validated, nor has its reliability been established. Its purpose is only to give a numerical value to your diet to serve as an index to how well you are eating.

Each item has a scale attached to it. Answer the question as honestly as you can and circle the numerical value associated with the answer. For example, if citrus fruits are consumed 5 to 6 times a week, the numerical value is three; if 7 or more times a week, the numerical value is four, etc.

Total the points. This score is an approximation of your diet. You should score about forty points; forty-five would be better.

It is not necessary to get a perfect diet every day of the week to score forty or forty-five points. A diet approximately 80 percent of ideal should score forty to forty-five points.

Read over each of the items and circle the points associated with each of the food items as it reflects your eating habits.

How many times a week do you have the following for breakfast?

Citrus fruits (fresh or juices)	times/wk	(7+)	(5-6)	(3-4)	(1-2)	(0)
	points	4	3	2	1	0
Whole grain cereals, hot or cold	times/wk	(7)	(5-6)	(3-4)	(1-2)	(0)
	points	4	3	2	1	0
Eggs, plain or with sausage, bacon, or ham (each egg counts as one time)	times/wk	(7+)	(5-6)	(3-4)	(1-2)	(0)
	points	0	2	3	2	1
Pancakes or waffles	times/wk	(7)	(5-6)	(3-4)	(1-2)	(0)
	points	0	0	1	2	1
Milk (2%, whole, skimmed, or yoghurt)	times/wk	(11-13)	(8-10)	(5-7)	(2-4)	(0)
	points	4	3	2	1	0

How many times a week do you have any of the following for your lunches and dinners?

Red meats (beef, pork, lamb) and organ meats (liver, kidney, heart)		(7+)	(5-6)	(3-4)	(1-2)	(0)
	times/wk	(7+)	(5-6)	(3-4)	(1-2)	(0)
	points	1	2	3	1	0

Poultry (chicken or turkey)		(7+)	(5-6)	(3-4)	(1-2)	(0)
	times/wk	(7+)	(5-6)	(3-4)	(1-2)	(0)
	points	2	3	3	1	0

Fish		(7+)	(5-6)	(3-4)	(1-2)	(0)
	times/wk	(7+)	(5-6)	(3-4)	(1-2)	(0)
	points	2	3	3	1	0

How many times a week do you eat:

White bread or rolls		(7+)	(5-6)	(3-4)	(1-2)	(0)
	times/wk	(7+)	(5-6)	(3-4)	(1-2)	(0)
	points	2	3	2	1	0

Whole wheat breads		(7+)	(5-6)	(3-4)	(1-2)	(0)
	times/wk	(7+)	(5-6)	(3-4)	(1-2)	(0)
	points	4	3	2	1	0

Vegetables of all types		(7+)	(5-6)	(3-4)	(1-2)	(0)
	times/wk	(7+)	(5-6)	(3-4)	(1-2)	(0)
	points	4	3	2	1	0

Cheese		(7+)	(5-6)	(3-4)	(1-2)	(0)
	times/wk	(7+)	(5-6)	(3-4)	(1-2)	(0)
	points	1	2	3	2	0

Fruits		(7+)	(5-6)	(3-4)	(1-2)	(0)
	times/wk	(7+)	(5-6)	(3-4)	(1-2)	(0)
	points	4	3	2	1	0

Legumes		(7+)	(5-6)	(3-4)	(1-2)	(0)
	times/wk	(7+)	(5-6)	(3-4)	(1-2)	(0)
	points	4	3	2	1	0

Nuts		(7+)	(5-6)	(3-4)	(1-2)	(0)
	times/wk	(7+)	(5-6)	(3-4)	(1-2)	(0)
	points	4	3	2	1	0

Margarine		(7+)	(5-6)	(3-4)	(1-2)	(0)
	times/wk	(7+)	(5-6)	(3-4)	(1-2)	(0)
	points	1	2	3	2	1

		(7+)	(5-6)	(3-4)	(1-2)	(0)
Butter	times/wk	(7+)	(5-6)	(3-4)	(1-2)	(0)
	points	-1	0	2	2	0
Vegetable Oils, Salad Dressings	times/wk	(7+)	(5-6)	(3-4)	(1-2)	(0)
	points	2	3	2	1	0
Cookies	times/wk	(7+)	(5-6)	(3-4)	(1-2)	(0)
	points	0	1	2	2	2
Snacks — potato or corn chips, pretzels	times/wk	(7+)	(5-6)	(3-4)	(1-2)	(0)
	points	0	1	2	2	2

Do you add salt to your food?		(every meal)	(once a day)	(no)
	points	-1	0	1

Do you take vitamin supplements?

Vitamin C		(every day)	(every other day)	(only when sick)	(no)
	points	0	0	0	2
Vitamin A or D		(every day)	(every other day)	(only when sick)	(no)
	points	-2	-1	0	2

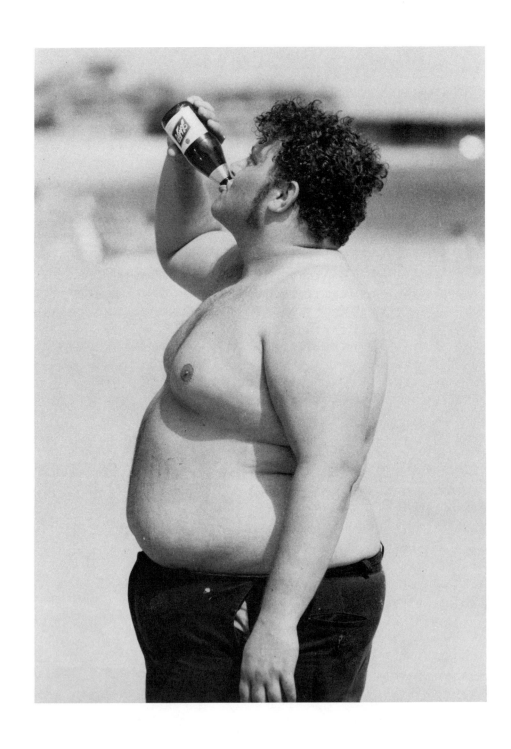

8
Overweight and Obesity: Girth Control

One of the nation's leading health problems, obesity affects more than one-fourth of all American adults. It has been implicated as the leading or contributing cause in a number of diseases and disorders.[1]

The Calorie

If you are overweight, you are probably well acquainted with the word *calorie*. However, many do not understand what a calorie is and how it functions in weight loss and control. A calorie is one unit of energy that is used to measure the "fuel value" contained in food; the body requires a certain amount of this energy (or fuel) to carry on the basic functions of living (such as standing, which uses almost two calories a minute, and

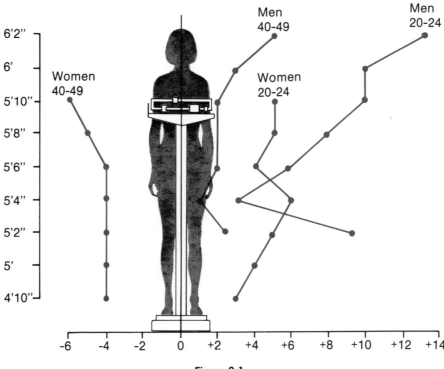

CHANGE IN AVERAGE WEIGHT
OF AMERICANS, 1959-1981

Men 40-49

Men 20-24

Women 40-49

Women 20-24

Figure 8-1.

sleeping, which uses one calorie a minute) and to enable the body to work and exercise. It takes three and one-half calories per minute to shower and the same to dress or undress. Brushing teeth and hair, washing your face and hands, or shaving require about two calories per minute. Even eating itself requires an energy level of one and one-half calories a minute.

As long as the caloric intake remains equal to the body's energy needs, current weight will be maintained. If too little fuel is taken in — as happens when you cut calories on a reducing diet — the body turns to its stored fat, breaks down fat tissue, and reclaims the energy that it stored there. The result is lost weight and tissue. When you take in more calories than your body's energy requires — as happens when you eat too much or exercise too little — the body stores the excess energy in the tissues in the form of fat. The result is extra tissue and added weight.

286

It takes 3,500 calories to form one pound of fat. It is an insidious process: eating only 100 excess calories daily — the equivalent of one banana or one glazed doughnut — can make you gain ten pounds of fat in one year and more than fifty pounds of fat in just five years!

Causes of Obesity

Obesity is clearly a multifaceted problem involving physiological, psychological, and cultural factors, all of which are extremely resistant to current therapeutic efforts. "Obesity" is the precise term to use in referring to gain of excess fat tissue. "Overweight" is a more general term referring to increased weight gain in all body tissues and compartments. The obese person is overweight, but the overweight person is not necessarily obese, and being overweight is not always undesirable.

Obesity may occur in two ways: *existing adipocytes (fat cells) may enlarge or "hypertrophy"*; or the number of fat cells may increase in a process called "hyperplasia." All obese individuals experience hypertrophy, but not all

BEST WEIGHT (in indoor clothing)

Men

Height	Age 20-29	Age 30-39	Age 40-49	Age 50-59	Age 60-69
5'3"	125 lbs.	129 lbs.	130 lbs.	131 lbs.	130 lbs.
5'6"	135 lbs.	140 lbs.	142 lbs.	143 lbs.	142 lbs.
5'9"	149 lbs.	153 lbs.	155 lbs.	156 lbs.	155 lbs.
6'0"	161 lbs.	166 lbs.	167 lbs.	168 lbs.	167 lbs.
6'3"	176 lbs.	181 lbs.	183 lbs.	184 lbs.	180 lbs.

Women

Height	Age 20-29	Age 30-39	Age 40-49	Age 50-59	Age 60-69
4'10"	97 lbs.	102 lbs.	106 lbs.	109 lbs.	111 lbs.
5'1"	106 lbs.	109 lbs.	114 lbs.	118 lbs.	120 lbs.
5'4"	114 lbs.	118 lbs.	122 lbs.	127 lbs.	129 lbs.
5'7"	123 lbs.	127 lbs.	132 lbs.	137 lbs.	140 lbs.
5'10"	134 lbs.	138 lbs.	142 lbs.	146 lbs.	147 lbs.

Source: Pacific Mututal Life Insurance Company
Reprinted from *Medical Times*, Vol. 107, No. 7, p. 76.

have abnormal amounts of fat cells. Hyperplastic obesity is also called "juvenile-onset" because development of extra adipocytes occurs during early or late childhood.

The earlier a child becomes obese, the less likely the child is to lose weight. Overfeeding of infants and children by forcing them to finish the bottle or using food as a mechanism for reward, punishment, or a soothing balm for physical and emotional aches and pains encourages hyperplasia to develop. Such use of food is carried into adult life where hypertrophy may occur. Once the adipocytes are developed, lipid accumulation occurs more readily than lipid breakdown, promoting a lifetime of obesity with alternating excess food intake and rigid dieting.

The exact mechanism that causes obesity is not known, but obesity most often stems from excess caloric intake combined with inadequate activity. Other contributing factors include metabolic and genetic differences: psychological, social and environmental problems: and sometimes disease. *In pinpointing the cause of all obesity, it is probably more accurate to describe a combination of factors,* since obesity is not one homogeneous entity.

Inactivity

Activity decreases as the mechanization of work and of transportation increases. Mayer describes obesity as a "disease of civilization." Many people today are sedentary enough to store rather than use the calories eaten.[2] It has not yet been determined whether the obese gain so much weight because they do not exercise, or if they do not exercise because they are obese. At any rate, inactivity is definitely a major factor that makes obesity self-perpetuating.

The tendency to be inactive and overweight appears early in life. Fat babies tend to be inactive babies with very moderate appetites, while active babies eat more but are thinner and lighter.[3] Later on in life, "inactivity is indeed the major factor in perpetuating obesity in many, if not most, overweight youngsters." In general, obese children and adolescents tend to avoid activity whenever possible and tend to be less mobile when they do engage in physical activity. Physical inactivity is common among babies and children who are confined to play pens, cribs, or strollers to keep them out of mischief. Young children are camped in front of television sets for hours at a time. Children are driven to and from school. Instead of being allowed to explore their environment and discover and develop their physical capabilities, children are encouraged to remain inactive. Not every child needs to participate in competitive sports, but all children (and adults) should vigorously exercise regularly.[4]

288

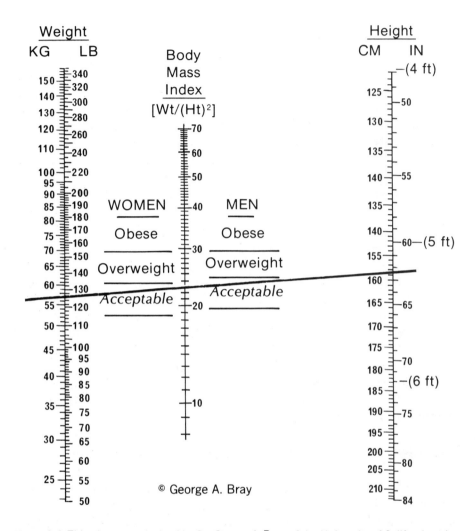

Figure 8-2. This chart was devised by Dr. George A. Bray of the University of California at Los Angeles Medical School. Find your weight in the left column; find your height in the right column. Using a ruler, draw a straight line between the two. The line will intersect the middle column at what is called your "body mass index," and will indicate whether your weight is normal for your height.

Metabolic and Glandular Disorders

Much obesity has been blamed on glandular or endocrine imbalance. Abnormal endocrine function may encourage increased food intake or decreased energy output and in this way contribute to weight gain. However, only about 2 to 5 percent of all obesity results directly from endocrine problems.

One of the most familiar problems is that of thyroid gland malfunction, in which either too much or too little thyroxine is secreted. Too little thyroxine (hypothyroidism) causes the metabolism to slow and fat to accumulate. Too much thyroxine (hyperthyroidism) and the reverse is true.

Effects of Heredity and Genetics

Seventy-five percent of overweight children have at least one overweight parent. Many have thought that this is due to environmental conditioning and that the child learns eating patterns that cause him or her to overeat and become obese. Supporting this theory are studies of identical twins separated at birth. This research showed that the twin reared by overweight parents who pushed food on him usually was overweight, while the identical brother or sister reared by normal weight parents was of normal weight.[5] However, the fact that children adopted at birth do not always show an association with the weight of their foster parents indicates that the genetic component is involved.[6] The implication is that it is possible to counteract genetic tendency to fatness with careful eating habits.

The Newly Emerging Brown Fat Theory of Obesity

Even though the adult-onset and juvenile-onset theories of obesity still tend to be considered the predominant theories of the cause of obesity, a new theory has developed recently that may, through further research, become a revolutionary explanation of some types of obesity. This brown fat theory maintains that body weight may not be directly related to what a person eats. Instead, it is thought that some obesity may result as an inability by the body to burn off excess calories as heat.

The body has a small store of heat-producing fat cells called brown fat (because of their high cytochrome content, which gives them a brownish coloration). "The tissue (brown fat cells) makes up only about 1 percent of a body mass in humans, but when it gets revved up it can produce an amount of heat equal to what the rest of the body can produce."[7] Overfeeding induces thermogenesis (heat production) in brown

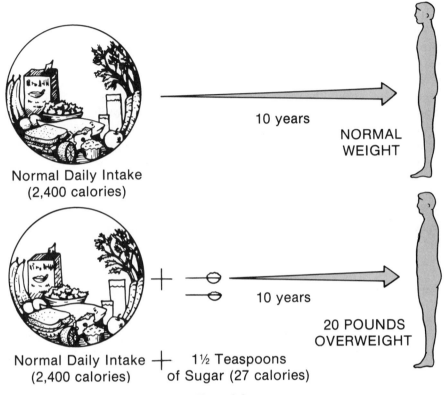

Normal Daily Intake
(2,400 calories)

10 years

NORMAL
WEIGHT

Normal Daily Intake + **1½ Teaspoons**
(2,400 calories) **of Sugar (27 calories)**

10 years

20 POUNDS
OVERWEIGHT

Figure 8-3.

fat, which may burn off excess dietary intake and help to maintain a normal weight. This may explain why food energy intake varies among people of the same body weight, and it also might explain why some people can overeat and stay slim.

Risks of Obesity

Obesity has not been shown to cause disease, but it may predispose and complicate numerous serious health problems, including diabetes, digestive diseases, arthritis, cerebral hemorrhage, difficulty in breathing, angina pectoris, circulatory collapse, varicose veins, hypertension, and dermatologic problems. Obesity lowers sexual drive and is connected with complications of pregnancy and premature aging.

Mortality

According to a Metropolitan Life study of 50,000 people, the death rate of obese men is 79 percent higher than for men of normal weight. It is unlikely that obesity in itself causes death, but it does contribute to other unhealthy conditions that cause death and it highly complicates diseases that should be more successfully managed if the individual were of desirable weight. The fat man is twice as likely to get diabetes and high blood pressure. He is a poor surgical risk; he is far more likely to develop arthritis or heart and kidney ailments; and he is abnormally subject to cancer. Overweight women are less likely to conceive, have a 35 percent chance of more complications in pregnancy, and bear fewer healthy babies. Stout women past the age of forty are also more likely to get gallstones.[8] The statement has been made that to be eleven pounds overweight carries with it a greater health risk than smoking twenty-five cigarettes a day.[9]

Respiration

The process of breathing is more difficult for an obese person because of the added weight on the chest wall. It takes more work to supply oxygen to the blood so that it, in turn, can supply oxygen to the brain and extra tissue. In gross obesity, breathing decreases, resulting in less oxygen taken into the bloodstream. Carbon dioxide builds up, and the person becomes sluggish and lethargic.[10] In overweight people, an increased body volume must be supplied with oxygen by the lungs that have not correspondingly increased in their size.

Arthritis

An obese arthritic is likely to suffer more than a thin one. As joints stiffen, any additional weight or strain naturally increases wear and strain in affected joints. While weight reduction cannot cure arthritis, it can lessen the discomfort.

A vicious cycle is set up in overweight persons with arthritis of the hip, knees, or feet or in those who suffer from a ruptured intervertebral disc. Increased weight leads to greater wear and tear on these joints,

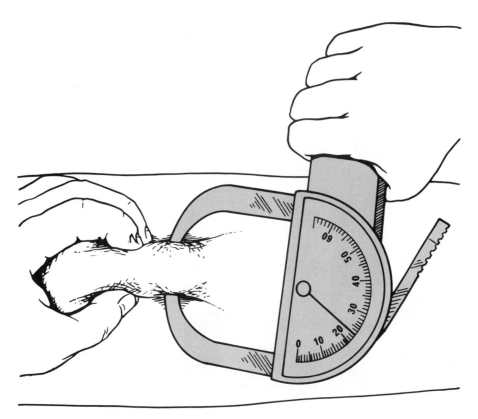

Figure 8-4. Measurement of skin fold thickness by calipers appears to be the simplest and best method for the evaluation of obesity.

which may become more irritated and painful. The increased discomfort forces the person to become less and less active, thereby favoring further weight gain.[11]

High Blood Pressure

High blood pressure (hypertension) is more common among the obese. It is the most potent risk factor for coronary heart disease. Obesity places a hydraulic load on the heart by increasing the amount of tissue that must be supplied with blood.[12] For every pound of fat tissue, three-fourths of a mile of capillaries are required to maintain it; hence, more strain is placed on the heart. Weight loss should lessen this load and result in a decrease in blood pressure. Blood pressure is better correlated with body weight than with body fat.

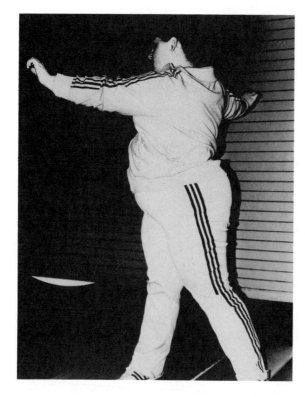

Obesity is easier to prevent than treat.

Coronary Heart Disease

Atherosclerosis is the deposit of fatty material in the lining of the arterial wall. It can result in rupture of the blood vessel or in narrowing of these vessels, which may lead to stroke or heart attack. Studies show that there is a marked increase in the occurrence of atherosclerosis in overweight people.[13]

No predictive value of body fatness for coronary heart disease has been shown. Only angina pectoris and sudden death have been predicted, and these vary with age.[14]

Diabetes, Gall Bladder, and Hernia

Diabetes is more common in overweight individuals than in those of normal weight. Most patients with maturity-onset diabetes are or have been obese. Weight control can not only delay maturity-onset diabetes but is essential in regulating insulin intake and blood sugar levels. In one group of studies, 70 to 85 percent of diabetics had a history of obesity.[15]

The incidence of gall bladder disease is significantly higher in overweight people as compared to those of normal weight. In one study, 88 percent of the 215 patients operated on for gallstones were found to be overweight.[16]

Some types of hernias also seem to be more common in overweight individuals, particularly hernias involving displacement of the stomach into the chest cavity.

Sexual Response

Sexual drives diminish in a grossly overweight individual. Obesity can present aesthetic and purely physical barriers to normal sexual relations. Obese women more frequently develop menstrual irregularity than do their slim counterparts.[17]

Pregnancy and Weight Gain

Overweight can be a factor in producing difficult and prolonged labor due to abnormal positioning of the fetus. This can cause fetal distress, which, in turn, may complicate labor and delivery. These difficulties during pregnancy, labor, and delivery may cause an increased occurrence of maternal and infant deaths.[18]

WEIGHT CONTROL FADS AND FALLACIES

Now, after reading about the harmful effects of obesity, are you considering the possibility of taking off a few pounds? Never fear, the weight reduction industry will gladly step in with pills, diets, and painless plans designed especially for you. People in the United States spend over $100 million a year buying dietetic foods, appetite suppressants, and exercise devices and attending reducing clinics.

CALORIC VALUES FOR COMMON SNACKS

Food	Amount or Average Serving	Calories
"Just a Little Sandwich"		
Hamburger on bun	3-in. patty	330
Peanut butter	1 tbsp. p.b.	330
Cheese	1-oz.	280
Ham	1-oz.	320
Pizza, cheese	⅛ pie	180
Beverages		
Carbonated drinks, soda, root beer, etc.	6-oz. glass	80
Pepsi-Cola	12-oz. glass	150
Club soda	8-oz. glass	5
Chocolate malted milk	10-oz. glass	500
Ginger ale	6-oz. glass	60
Tea or coffee, straight	1 cup	0
Tea or coffee, with 2 tbsp. cream and 2 t. sugar	1 cup	90
Alcoholic Drinks		
Ale	8-oz. glass	155
Beer	8-oz. glass	110
Highball (with ginger ale)	8-oz. glass	185
Manhattan	average	165
Martini	average	140
Wine, muscatel or port	2-oz. glass	95
Sherry	2-oz. glass	75
Scotch, bourbon, rye	1½-oz. jigger	130
Fruits		
Apple	1 medium	70
Banana	1 small	85
Grapes	30 medium	75
Orange	1 medium	70
Pear	1	65
Salted Nutes and Potato Chips		
Almonds, filberts, hazelnuts	12-15	95
Cashews	6-8	90
Peanuts	15-17	85
Pecans, walnuts	10-15 halves	100
Potato chips	1 serving	108
Candies		
Chocolate bars		
Plain, sweet milk	1 bar (1 oz.)	155
With almonds	1 bar (1 oz.)	140

CALORIC VALUES FOR COMMON SNACKS (continued)

Food	Amount or Average Serving	Calories
Candies (continued)		
Chocolate-covered bar	1 bar	270
Chocolate cream, bonbon, fudge	1 piece 1-in. sq.	90-120
Caramels, plain	2 medium	85
Hard candies, Lifesaver type	1 roll	95
Peanut brittle	1 piece 2½ × 2½ × ⅜ in.	110
Desserts		
Pie		
Fruit	1/6 pie	375
Custard	1/6 pie	265
Mince	1/6 pie	400
Pumpkin with whipped cream	1/6 pie	460
Cake		
Chocolate layer	3-in. section	350
Doughnut, sugared	1 average	150
Sweets		
Ice cream		
Plain vanilla	1/6 qt.	200
Chocolate and other flavors	1/6 qt.	260
Orange sherbet	½ cup	120
Sundaes, small chocolate nut with whipped cream	average	400
Ice-cream sodas, chocolate	10-oz. glass	270
Midnight Snacks for Icebox Raiders		
Cold potato	½ medium	65
Chicken leg	1 average	88
Milk	7-oz. glass	140
Roast beef	½ in. × 2 in. × 3 in. piece	130
Cheese	¼ × 2 in. × 3 in. piece	120
Leftover beans	½ cup	105
Brownie	¾ in. × 1¾ in. × 2¼ in.	140
Cream puff	4-in. diam.	450

Source: Adapted from Helen S. Mitchell et al., *Cooper's Nutrition in Health and Disease*, 15th ed. (Philadelphia: J. B. Lippincott Co., 1968), pp. 232-83. Data provided by Smith, Kline and French Laboratories.

Many people do need to slim down and really want to reduce. Yet, despite the money and time invested in reducing programs and gimmicks, no nationwide decrease in obesity has been reported. Studies on the long-range effects of dieting show that within a year, about 90 percent of individuals who lose weight gain it back. By ignoring the fundamental rules of weight reduction, they are doing little more than slenderizing their pocketbooks.

It is simply foolish for anyone who has spent years building up a storage of fat to believe that he or she can safely get rid of those stores overnight. The best way for the public to avoid being taken in by inaccurate or fraudulent claims is to have accurate information concerning the nature and causes of obesity: know the role of diet, drugs, exercise, and psychological factors in weight control management; know the difference between "fad" programs and sound diet management; and know how to recognize legitimate sources of information concerning weight loss.

Popular Commercial Diets

There is a constant parade of "miracle diets" and "reducing formulas" worded to appeal to fat people from every walk of life. Testimonials such as "I thank you for my new body" or "my husband asked me for a date" play upon emotions rather than appeal to intelligence.

For long-term weight control, commerical diets and fad reducing plans are ineffective and may be physically harmful. Nearly all diets, balanced or unbalanced, will produce initial weight loss if the total number calories consumed in twenty-four hours is less than the individual's caloric requirement for maintaining weight. But there is more to proper dieting than just losing weight. A sensible diet should use common foods and provide for proper nutrition to maintain health. It must involve permanent changes in eating habits to be safe and effective.

When choosing a diet, consider the safety factors involved. Adherence to a faulty diet can upset a person's nutritional equilibrium and produce malnutrition. Concentration on one or two nutrients to the exclusion of others can upset body metabolism. Inadequate levels of carbohydrates and essential amino acids, for example, can result in fatigue and depression, which, in turn, helps the dieter return to old habits of overeating. A crash diet program may cause high blood pressure, psychiatric disorders, and depression, especially in persons with previous mental illness.[19]

298

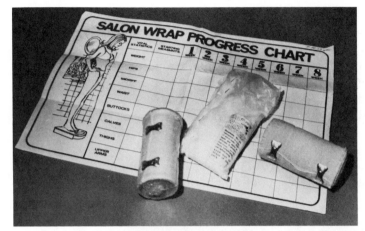

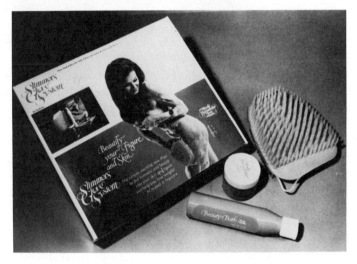

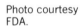

Prescription Reducing Drugs

In a medication-oriented society, drug abuse is common in all health areas. Obesity therapy is no exception. Everyone seems to be searching for a magic pill that will make up for lack of self-control to lose weight. Anorectics used to suppress appetite and aid in weight loss are not as effective as advertised and are potentially dangerous to health. Anorectics should be used only under the direction of a physician on a short-term basis as adjunctive aids in obesity treatments where diet control is the prime factor. Most such drugs contain amphetamines, a psychoactive, habit-forming drug that can cause psychotic behavior, drug dependence, and withdrawal if sufficiently abused.

The amphetamines are the most important group of appetite suppressant drugs from a commercial standpoint. Because of the potent effects of such stimulants, the majority are classified under the Drug Abuse Prevention and Control Act. A panel of medical consultants advised the FDA that the value of amphetamine-related diet drugs was "clinically trivial" and that, in view of their potential for misuse, such drugs should be brought under tighter controls.[20]

NONPRESCRIPTION DIET PRODUCTS ━━━━━━━━

Beginning with the Metrecal 900-calorie formula, diet foods have become standard items in supermarkets. They include ready-to-use liquids in cans and powder envelopes to be mixed with milk, and cookies, wafers, and soups.

Diet formulas are convenient and easy to prepare, and nearly everyone who restricts caloric intake to 900 calories daily can expect to lose weight, even without exercise. For many, it is easier to use a formula diet than to juggle regular foods to prepare a balanced diet low in calories. However, few persons can stay on such a drastic and monotonous diet for more than a few weeks, and thus, these diets fail to provide long-term maintenance of reduced weight.

Diet formulas may induce gastrointestinal side effects (gas, diarrhea, or constipation) and, rarely, emotional disturbances. Synthetic diets also run the risk, especially when used as sole nourishment for long periods, of inadvertently omitting essential nutrients usually supplied in regular meals.

Some mislabeling is found in formula diet products, but for the most part, the products are what they purport to be. The biggest problem is that many dieters do not understand the correct use of such products and so do not use them safely. The FDA now requires diet food labels to contain this statement: "Weight control by diet requires limiting total intake of calories." The purpose of this statement is to remind consumers that the product is useful for weight control only when considered with the total diet.

In addition to diet formulas, over-the-counter diet pills and capsules and candies have become popular. Before-meal candies, bulk producers, medications with phenylpropanolamine and benzocaine, and diuretic compounds have flooded the market. These diet aids, however, should be used with caution. They should not be used over an extended period of time, and use should be discontinued if any side effects or unusual conditions arise.

It should also be noted that such diet preparations may not be entirely effective in helping you achieve the weight loss that you desire. These products do not provide a magic nor painless means of losing weight, because they do not cause permanent change in life-style or diet.

Recognizing Good and Fad Diets

Despite the abundance of fad reducing regimens, you can locate a sound diet and exercise program if you are willing to spend a little time and effort. Consider the following characteristics of reduction programs when evaluating a new diet or exercise gadget:

Earmarks of a Sound Diet

1. Based on a negative caloric balance.
2. Is a long-term program. Once ideal weight is achieved, the diet can be adjusted slightly to maintain the weight for life.
3. Limits calories but maintains balance of daily nutrient requirements.
4. Based on slow, regular weight loss.
5. Emphasizes self-control. There is no guaranteed success.
6. Includes an exercise program.
7. Is an emphasis of proper eating habits with food that you normally eat.
8. Provides for social, cultural, and psychological needs relating to overeating.
9. Is adjusted to the individual's percent of body fat and metabolism.

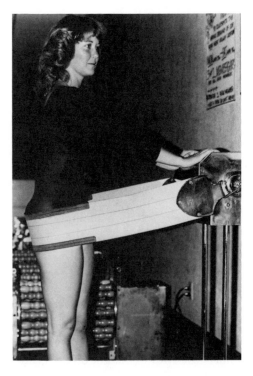

A common type of quackery involves programs and gadgets for spot reducing.

Earmarks of a Fad or Fraudulent Diet

1. Claims that calories do not count.
2. Promises quick, easy weight loss but does not provide a permanent program for maintenance of ideal weight.
3. Alters proportions or omits certain nutrients. Claims that some foods are naturally more fattening than others.
4. Guarantees sudden weight loss or spot reduction.
5. Promises weight control without effort.
6. Recommends diet or exercise but not both.
7. Recommends drastic change in the types of foods that you are used to eating.
8. Ignores emotional and psychological factors involved in overeating.
9. Promises cures for disease through diet.
10. Carries spectacular advertising appealing to the emotions.
11. Guarantees success for everyone.

ANOREXIA NERVOSA

Most normal dieters plan to reduce to a selected normal weight and maintain the weight loss. As the dieter loses weight, the usual battles with willpower and perhaps lethargy or apathy are experienced if a large amount of weight is lost. However, weight loss is usually accompanied by increased sociability and happiness as the dieter nears his or her goal.

There is a rare and severe psychological illness called anorexia nervosa, a condition that begins with food aversion in the initial stages of dieting but continues to the point of starvation. Anorexics try to lose weight to a level way below normal. In addition to starving themselves, they take enormous amounts of laxatives or diuretics or go on eating binges and then self-induced vomiting. Some individuals exist on a 200-calorie-per-day regimen and claim that they are not hungry. In the advanced stages of the disease, severe emaciation, isolation, annoyance, and resentment within the family often develop. When signs of starvation appear, anorexics still look at their skeletonlike bodies in the mirror and believe that they are grossly overweight. They feel as though they are reaching an aesthetic ideal by losing more and more weight. These distorted thoughts and compulsions are purely delusional. About 10 percent of anorexics are successful in starving themselves to death.[21]

Many anorexics are young, middle-class females attempting to assert their autonomy to gain identity apart from their parents or close associates. Starving themselves is their declaration of independence. In other young women, the beginnings of anorexia nervosa may be concurrent with the onset of the first menstrual period. To these girls, the onset of menstruation signals adulthood, which elicits a fear of maturity and its new responsibilities. Obesity to them is a problem that is visible and manageable, so an intense effort is directed at control of obesity (even though the girl may not be overweight).[22]

The origin of the disease appears to be cultural and psychological. The need to be accepted, upwardly mobile, and fashionable can bring on anorexia nervosa. There is no organic cause for the disease; however, whenever severe malnutrition exists for any length of time, an enormous range of functional disturbances appear, and secondary physiological damage may complicate the disorder.[23]

Anorexia nervosa is seldom recognized during the early stages, because it so closely resembles regular dieting. Parents should become concerned if a youngster has lost about ten pounds in a month or if a smaller weight loss occurs and other evidence is present:

1. The person is less than twenty-five years of age.
2. There is a distorted attitude toward eating, food, or weight control that overrides hunger and reason. These attitudes might include a denial of pleasure associated with eating, increased pleasure in losing weight, desired body image of thinness, or unusual hoarding or handling of food.
3. The person has begun a bizarre diet (too often looked on as good by parents anxious for the son or daughter to lose weight or considered "typical" behavior for a teenager).
4. Two or more of the following: increased sensation of hunger, increased growth of downy hair over certain areas of the body (typically the face), stoppage of menstruation, periods of overactivity, slowed heart rate (less than sixty beats per minute), vomiting, dryness of skin, subnormal body temperature, slower than normal basal metabolic rate.
5. Deterioration of social relationships (person becomes withdrawn, complains about silly or immature friends, uninterested in going out with boys).
6. No known medical illness that accounts for weight loss or anorexia.
7. Usually no other psychiatric illness.[24]

SENSIBLE PROCEDURES OF WEIGHT CONTROL

The problem with losing weight is that, although many individuals repeatedly succeed in doing it, they invariably put it on again. Their experience resembles that of Mark Twain in giving up smoking, which he found very easy, having done it hundreds of times.[25]

To many people, the idea behind weight loss has nothing to do with permanent, ideal weight control. They plan diets for special occasions, and as soon as they lose the desired poundage, they return to their old eating habits with little thought of the consequences. To some, the inconvenience in spot dieting and seesawing up and down on the weight

How much exercise is needed to burn off a given number of calories.* For example, it would take 19 minutes of walking (at 3.5 mph) or 5 minutes of running to burn off the calories contained in an apple.

Food	Calories	Walking (3.5 mph) 5.2 calories per min.	Bike Riding 8.2 calories per min.	Swimming 11.2 calories per min.	Running 19.4 calories per min.
		Minutes of Activity			
Apple, large	101	19	12	9	5
Bacon, 2 strips	96	18	12	9	5
Banana, small	88	17	11	8	4
Beer, 1 glass	114	22	14	10	6
Bread and butter	78	15	10	7	4
Cake, 2-layer, 1/12	356	68	43	32	18
Carbonated beverage, 1 glass	106	20	13	9	5
Carrot, raw	42	8	5	4	2
Cereal, dry, ½ c. with milk, sugar	200	38	24	18	10
Chicken, fried, ½ breast	232	45	28	21	12
Cookie, plain	15	3	2	1	1
Egg, fried	110	21	13	10	6
Ham, 2 slices	167	32	20	15	9
Ice Cream, 1/6 qt.	193	37	24	17	10
Malted milk shake	502	97	61	45	26
Milk, 1 glass	166	32	20	15	9
Milk, skim, 1 glass	81	16	10	7	4
Orange juice, 1 glass	120	23	15	11	6
Pancake with syrup	124	24	15	11	6
Peach, medium	46	9	6	4	2
Pie, apple, 1/6	377	73	46	34	19
Pizza, cheese, 1/8	180	35	22	16	9
Pork chop, loin	314	60	38	28	16
Club sandwich	590	113	72	53	30
Hamburger sandwich	350	67	43	31	18
Shrimp, French fried	180	35	22	16	9
Spaghetti, 1 serving	396	76	48	35	20
Steak, T-bone	235	45	29	21	12
Strawberry shortcake	400	77	49	36	21

Adapted from F. J. Konishi, *J. Am. Dietetic Assn.* 46:186, 1965. Copyright The American Dietetic Association. Reprinted by permission from *Journal of the American Dietetic Association.*

Calories Burned in Various Physical Activities*

Activity — Work Tasks	Calories per minute	Activity — Recreation	Calories per minute
Carpentry	3.8	Archery	5.2
Chopping wood	7.5	Badminton	5.2-10.0
Cleaning windows	3.7	(recreation-competition)	
Clerical work	1.2-1.6	Baseball (except pitcher)	4.7
Dressing	3.4	Basketball - Half-full court	6.0-9.0
Driving car	2.8	(more for fastbreak)	
Driving motorcycle	3.4	Bowling (while active)	7.0
Farming		Calisthenics	5.0
Chores	3.8	Canoeing (2.5-4.0 mph)	3.0-7.0
Haying, plowing		Cycling (5-15 mph -	5.0-12.0
with horse	6.7	10-speed bicycle)	
Planting, hoeing, raking	4.7	Dancing	
Gardening		Modern: moderate-vigorous	4.2-5.7
Digging	8.6	Ballroom: waltz-rumba	5.7-7.0
Weeding	5.6	Square	7.7
Hiking		Football (while active)	13.3
Road-field (3.5 mph)	5.6-7.0	Golf (foursome-twosome)	3.7-5.0
Snow: hard-soft		Handball and squash	10.0
(3.5-2.5 mph)	10.0-20.0	Horseshoes	3.8
Downhill: 5-10% grade		Judo and karate	13.0
(2.5 mph)	3.5-3.6	Mountain climbing	10.0
Downhill: 15-20% grade		Pool or billiards	1.8
2.5 mph)	3.7-4.3	Rowing (pleasure-vigorous)	5.0-15.0
Uphill: 5-15% grade		Running	
(3.5 mph)	8.0-15.0	12-min mile (5 mph)	10.0
40-lb. pack: (3.0 mph)	5.0	8-min mile (7.5 mph)	15.0
40-lb. pack: 36% slope		6-min mile (10 mph)	20.0
(1.5 mph)	16.0	5-min mile (12 mph)	25.0
House painting	3.5	Skating	5.0-15.0
Ironing clothes	4.2	(recreation-vigorous)	
Making beds	3.4	Skiing	
Metal working	3.5	Moderate to steep	8.0-12.0
Mixing cement	4.7	Downhill racing	16.5
Mopping floors	4.9	Cross-country (3-8 mph)	9.0-17.0
Pick-and-shovel work	6.7	Snowshoeing (2.5 mph)	9.0
Plastering walls	4.1	Soccer	9.0
Pulaski (depends on rate	7.8	Swimming	
of work and other factors)		Pleasure	6.0

*Calories burned depends on efficiency and body size. Add 10 percent for each 15 pounds above 150; subtract 10 percent for each 15 pounds under 150.

Calories Burned in Various Physical Activities (continued)

Activity	Calories per minute	Activity	Calories per minute
Work Tasks		**Recreation**	
Repaving roads	5.0	Swimming (cont.)	
Sawing		Crawl (25-50 yd/min)	6.0-12.5
Chain saw	6.2	Butterfly (50 yd/min)	14.0
Crosscut saw	7.5-10.5	Backstroke	6.0-12.5
Shining shoes	3.2	(25-50 yd/min)	
Shoveling (depends on	5.4-10.5	Breaststroke	6.0-12.5
weight of load, rate of		(25-50 yd/min)	
work, height of lift)		Sidestroke (40 yd/min)	11.0
Forest Service data	8.0	Skipping rope	10.0-15.0
(average)		Table tennis	4.9-7.0
Showering	3.4	Tennis	7.0-11.0
Stacking lumber	5.8	(recreation-competition)	
Standing, light activity	2.6	Volleyball	3.5-8.0
Stone masonry	6.3	(recreation-competition)	
Sweeping floors	3.9	Water skiing	8.0
Tree felling (ax)	8.4-12.7	Wrestling	14.4
Truck and auto repair	4.2		
Walking			
Downstairs	7.1		
Indoors	3.1		
Upstairs	10.0-18.0		
Washing clothes	3.1		
Washing and dressing	2.6		
Washing and shaving	2.6		

scales is preferable to maintaining a sound lifetime diet, or perhaps they lack the self-control to maintain sound eating habits.

The goal of an effective weight loss regimen is not merely to prescribe a diet. Weight control requires a lifelong commitment; an understanding of your eating habits, motivation, and willingness to change them; a clear concept of the weight that you desire and what the rate of weight loss must be to safely obtain the desired weight; a consideration of past weight history, personality, and body type; and a recognition of obesity-related medical conditions. Moderate, frequent exercise is necessary, and accomplishment must be reinforced to sustain motivation. Crash dieting, the use of chemical crutches, and magical formulas are ineffective.

Behavior Modification

Too many people regard a diet as a short-term tool by which to lose weight; they figure that they can exist on cottage cheese and clear broth and green salad for a month or two, because after the torture is over they can once again enjoy pizza and chocolate doughnuts and french fries with their hamburgers.

Diet is not temporary; diet — the kind of diet that allows you to maintain your ideal weight and your optimum health — is a continual pattern of eating habits. Every day, every month, every year you need to eat in a way in which you can maintain healthy weight and fulfill your nutritional needs. It is a permanent, gradual process.

Behavior therapy, or modification, is a new concept in weight control that focuses on helping change habits and life-style on a long-term basis. Behavior control tries to guide people away from the all-or-nothing approach to losing weight. Modifying eating habits is not necessarily a drastic procedure. The focus is not solely on eating, but also on the patient's knowledge, misconceptions, activity, time management, and life stresses. The program stresses control of the hows, whys, and whens of eating.

The theoretical underpinnings of behavior therapy come from the findings of Dr. Albert Stunkard, who claims that overweight and obese people are very susceptible to food cues. "Put a cue — say, a bowl of potato chips — in front of a normal-weight person who's just eaten, and he will ignore them. But put the bowl in front of an obese individual and he will devour them, even if he's just gotten up from a large meal." A decrease in weight alone does not lead to a decrease in susceptibility to cues. "In all our studies, we observed that formerly obese people reacted to cues the same way currently obese individuals did."[26]

Cues that can stimulate desire include pizza shops, baker's windows, everybody else's leftovers, a last piece of cheesecake, watching television, or reading.

Many physicians utilize a behavior assessment evaluation to identify specific behavior patterns and what influences these patterns, and to help the patient recognize and control cues or make them less tempting. Here is an outline of one program:

1. **Keep a Food Intake Sheet.** Keep track of what you eat for two weeks. Your record should be very detailed, including a remark on

where you ate, when, your emotional state while eating, etc.

2. **Try to Pinpoint Your Eating Problems.** Check your eating speed. This may prove vital. Also check places where you ate, how you felt when you ate, and when.

3. **Make Eating a Pure Experience.** Learn to eat just for the joy of eating. Sit in the same place each time that you eat, and just eat. No television, no newspaper, nothing else. Eat more slowly by beginning after others or cutting your food into smaller pieces or putting your fork down after every third bite; for snacking problems, create an alternative set of activities at the time that you usually snack, i.e., walking, hobbies.

4. **Reduce Temptations.** Make a shopping list, and purchase only those items that are on your list. Snacking is much less likely if you have to spend fifteen to twenty minutes preparing the snack.

5. **Enlist Your Family's Support.** Explain your plans to them, and ask for their moral support. Requesting that they have fewer snack foods around would also help.

6. **Cope with Emotions.** Do not eat when you get upset or angry; try jogging instead.

7. **Take It Slowly.** Aim at a gradual weight loss; keep a record, but do not starve yourself.

8. **Get More Exercise.** You are more likely to do this (jogging, calisthenics, etc.) if you have a partner to do it with.

9. **Special Situations.** If you are going to a wedding, party, or church social, eat something substantial before you leave the house so that you will not arrive at the function hungry. To avoid temptation while you are there, dance a lot, engage in conversation. In short, keep yourself busy.[27]

These general rules apply to everyone, but authorities emphasize that habit changes should be individually worked out and applied. For example, some persons can easily eliminate all between-meal snacking, while others cannot.

The constant eater should be advised to satisfy his or her need with a handy, plentiful supply of high-bulk, low-calorie foods (celery, carrots, cucumber sticks, lettuce, raw cauliflower, radishes, green peppers, apples, fruit sticks, etc.). This person will not be very hungry at mealtime and can round out meals with leafy salads to get a filled feeling without eating lots of high-calorie foods.

Caloric Values for Representative Foods, Classified by Food Groups

Food*	Weight or Approximate Measure	Calories
Milk Group		
Cheese, Cheddar	1⅛ in. cube	115
Cheese, cottage, creamed	¼ cup	60
Cream	1 tbsp.	35
Milk, fluid, skim (buttermilk)	1 cup	90
Milk, fluid, whole	1 cup	165
Meat Group		
Beans, dry, canned	¾ cup	250
Beef, pot roast	3 oz.	245
Chicken	¼ small broiler	185
Egg	1 medium	80
Frankfurter	1 medium	155
Haddock	1 fillet	135
Ham, luncheon meat	2 oz.	170
Liver, beef	2 oz.	120
Peanut butter	1 tbsp.	90
Pork chop	1 chop	260
Salmon, canned	½ cup	120
Sausage, salami	1 slice	135
Vegetable Group		
Beans, snap, green	½ cup	15
Broccoli	½ cup	20
Cabbage, shredded, raw	½ cup	10
Carrots, diced	½ cup	20
Corn, canned	½ cup	85
Lettuce leaves	2 large or 4 small	5
Peas, green	½ cup	55
Potato, white	1 medium	90
Spinach	½ cup	20
Squash, winter	½ cup	50
Sweet potato	1 medium	155
Tomato juice, canned	½ cup (small glass)	25
Fruit Group		
Apple, raw	1 medium	70
Apricots, dried, cooked	½ cup	135
Banana, raw	1 small	85
Cantaloupe	½ melon	40
Grapefruit	½ medium	50
Orange	1 medium	70

Orange juice, fresh	½ cup (small glass)	60
Peaches, canned	2 halves with juice	90
Pineapple juice, canned	½ cup (small glass)	60
Prunes, dried, cooked	5 with juice	160
Strawberries, raw	½ cup	30

Bread-Cereal Group

Bread, white, enriched	1 slice	60
Cornflakes, fortified	1⅓ cup	110
Macaroni, enriched, cooked	¾ cup	115
Oatmeal, cooked	⅔ cup	100
Rice, cooked	¾ cup	150

Fats Group

Bacon, crisp	2 strips	95
Butter or fortified margarine	1 tbsp.	100
Oils, salad or cooking	1 tbsp.	125

Sweets Group

Beverages, cola type	6 oz.	80
Sugar, granulated	1 tbsp.	50

*Foods on this list are in forms ready to eat. All meats and vegetables are cooked unless otherwise indicated.

Source: Adapted from Ethel A. Martin, *Nutrition in Action,* 2nd ed. (New York: Holt, Rinehart, and Winston, Inc., 1965), p. 61.

Changing Eating Habits

Many of us overeat because we eat too fast. The feeling of fullness comes on slowly.

1. Eat in slow motion.
2. Sip your beverages, do not gulp.
3. After each mouthful, place your utensils on the plate until you have swallowed that mouthful.
4. Before your main meal, drink a low-calorie drink or a cup of boullion to help to take the edge off your appetite.
5. If invited out, eat a few low-calorie snacks before going.
6. Eat the salad before the rest of the meal.
7. Get in the habit of leaving at least two forkfuls of food on the plate at the end of the meal.

8. Eat foods that take time to eat — such as an orange that has to be peeled instead of an apple.

9. Put scraps of food directly in the garbage.

10. If sweets must be kept around the house, put them in a seldom-used cupboard or in an unlikely place, e.g., broom closet, and let others get their own sweets.

11. When the meal is over, do not linger at the table unless all food has been cleared.

12. Make small portions of food appear larger on the plate by using smaller plates and spreading your food on the plate.

13. Put your own portions on your plate — preferably in the kitchen.

14. Resist the temptation to eat what others have left when you are cleaning up after a meal.

15. If you envy a food that someone else is eating, take one small bit of it to satisfy yourself.

16. Reduce or eliminate use of salt at the table.

Changing Shopping Habits

You can also modify your shopping habits to help yourself lose weight.

1. Shop only from a prepared list, and stick to it.

2. Do not buy foods that later may be a problem to resist.

3. Shop after eating, or at least when you are not hungry.

4. Resist the free snacks offered at supermarkets.

5. Buy tuna fish that has been packed in water instead of oil.

6. Buy fruit that is fresh or canned without sugar.

7. Choose canned or frozen vegetables that are plain instead of those containing rich sauces; avoid using the frozen-in-butter vegetables that come in plastic pouches.

8. Do not trust a product's claim of being low-calorie. Compare the ingredients to those in the regular product — often there is only a minor difference!

Changing Cooking Habits

The way in which you prepare and serve food can also be modified to make your dieting easier.

312

1. Trim all fat from meat before cooking.
2. Broil meat that you normally would fry, even as a first step to stews and other dishes.
3. Broil, boil, or roast meat without added sauces, flour, or fat.
4. Marinate or baste poultry or meats using a bottled, low-calorie dressing. This also eliminates the need to use fat.
5. When broiling or baking fish, use lemon juice or boullion instead of butter.
6. Use lean meat in all recipes. When you buy ground beef, specify lean round or sirloin; these cuts are usually just as economical because they have no excess fat and so do not "shrink" when cooked.
7. Before cooking chicken, remove the skin and any loose fat.
8. Cook vegetables in a small amount of water with herbs or in boullion instead of with butter.
9. Use whipped butter or whipped margarine for spreads. The air or water that they contain reduces the fat content and cuts their calories almost in half.
10. Learn which are the low- or no-calorie foods, and serve them often in meals and for snacks. Some are green beans, green peppers, leeks, celery, cauliflower, carrots, water cress, zucchini, lettuce, and cucumbers.
11. Experiment with seasonings. Here are a few ideas: mint on carrots, basil on tomatoes, parsley or chives on boiled potatoes, Italian seasoning on green beans. Juicy lemon wedges, herb vinegar, pickle relish, soy and Worcestershire sauces, and seasoned salt all add zip while adding few, if any, calories.
12. Go all out on garnishes, for they brighten any plate, taste good, and cost little in calories.[28]

Eating Out at Restaurants

Eating out can cause problems if you do not plan ahead and consider alternatives. If you know that you are going to eat out, trim calories in the other two meals of the day. Try not to eat less — just eat foods that are less fattening. Half an hour before going to the restaurant, enjoy a tall glass of mineral water or water; it will help dull the appetite.

Look for low-calorie items on the menu. Salads, fresh fruit, fresh vegetables, and broiled or grilled foods are generally good choices. If you are extremely hungry, order a low-calorie appetizer to take the edge off your appetite. Read menus carefully, and do not be afraid to ask the waiter questions. Avoid foods that have breading, sauces, or gravies. Ask that salad dressing be served on the side, or ask for lemon or vinegar instead of salad dressing.

If they are available, order smaller portions — a luncheon steak instead of a dinner steak, for instance. If you are at a cafeteria or a buffet where you serve yourself, select a smaller plate — perhaps a salad plate — so that you cannot take as much food.

Do not take seconds. Make it an ironclad rule at your house, and learn to say no to others. Avoid fast-food restaurants, snack trays at parties, and desserts — unless you can get fresh fruit in its own juice.

Dieting for weight control cannot be effective unless an active exercise program is adopted. The first step is to make the decision to develop such a program.

The following tips may help you begin and continue that exercise program that will help in weight control:

1. Accept the importance of physical activity in spite of whatever else you have to do. If you really want to do it, you will find the time.
2. Schedule a time for physical activity in spite of all else you do. Make it a high priority in your life, and be consistent.
3. Find activities that you enjoy doing. You will be more likely to continue exercising.
4. "Don't lie down when you can sit down. Don't sit when you can stand. Don't stand when you can move."[30]
5. Set specific long-term goals in your exercise program in the areas of intensity, duration, and frequency.
6. Use variety in your exercise program. It will make exercise more interesting and enjoyable.
7. Encourage others to participate in exercise with you.
8. Choose exercises befitting your age, health condition, and body type.
9. Choose activities that can be done year round.
10. Activities that are rhythmic, repetitive, and challenging offer the best rewards in terms of weight loss.
11. Don't ever begin a "crash" exercise progam. Gradual increases in exercise are best and most healthful.
12. Change your attitude toward exercise. Exercise can be fun — don't be too sober about it.

314

Sample of How Calorie Intake Can Be Reduced through Sensible Substitution

For This		Substitute This	
Breakfast			
From	Calories	To	Calories
½ glass (4 oz.) orange juice	50	½ glass (4 oz.) orange juice	50
1 scrambled egg	120	1 boiled egg	78
2 slices bacon	100	1 slice bacon	50
2 slices white bread	126	2 slices gluten bread (white) 35 calories per slice	70
2 pats butter	100	Low-calorie margarine, 17 calories per pat	34
2 cups coffee, each with sugar (2 lumps) and cream (2 tbsp)	220	2 cups coffee with no-calorie sweetener and nondairy cream, 11 calories per tbsp.	22
Total Calories	716	Total Calories	304
Midmorning Snack			
From	Calories	To	Calories
1 cup coffee with sugar (2 lumps) and cream (2 tbsp.)	110	1 cup coffee with no-calorie sweetener and nondairy cream	11
1 small Danish pastry	140	2 low-calorie cookies, 25 calories per cookie	50
Total Calories	250	Total Calories	61
Lunch			
From	Calories	To	Calories
Hamburger	350	Hamburger	350
1 slice apple pie	338	Low-calorie pudding	123
1 glass (8 oz.) whole milk	165	1 glass (8 oz.) skim milk	80
Total Calories	853	Total Calories	553
Midafternoon Snack			
From	Calories	To	Calories
1 bottle cola beverage	105	Low-calorie cola	
1 custard (4 oz. cup)	205	2 low-calorie cookies	52
Total Calories	310	Total Calories	52
Dinner			
From	Calories	To	Calories
½ glass (4 oz.) tomato juice	25	Consomme, 1 cup	10
6 oz. meat loaf	680	6 oz. club steak, broiled, lean	320
with 4 tbsp. gravy (41 calories per tbsp.)	164		
½ cup mashed potatoes	123	1 medium potato, baked	100

(continued)

*Reprinted with permission from Riker Laboratories.

Sample of How Calorie Intake Can Be Reduced through Sensible Substitution (continued)

For This		Substitute This	
Dinner (continued)			
½ cup green peas	72	12 spears asparagus	40
2 slices French bread	160	2 pats low-calorie margine	34
with 2 pats butter	100		
Tossed Salad	20	Hearts of lettuce	20
with 1½ tbsp. Roquefort cheese		with low-calorie salad dressing	15
dressing (100 calories per tbsp.)	150		
Iced plain layer cake	290	1 cup low-calorie whipped dessert	123
1 cup coffee with sugar (2		1 cup coffee with no-calorie	
lumps) and cream (2 tbsp.)	110	sweetener and nondairy cream	11
Total Calories	1894	Total Calories	673
Total Calories for Day	4023	Total Calories for Day	1643
		A Saving of 2380 Calories	

Beverages	Calories		Calories	Calories Saved
Milk (whole), 8 oz.	165	Milk (buttermilk, skim) 8 oz.	80	85
Prune juice, 8 oz.	170	Tomato juice, 8 oz.	50	120
Soft drinks, 8 oz.	105	Diet soft drinks, 8 oz.	1	104
Coffee (with cream and		Coffee (black with		
2 tsp. sugar)	110	artificial sweetener)	0	110
Cocoa (all milk), 8 oz.	235	Cocoa (milk and		
		water), 8 oz.	140	95
Chocolate malted milk		Lemonade (sweetened),		
shake, 8 oz.	500	8 oz.	100	400
Beer (1 bottle), 12 oz.	175	Liquor (1½ oz.), with soda		
		or water, 8 oz.	120	55
Breakfast Foods				
Rice flakes, 1 cup	110	Puffed rice, 1 cup	50	60
Eggs (scrambled), 2	220	Eggs (boiled, poached), 2	160	60
Butter and Cheese				
Butter on toast	170	Apple butter on toast	90	80
Cheese (Blue, Cheddar,		Cheese (cottage,		
Cream, Swiss), 1 oz.	105	uncreamed), 1 oz.	25	80
Desserts				
Angel food cake, 2″ piece	110	Cantaloupe melon, ½	40	70
Cheesecake, 2″ piece	200	Watermelon, ½″ slice		
		(10″ diam.)	60	140
Chocolate cake with icing,		Sponge cake, 2″ piece	120	305
2″ piece	425			
Fruit cake, 2″ piece	115	Grapes, 1 cup	65	50

(continued)

Sample of How Calorie Intake Can Be Reduced through Sensible Substitution (continued)

For This		Substitute This		
Pound cake, 1-oz. piece	140	Plums, 2	50	90
Cupcake, white icing, 1	230	Plain cupcake, 1	115	115
Cookies, assorted		Vanilla wafer (dietetic), 1	25	95
(3" diam.), 1	120			
Ice cream, 4 oz.	150	Yoghurt (flavored), 4 oz.	60	90
Pie				
Apple, 1 piece (1/7 of		Tangerine (fresh), 1	40	305
a 9" pie)	345			
Blueberry, 1 piece	290	Blueberries (frozen,		
		unsweetened), ½ cup	45	245
Cherry, 1 piece	355	Cherries (whole), ½ cup	40	315
Custard, 1 piece	280	Banana, small, 1	85	195
Lemon meringue, 1 piece	305	Lemon-flavored gelatin, ½ cup	70	235
Peach, 1 piece	280	Peach (whole), 1	35	245
Rhubarb, 1 piece	265	Grapefruit, ½	55	210
Pudding (flavored), ½ cup	140	Pudding (dietetic, non-fat		
		milk), ½ cup	60	80
Fish and Fowl				
Tuna (canned), 3 oz.	165	Crabmeat (canned), 3 oz.	80	85
Oysters (fried), 6	400	Oysters (shell w/sauce), 6	100	300
Ocean perch (fried), 4 oz.	260	Bass, 4 oz.	105	155
Fish sticks, 5 sticks or 4 oz.	200	Swordfish, (broiled), 3 oz.	140	60
Lobster meat, 4 oz.		Lobster meat, 4 oz.		
with 2 tbsp. buter	300	with lemon	95	205
Duck (roasted), 3 oz.	310	Chicken (roasted), 3 oz.	160	150
Meats				
Loin roast, 3 oz.	290	Pot roast (round), 3 oz.	160	130
Rump roast, 3 oz.	290	Rib roast 3 oz.	200	90
Swiss steak, 3½ oz.	300	Liver (fried), 2½ oz.	210	90
Hamburger (av fat, broiled)		Hamburger (lean, broiled)		
3 oz.	240	3 oz.	145	95
Porterhouse steak, 3 oz.	250	Club steak, 3 oz.	160	90
Rib lamb chop (med.), 3 oz.	300	Lamb leg roast (lean only)		
		3 oz.	160	140
Pork chop (med.), 3 oz.	340	Veal chop (med.), 3 oz.	185	155
Pork roast, 3 oz.	310	Veal roast, 3 oz.	230	80
Pork sausage, 3 oz.	405	Ham (boiled, lean), 3 oz.	200	205
Potatoes				
Fried, 1 cup	480	Baked (2½" diam.)	100	380
Mashed, 1 cup	245	Boiled (2½" diam.)	100	145

(continued)

Sample of How Calorie Intake Can Be Reduced through Sensible Substitution (continued)

For This		Substitute This		
Salads				
Chef salad with oil dressing, 1 tbsp.	180	Chef salad with dietetic dressing, 1 tbsp.	40	120
Chef salad with mayonnaise, 1 tbsp.	125	Chef salad with dietetic dressing, 1 tbsp.	40	85
Chef salad with Roquefort, Blue, Russian, French dressing, 1 tbsp.	105	Chef salad with dietetic dressing, 1 tbsp.	40	65
Sandwiches				
Club	375	Bacon and tomato (open)	200	175
Peanut butter and jelly	275	Egg salad (open)	165	110
Turkey with gravy, 3 tbsp.	520	Hamburger lean, (open), 3 oz.	200	320
Snacks				
Fudge, 1 oz.	115	Vanilla wafers (dietetic), 2	50	65
Peanuts (salted), 1 oz.	170	Apple, 1	100	70
Peanuts (roasted), 1 cup, shelled	1375	Grapes, 1 cup	65	1305
Potato chips, 10 med.	115	Pretzels, 10 small sticks	35	80
Chocolate, 1 oz. bar	145	Toasted marshmallows, 3	75	70
Soups				
Creamed, 1 cup	210	Chicken noodle, 1 cup	110	100
Bean, 1 cup	190	Beef noodle, 1 cup	110	80
Minestrone, 1 cup	105	Beef bouillon, 1 cup	10	95
Vegetables				
Baked beans, 1 cup	320	Green beans, 1 cup	30	290
Lima beans, 1 cup	160	Asparagus, 1 cup	30	130
Corn (canned), 1 cup	185	Cauliflower, 1 cup	30	155
Peas (canned), 1 cup	145	Peas (fresh), 1 cup	115	30
Winter squash, 1 cup	75	Summer squash, 1 cup	30	45
Succotash, 1 cup	260	Spinach, 1 cup	40	220

Notes

1. Alfred A. Rimm and Philip L. White, "Obesity: Its Risks and Hazards," in *Obesity in America*, George A. Bray, ed., Department of Health, Education, and Welfare, Public

Health Service, National Institutes of Health, November 1979, NIH Publication No. 79-359, pp. 103-24.

2. Hearings before the Select Committee on Nutrition and Human Needs of the U.S. Senate, *Nutrition and Disease* — 1974, Part 4, February 26, 1974, pp. 431-435, as submitted by Dr. George A. Bray.

3. Jean Mayer, "Hidden Bonds," *World Health*, February/March 1974, pp. 21-27.

4. Ruth Huenemann, "Food Habits of Obese and Nonobese Adolescents," *Postgraduate Medicine*, May 1972, pp. 109-112.

5. Thomas J. Coates and Carl C. Thousen, "Treating Obesity in Children and Adolescents, A Review," *American Journal of Public Health*, February 1978, vol. 68, no. 2, p. 145.

6. Mayer, "Hidden Bonds," p. 21-27.

7. John Elliott, "Blame It All on Brown Fat Now," *JAMA*, May 23-30, 1980, p. 1983.

8. Henry A. Jordan, "In Defense of Body Weight," reprint from *Journal of the American Dietetic Association*, January 1973.

9. "Obesity: The 20th Century Disease," *Feel Younger — Live Longer*. New York: Rand-McNally and Company, 1976, p. 52.

10. Neil Soloman, "Health Hazards of Obesity," *Obesity/Bariatric Medicine*, May/June 1972.

11. Sandoz Laboratories, "Overweight Can Hurt More Than Just Your Looks," wall chart, 1974.

12. George Mann, "The Influence of Obesity on Health," *The New England Journal of Medicine*, July 25, 1974.

13. "Overweight Can Hurt More Than Just Your Looks."

14. Mann, "Influence of Obesity."

15. "Overweight Can Hurt."

16. Ibid.

17. Soloman, "Health Hazards of Obesity."

18. Van Itallie and Campbell, "Multidisciplinary Approach to the Problem of Obesity," paper to American Dietetic Association, October 7, 1971.

19. N. Allon, "The Stigma of Overweight in Everyday Life," in *Obesity in Perspective*, George A. Bray, ed. Bethesda, Maryland: National Institutes of Health, DHEW Publication No. (NIH) 75-708, 1975, pp. 84-92.

20. Phillip L. White, "The Dangers in Diet Advice," *Medical Insight*, July/August 1973.

21. "Dieting to Death," *Emergency Medicine*, October 1976, p. 127.

22. William A. Nolen, "Anorexia Nervosa: The Dieting Disease," *McCall's*, June 1977, p. 72.

23. "Dieting to Death," p. 127.

24. Ibid., and Thomas F. Richardson, "Anorexia Nervosa: An Overview," *American Journal of Nursing*, August 1980, p. 1470.

25. Thaddeus S. Danowski, "The Management of Obesity," *Hospital Practice*, April 1976, pp. 39-46.

26. John Kelly, "Who Controls Your Eating Habits," *Family Health*, vol. 5, April 1973, pp. 36-37.

27. Excerpts from "Who Controls Your Eating Habits," by John Kelly, *Family Health Magazine*, April 1973, pp. 36-37.

28. Taken from *Slim Ideas*, a pamphlet by Riker Laboratories.

29. For the complete survey, write to Dr. Richard Kozlenko, Health Evaluation System, 150 Shoreline Highway, Suite 31, Mill Valley, California 94941.

30. Laurence E. Morehouse and Leonard Gross, *Total Fitness in 30 Minutes a Week* (New York: Pocket Books, 1976), p. 185.

Self-Evaluation

Your Emotional Investment in Eating

Hunger, scientists tell us, is physiological: a sensation that occurs when the blood sugar begins to drop and the stomach contracts. But we are all aware that many people eat for unconscious and emotional reasons as well.

Richard Kozlenko, a physician trained in biochemistry who cofounded the Wholistic Health and Nutrition Institute in Mill Valley, California, cites an example of what he calls mouth hunger: "the feeling that comes when you see a cake in a shop window and your mouth begins to water." Some people crave the taste of food in their mouths even after they have eaten much more than is necessary to fulfill their bodies' physical needs. Too often, Kozlenko says, the dictates of emotion overpower the subtle cues from within, signaling that the body has had enough.

He believes, further, that "emotional directives" often lead to poor eating habits that, in turn, can affect the normal functioning of the body and whether we feel alive or listless. Gorging, continual snacking, or eating at the wrong times can result in bloating or "gas," and, ultimately, in obesity. Eating too fast or eating too much, even chewing improperly, can tax the digestive enzymes and interfere with the assimilation of nutrients. The poor digestion that results, says Kozlenko, can make it easier for food to be broken down into substances harmful to the body. (Excess protein, for example, if poorly digested, is converted into toxic amines.)

Kozlenko, a noted spokesman for the holistic health movement, has developed an inventory of eating habits that helps his patients at the institute become more aware not only of their eating behavior but also of their emotional investment in food. Kozlenko asks them to experiment with various diets and to repeat the survey at intervals. He claims that by concentrating on changing one dimension of eating behavior, a person can drastically alter the way he or she feels physically. (For example, by eating dinner an hour earlier each day, you may give your food more chance to metabolize before you go to bed.)

For those readers who wish some indication of how well attuned they are to their own habits and the "emotional interference" in their eating, we include a portion of Richard Kozlenko's survey, followed by a scoring key.[29]

Check the statements according to the appropriate frequency.

VERY FREQUENT — Roughly 50% to 90% of the time or almost every to every other day

OFTEN — Roughly 20% to 50% of the time or 1 to 3 times weekly

320

OCCASIONALLY — Roughly 10% of the time or 2 to 3 times monthly
SELDOM — Roughly 1% to 3% of the time or from 4 times yearly to once a
month
NEVER — Essentially total avoidance

	Very Frequently 4	Often 3	Occasionally 2	Seldom 1	Never 0
1. Eat excessively when bored or depressed.					
2. Insomnia					
3. Eat foods you know are "bad" for you					
4. Prefer eating alone					
5. Feel conspicuous or embarrassed when eating with others					
6. Parents used, made available, or encouraged sweets					
7. Fear weight gain					
8. "Hell with it all" feeling					
9. Will sneak or hide food					
10. Alcoholic beverages					
11. Eat foods discouraged by parents					
12. Eat or drink in secrecy					
13. Drugs (tranquilizers, sleeping pills, appetite suppressants, etc.)					

	Very Frequently 4	Often 3	Occasionally 2	Seldom 1	Never 0
14. Self-conscious of how my body looks					
15. I mistreat myself					
16. Wish I looked different					
17. Feelings (diet or otherwise) of being "rushed" or sense of time urgency					
18. Waves of anger or hostility					
19. Feelings of being in the midst of "struggle" (over diet or otherwise)					
20. Fatigue or "wiped out" feelings					
21. Uncontrollable hunger urges					
22. Gulp my food					
23. Stuff myself					
24. Indulge in sweets					
25. Eat when not hungry					
26. Eat and "run"					
27. Cravings for sweets					
28. Meals or heavy snacks after 7 p.m.					
29. Eat within an hour of retiring					
30. Eating binges					

SCORING:

60 and below: Good relationship with your body, sensitive to physical needs.

61-80: Average range, for normally healthy people.

81-95: Eating is based somewhat too much on emotional directives.

95 and above: Excessive emotional interference in eating habits.

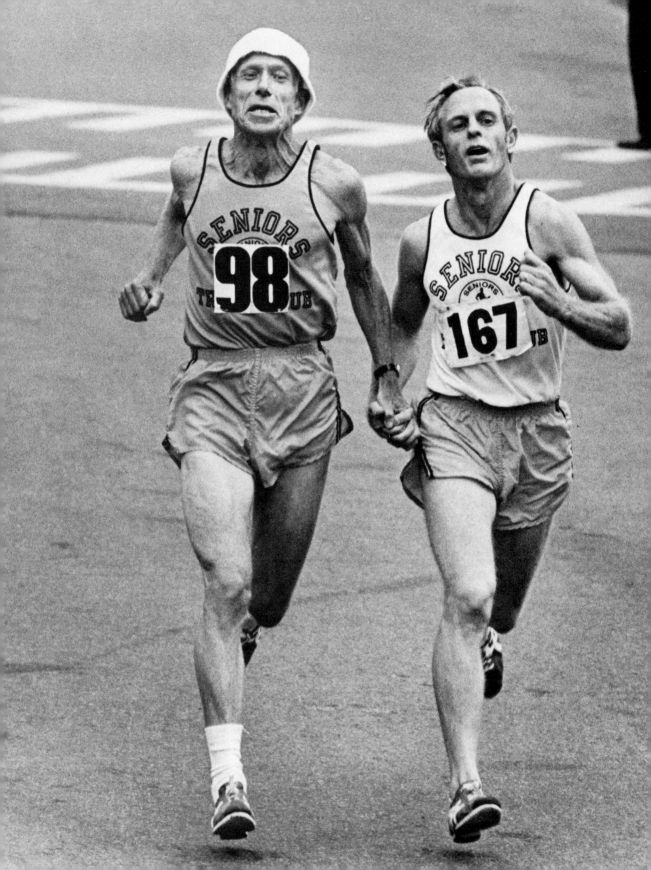

9
Fitness: Keep Moving

Physical fitness: it is a state of being that guarantees that you are healthy enough and fit enough to actively adjust to all of the physical, mental, emotional, and social demands of your environment. It means that your body is trim and firm; it means that you have the strength and flexibility to function well physically; it means that you are not plagued by disease. It means that your heart and other organs work together smoothly as a system to support your body in meeting the demands placed on it.

Just because you are trim does not mean that you are necessarily fit — and fitness depends on much more than just looks. One of the greatest keys to fitness — to your body's ability to work to its peak — is exercise.

ASSESSING YOUR OWN PHYSICAL FITNESS

Physical fitness — the ability to carry out daily tasks with vigor and alertness, without undue fatigue, and with ample energy to enjoy leisure-time pursuits — is composed of three major elements:

1. **Muscular strength and endurance.** The strength of the muscles has to do with their contraction power. This is important not only to your ability to perform manual labor or participate in your favorite sports activity: the body is dependent for survival on the strength of the muscles in the heart, respiratory system, digestive system, and organs of elimination. The ability of the muscles to perform work is an indication of their endurance; how quickly you tire out is directly related to the amount of endurance that you have.
2. **Cardio-respiratory endurance.** The heart is the best gauge of physical fitness: how quickly does it adapt to stress, working with the respiratory system to pump fresh oxygen to the body tissues during time of physical labor and activity?
3. **Flexibility.** The range of motion of a joint is a matter of flexibility; the greater the range of motion, the more flexibility you have in muscle, tendons and ligaments.

A number of tests are available to help you assess your own physical fitness — but, sadly, most of them ignore the most important index of fitness: the cardiovascular system. A good key to fitness is to measure your resting pulse rate and compare it against your pulse rate after you engage in several different kinds of activities — a measurement of how well your heart is adapting, and how fit your cardiovascular system is.

Measuring the Resting Pulse Rate

To measure your resting pulse rate, use the artery in your wrist (the best place), or in your neck just next to the Adam's apple. Your pulse is slowest after you have been asleep for six hours — so take your pulse in the morning when you first wake up, before you get out of bed, eat, or perform any kind of movement (even the act of walking across the room will increase your pulse rate and give a false reading). Count the pulsations for one full minute to obtain your resting pulse rate. According to the American Heart Association, a normal resting heart rate is between sixty and eighty beats per minute — and the "normal" for you is dependent on your age, weight, and level of fitness.

Once you have obtained a resting heart rate, measure it against your pulse after you perform different kinds of activities. Choose a specific kind of exercise or activity, and perform it for a few minutes. Take your pulse immediately after you stop: measure your pulse for ten seconds,

Figure 9-1.

HOW TO READ AND RECORD YOUR HEART RATE

The action of your heart is the best gauge of your physical fitness. An accurate record of your heart rate (beats per minute) under various conditions over a period of time will enable your physician to gauge your progress. Accordingly, you'll need to learn to take your pulse under these conditions:

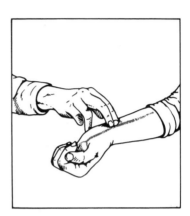

- At rest; for example, when you first awaken in the morning, before rising or exercising.
- After a specific period of exercise, as directed by your physician.
- After you have performed your regular work for a specific period, as directed by your physician.

Taking your pulse is, for these purposes, the same as counting the number of times your heart beats per minute. Don't be concerned that your heart rate seems fast at one reading or slow at another, many factors, including sex and age, affect the heart rate under various circumstances. To get an accurate measurement for your physical fitness program, follow the simple steps below:

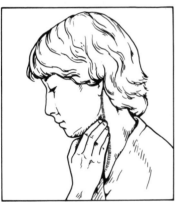

1. Experiment a bit and select the best body site to take your pulse. In some sites the pulse is prominent at rest; in others, after exercise. The best locations are typically at the wrist, just below the base of the thumb; at the neck, just over the collar line and to the right or left of the windpipe; and at the inside of the elbow, just above the skin crease.
2. When taking your pulse at rest, simply count the number of pulsations for a full minute, using a watch with a second hand for accuracy.
3. *Immediately* after exercise count the beats for the first 10 seconds *only*; then mutiply this number by six to get a per minute reading. Don't try to take your pulse during exercise, but start *immediately* after the prescribed exercise. The reason for this is that the heart rate rapidly slows after the stress of exercise; in fact, the faster it slows the more fit you are, as a rule. If you do take a full minute's count, you'll notice a significant difference in the number of heartbeats during the first 10 seconds of the minute and the last 10 seconds.
4. One of the reasons for testing your heart rate is to find out what normal work activity does to your heart. Select an activity that is ordinary and usual — both in the stress it creates and the muscular power it requires. Take a resting pulse count just before doing the activity, then take a post-activity count for 10 seconds and multiply by six.
5. Write down the count of your pulse immediately after taking it. Keep a small notebook for the purpose, and enter the date, time, and kind of reading (resting, postexercise, postwork) for each count.

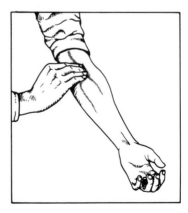

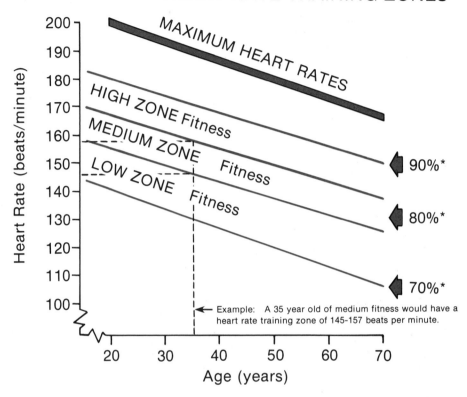

HEART RATE TRAINING ZONES

*Percent of maximum heart rate.

Figure 9-2. The chart illustrates average maximum heart rates as well as heart rate training zones for those in low, medium, and high fitness categories. The heart rate training zone tells you how intense your exercise must be to gain a training effect.

and multiply the number by six to obtain an accurate measurement. (The heart rate slows rapidly once you stop exercising, and to count the pulsations for a full minute would give a false reading.)

THE ELEMENTS OF FITNESS ━━━━━

As mentioned earlier, the major elements of fitness include muscular strength, endurance; and flexibility.

328

Strength

Muscular strength is usually developed through two different kinds of physical exercise: isometrics and isotonics. Both exercises work on the notion that strength is developed by overcoming resistance (such as a partner, equipment, or a heavy object). Your ability to perform adequately in any physical capacity depends on the strength of your muscles, and your ability to maintain health depends on the strength of the muscles of your various body systems.

Isometrics

In isometrics, one set of muscles is used to push or pull against another set of muscles (or, in some cases, against an object that cannot be moved). Done routinely and consistently several times a week, isometrics can increase the strength and size of the muscles that are exercised. While isometrics increase the strength of the muscles that are exercised, they do not increase the heart's capacity to pump freshly oxygenated blood, nor do they increase the function of the respiratory system. Vigorous isometric exercise is dangerous for people who suffer from heart disease, since it can increase the blood pressure substantially if overdone.

Figure 9-3.

ISOMETRIC VS ISOTONIC EXERCISE

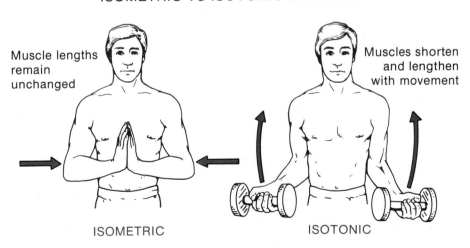

Muscle lengths remain unchanged

Muscles shorten and lengthen with movement

ISOMETRIC

ISOTONIC

If you are not in good physical health, or if you have had heart disease of any kind, you should receive your doctor's approval before you begin a program of isometrics.

Isotonics

Most people prefer isotonics over isometrics: isotonics involve a group of muscles working against a moving object (such as weights). Isotonics also involve calisthenics, a series of body movements designed to increase muscular strength (sit-ups and push-ups are good examples of calisthenics). Like isometrics, isotonics do not exercise the heart or respiratory systems, but they are good as warm-ups to exercise that does work the cardiovascular system.

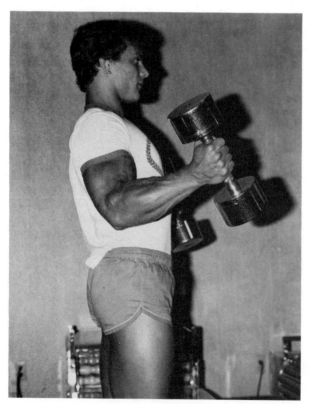

Weight lifting is an example of isotonic exercise.

Endurance

Muscular endurance basically gives an indication of how long you can sustain effort — it measures your basic stamina. Aerobic exercise — exercise that forces the body to increase its utilization of oxygen — tests and develops muscular endurance and is the most beneficial type of exercise for improving the strength of the cardiovascular system. Participating in aerobic exercise causes your heart to gradually strengthen and improve its capacity to pump freshly oxygenated blood to all the body tissues. Over a period of time, the heart muscle's increased strength results in a lower resting heart rate — and a healthier heart. The best aerobic exercises are swimming, bicycling, rapid walking, jogging, long-distance running, rowing, and tennis.

To be worthwhile, aerobic exercise has to really make you work — you need to place new demands on your heart and lungs. A leisurely stroll may be nice, but it does not force your system to improve itself. Aerobic exercises should always be preceded by a period of isotonic or calisthenic warm-ups to gently stretch the muscles and prepare them for the exercise, and all aerobic exercise programs should begin with slight

Swimming is an excellent form of aerobic exercise.

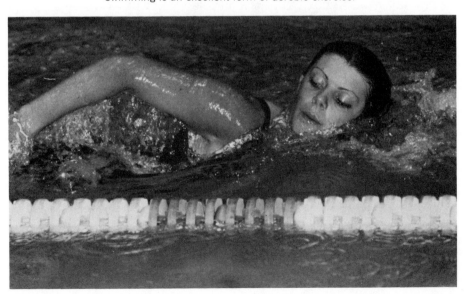

exercise and should increase gradually over time as your system strengthens. Even people in good health and good physical condition need to progress slowly; those who have been ill or who are overweight should get a doctor's approval.

Flexibility

To appreciate true flexibility, watch an infant — constantly in motion, he keeps his muscles and joints flexible. We were all like that once, but hours at desks and in front of television sets have rendered many of us inflexible so that even limited motion can become uncomfortable or painful.

Improving flexibility necessitates developing a program of slow, gentle stretching exercises designed to improve motion and flexibility. Keep the exercises slow and controlled, and start out with only a few — or you will get muscle soreness and stiffness instead of increased flexibility. Stretch slowly and carefully to the point of *mild* discomfort — and

Flexibility is one measure of fitness.

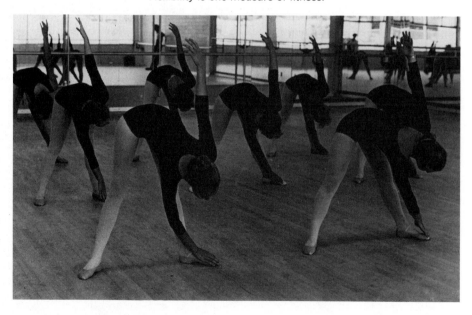

then stretch just a little more. Return to the normal position as slowly as you stretched out of it. Avoid the urge to do fast, jerky exercises.

Increasing flexibility has other benefits: your agility (ability to change position quickly) and your speed are generally increased along with an improvement in flexibility.

BENEFITS OF EXERCISE

Exercise, in a word, improves the overall condition of your body. Simply, it improves your health. Some of the specific benefits of exercise include the following:

1. **Body posture is improved.** As you exercise, the muscles, tendons, and ligaments that support your skeleton are strengthened, and your ability to stand erect with ease is improved. Good posture is important for reasons other than physical attraction, too — it guarantees a better blood supply to the brain and eases the process of returning venous blood to the heart.

2. **Stress is reduced.** As little exercise as walking for fifteen minutes has a more tranquilizing effect than even powerful drugs for relieving anxiety and muscle tension and stress. In addition, exercise improves your ability to deal with stress, provides an outlet for your hostilities, and improves your alertness. Researchers do not know exactly why exercise relieves stress, but several theories cite that exercise reduces the level of salts in the brain, promotes sound sleep, raises hormonal levels critical to the thinking process, sends more oxygen to the brain, and gives people a sense of accomplishment — something that simply makes them feel better about themselves and less prone to suffer from stress.

3. **Exercise increases bone mass.** Among those who do not exercise, the bones undergo an actual physical change — they get brittle and frail, more prone to injury, and they lose vital minerals, which requires more healing time if a break does occur. An hour of exercise three times a week is generally sufficient to promote bone mass and insure the health of the bones.

4. **Exercise improves the condition of the heart and the blood vessels,** contributing greatly to the health of the entire cardiovascular system. Regular exercise increases the strength of the heart, enabling it to be more effective in pumping blood and causing it to

pump more slowly while at rest (which means that it will wear out less quickly!). Because the heart muscle is strengthened, it returns to normal more quickly after exertion, lessening the danger of damage to the heart muscle resulting from participation in sports or other activities. And because the heart muscle is stronger, circulation is improved throughout the entire body. With a stronger heart, you run less of a risk of heart attack, but if you do suffer an attack, you will recover more fully and more quickly if you are in good condition.

5. **Exercise lowers the blood pressure.**

6. **Exercise enhances the production of red blood cells in the bone marrow,** expanding the ability of the blood to effectively circulate nutrients throughout the system.

7. **The lungs and the respiratory system are strengthened and improved.** During aerobic exercise, the lungs are expanded, and the muscles that cause the lungs to expand and contract are strengthened, making it easier for you to breathe. With regular exercise and its effects, you take in more oxygen and slough off more carbon dioxide. The blood itself becomes richer in oxygen content, which means that the heart has to pump more slowly to circulate the same amount of oxygen throughout the body.

8. **Exercise increases the efficiency of the digestive system.** Your appetite is increased, you eat more, the peristaltic motion of the system is speeded up, digestion is improved, and food is absorbed more completely and more quickly. For some, exercise results in a natural urge to eat better, more balanced foods. And there is another digestive benefit to exercise: the strengthening of all of the body's muscles tends to eliminate the problem of constipation.

9. **Regular exercise makes the degenerative process of aging less devastating to the body.** People who have exercised continuously throughout their lives maintain better muscle strength and flexibility into old age and have less of a tendency to develop arthritis or other afflictions involving the joints. Both physical and mental health are prolonged as a result of regular exercise.

10. **Regular exercise is one of the most effective ways of maintaining normal weight.** Exercise burns off calories and increases metabolism — which means that you will continue to burn more calories throughout the day, long after you have stopped exercising. Exercise should always be added to a program of calorie control — it

speeds the process of weight loss and firms and tones the body as the pounds are shed. Regular exercise also reduces the amount of cholesterol and lipids (fats) in the blood.

THE EFFECTS OF INACTIVITY

The many benefits of exercise are established even more when you consider the effects of inactivity — prolonged bed rest during an illness, sitting at a study desk day after day, choosing forms of recreation such as movies and television over sports participation or exercise.[1]

Inactivity — especially bed rest — causes loss of body water. More than 50 percent of your body weight is water; your muscles are composed of more than 70 percent water. Water in the body is essential to proper circulation of blood to the lower extremities, maintenance of blood supply to the brain, proper functioning of the kidneys, proper balance of blood constituents, and optimum functioning of every organ and system in your body.

Every day, your body destroys red blood cells; they are smashed to pieces from the action of tumbling through the vast network of arteries and veins in your body. But you do not run out of them, because your bone marrow consistently, under normal conditions, manufactures enough red blood cells to replace what has been lost. Because of increased activity, those who are exercising destroy more red blood cells; their bone marrow, as a result, produces more. Those who are inactive still suffer red blood cell loss due to the normal hazard of blood circulation, but studies reveal that even after only four weeks of inactivity, the bone marrow has been crippled in its ability to replace the cells that are lost.

Even eight days of inactivity can begin having its effect on the heart: the resting heart rate increases in that short a period. In other words, after only eight days of sitting around in a chair, it takes more work for your heart to circulate your blood; your heart has to pump harder to accomplish its job. Because blood tends to pool in the lower extremities and not circulate properly to the brain, inactivity increases your tendency to faint. Inactivity also reduces overall blood volume — another precursor to fainting.

As your periods of inactivity increase, your capacity for exercise decreases. The reasons include loss of muscle tone, impaired circulation, and limited delivery of oxygen to muscles and tissues.

Muscles decrease in size, strength, and tone as a result of inactivity. Important chemicals are not circulated to muscle masses if you are not getting regular exercise, and there is a gradual decrease in muscle mass. Your calorie intake, instead of being used for the energy demanded by exercise, goes instead to store fat in your body.

During periods of inactivity, calcium is literally mobilized out of your bones and is discarded. Studies have shown that progressive loss of calcium in as short a time as four weeks could only be remedied by exercise in an upright position. (This was a critical problem for some of those participating in long-term manned space flights.)

Inactivity has its effects on the joints of the body, too. If you do not exercise enough, you are likely to develop stiffness, soreness, and loss of motion, because the joints are not consistently used in their full range of motion. In some cases, tendons and ligaments that surround joints literally shorten from disuse, limiting your capacity to work and exercise.

One of the most critical results of inactivity is on the feet: they lose their muscle tone, flexibility, and strength, limiting the amount of time they can support you in even common activities such as standing and walking. In extreme cases, they can lose their weight-bearing abilities altogether.

Probably the most common result of inactivity and lack of exercise is the feeling of fatigue and sluggishness. You can reach a point where you are so inactive and so tired that resting and sleeping do not relieve your fatigue — they only make matters worse.

Basically, inactivity leads to widespread changes that limit your body's ability to function normally and to cope with your daily living patterns. Exercise can change all that.

DEVELOPING AN EXERCISE PROGRAM

There are many aspects of your health over which you do not have much control — such as your hereditary tendency to cancer of the colon, your body's rate of metabolism, the amount of air pollution in your city — but you have optimum control over how physically fit you are.[2] Even those with severe physical disabilities can do some activities to make themselves as physically fit as possible. Those without disability can take the initiative to exercise and bring their weight into control: and that includes the majority of us.

TRAINING EFFECTS
OF AEROBIC EXERCISE

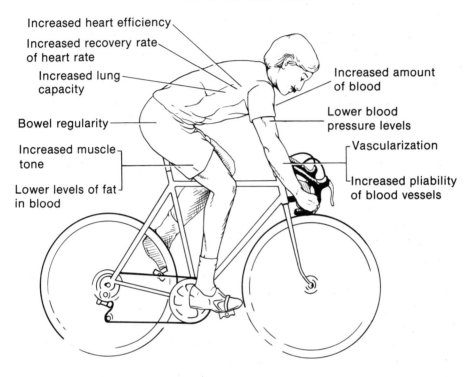

Increased heart efficiency

Increased recovery rate
of heart rate

Increased lung
capacity

Bowel regularity

Increased muscle
tone

Lower levels of fat
in blood

Increased amount
of blood

Lower blood
pressure levels

Vascularization

Increased pliability
of blood vessels

Figure 9-4.

Think about your own program of physical fitness — if you have one. If you think that you are too busy to exercise every day, reassess your values: physical fitness needs to be part of your life. Think about the reasons why you want to be physically fit — there are health reasons, appearance reasons, and personal reasons, and all of them are compelling reasons!

Do not think of physical fitness as being a short-term, crash program to correct or reverse years of inactivity. Go slowly at first, without stress; take the time and energy required to find a program that is just right for you — one you can stick with for the rest of your life with only a few modifications to accommodate aging and changes in environment.

Have fun with physical fitness. There are many ways to exercise: you can jog on a treadmill for an hour, staring into a full-length mirror, or you can play a rigorous game of tennis at the park, or swim for an hour at the community pool, or choose to do your jogging along a country road. And do not take yourself so seriously that the whole experience becomes grim — slow, steady improvement is what you are after. Do not get discouraged and quit your exercise program if you have not reached a certain self-set level of fitness in the first four weeks.

Try not to concentrate on what is going on inside your body while you exercise — forget how much you are huffing and puffing, forget how hard your heart is pounding, and just concentrate on slamming that racquetball across the court. There are certain warning and danger signs from your body that signal overexertion, and you need to be aware of those. Beyond that, have fun, and forget all the mechanics.

Get outside and into your environment as much as you can. The sunshine, fresh air, and change of scenery are good for your mind as well as your body. Try riding your bicycle, playing a game of golf (no carts!), walking briskly to the library, or some other form of activity that enables you to take advantage of the outdoors. If you dress for the weather, you will be comfortable and rejuvenated.

Remember moderation — a little exercise every day is much better for you than a lot of exercise once a week. It would be better to ride your bicycle to campus and back every day than to participate in a number of concentrated activities on Saturday after you have finished studying.

Set modest expectations for yourself. Set goals that you know you can reach. If you set heroic expectations for yourself, your fear of failure will quite likely cause you to abandon the whole effort altogether. You cannot expect to lose forty pounds by the time you go home for Christmas, but you can expect to be ten pounds lighter and a little more limber.

Do not dwell on past mistakes. It is never too late to start a fitness and weight control program. Maybe you never could do the required amount of sit-ups in junior high school gym class, and maybe you were the last chosen for the volleyball team in the sixth grade. You can start now — no matter what your age or condition — to make gradual, steady improvement. Even those who are fifty or sixty years of age or older can start to make improvements.

Get involved in your fitness activity! Make it more than mere exercise. Get some friends to join you, sign up for a team or league, subscribe to a magazine aimed at runners, or keep a record of your efforts and achievements. Make your activity — and your exercise — an important part of your day.

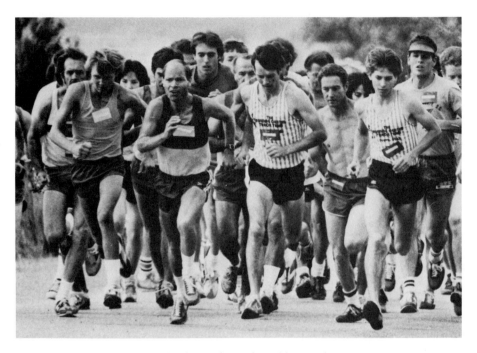

Running is one form of aerobic exercise.

Do not stick to just one activity. Maybe you have decided that bicycling will be your main fitness activity; you ride to campus each day, and a couple of times a week you and a few friends backpack to various sites in your county. Maybe you are even training to race. Get some variety into your fitness regime. Try swimming once at the university pool; challenge a friend to a game of tennis next Saturday. You might even try jumping rope in the dorm basement to release some of the tension when you are preparing for final exams. Variety cannot only alleviate boredom, but it helps guarantee that your fitness program is a well-rounded one that tones and conditions your entire body.

Part of becoming fit is changing your life-style — learning new habits. You will probably need to force yourself at first, so try writing yourself a contract. Make it cover a three-month period for starters. Agree with yourself to do a certain number of activities and to make a certain amount of progress within that time. Every week or so, review your contract. See how you are doing, how far you have come toward reaching your eventual goals. It will help you get into the habit of fitness, and it will provide you with positive reinforcement and a sense of achievement.

Perhaps most important, be sensible. If you are really out of shape, get a physical exam and talk your plans over with your doctor. Sudden exertion could shock your cardiovascular system and lead to serious complications. The goal of a fitness program is to help you — not hurt you. Pay attention to your body's warning signs, get your doctor's approval, and work into your program steadily but gradually. Avoiding illness and injury will make it easier to stick with any fitness program that you choose for yourself.

Warming Up

Whatever you decide to do, make sure that every time you exercise, you take a few minutes for "warming-up" exercises: exercises that slowly stretch your muscles and prepare them for the upcoming workout. Warming up helps prevent injury from exercising — and if you do not warm up, you can suffer heart irregularities, muscle cramps, and serious leg injuries.

Warming up is especially critical for those over the age of thirty, who may have lost some of the flexibility of the muscles. The key to any kind of warm-up exercise is to *stretch* — do not jerk. There are plenty of warm-up exercises available, and you can choose whichever ones work best for you. Take about ten minutes to warm up. Then begin your main exercise slowly, working up to regular pitch over the period of a few minutes. Taking these precautions can help you avoid serious injury from exercising.

Cooling Down

Many people remember to do warm-up exercises, but too many forget that it is just as important to take ten minutes to cool down once you have finished exercising. Do not just stop abruptly — it can be too stressful to the body. If you have been jogging or running, walk slowly and leisurely for about ten minutes. If you have been swimming vigorously, swim slowly. You can even repeat the exercises that you used for warming up.

Cooling down is important for several reasons. First, it prevents muscle stiffness because it allows time for the metabolic wastes to be worked out of your muscles. Second, it redistributes the blood that may be pooled in the extremities from a vigorous workout.

Cool down for about ten minutes, then take a lukewarm bath or shower to promote circulation and relaxation. Steer away from hot water — it reduces circulation and causes fatigue.

MAKING YOUR EXERCISE PROGRAM SUCCESSFUL

There are many things that you can do to make your exercise program a success — to help avoid the tendency to drop out after a couple of weeks.[3]

Before you start anything, see your doctor. You should have a physical examination to determine your strength, heart capacity, flexibility, and general condition. You should be prepared to discuss with your doctor your specific plans for a fitness program. Your doctor may be able to add to your ideas, or he may discourage you from several because of the harm that you may incur if you are out of shape. Whatever the outcome, your fitness plan can be tailored to your own needs and problems, and your doctor can help prevent illness or resulting injury.

Learn to count your pulse, and check your heart at various levels of activity.

Keep your condition in mind, and do not do too much at the start. (Your doctor can help with this.) Extreme soreness, stiffness, and fatigue can discourage even the most devoted beginners. Do what you reasonably can at first — even if it seems so little — and gradually add more as your condition improves.

Avoid competitive activities that require a sudden burst of energy — the anaerobic exercises. Rhythmic exercises — such as walking, cycling, rowing, or noncompetitive swimming — are excellent choices.

Depending on the condition of your heart (which your doctor can help assess), you will need to choose exercises that will increase your heart rate in order to improve your heart's capacity and develop your heart's strength. Your resting heart rate, if you are in excellent condition, should be about sixty to eighty beats per minute; you will want to choose

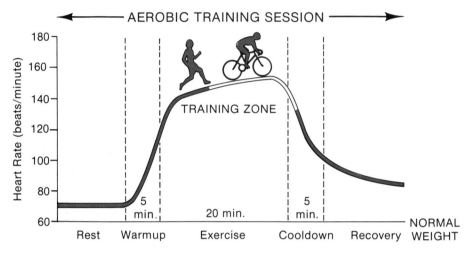

Figure 9-5. Warmup, aerobic exercise, cool down — these are the elements of the training session. This represents a medium training zone for a 35-year-old male.

a mild exercise that increases your heartbeat only slightly to begin with if you are not in good condition.

Cardiovascular fitness is realized when the stress load causes the heart rate to beat at 75 to 85 percent of its maximum. Maximum heart rate can be determined by subtracting your age from 220. Thus, a stress rate equal to 75 to 80 percent of maximum for a twenty-year-old would be 220 – 200 = 200 × .75 to .85 = 150 to 170 beats per minute.

The following heart rates can be obtained from the activities listed:[4]

- **100-110 beats per minute:** riding a bicycle at five miles per hour, ironing clothes, pitching horseshoes, polishing your car, or performing light calisthenics (isotonic exercise).
- **100-120:** bowling, archery, softball, walking about two and one-half miles per hour, or painting a house.
- **120-130:** ballroom dancing, canoeing at about two miles an hour, riding an exercycle, golfing (if you carry your own bag), sweeping the floor, or scrubbing the floor.
- **130-140:** climbing stairs, rowing a boat, swimming, playing table tennis, or doing pick-and-shovel work.

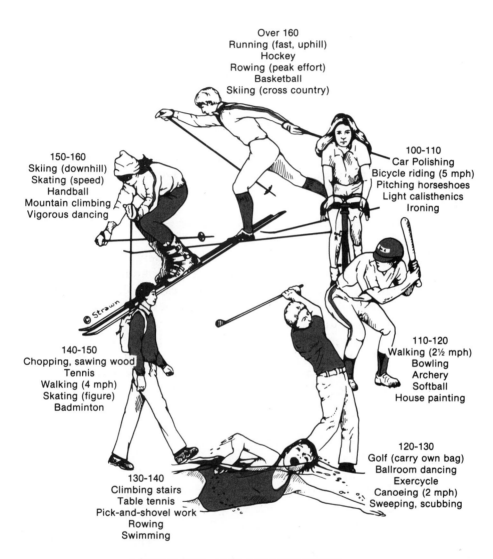

Over 160
Running (fast, uphill)
Hockey
Rowing (peak effort)
Basketball
Skiing (cross country)

100-110
Car Polishing
Bicycle riding (5 mph)
Pitching horseshoes
Light calisthenics
Ironing

150-160
Skiing (downhill)
Skating (speed)
Handball
Mountain climbing
Vigorous dancing

140-150
Chopping, sawing wood
Tennis
Walking (4 mph)
Skating (figure)
Badminton

110-120
Walking (2½ mph)
Bowling
Archery
Softball
House painting

120-130
Golf (carry own bag)
Ballroom dancing
Exercycle
Canoeing (2 mph)
Sweeping, scubbing

130-140
Climbing stairs
Table tennis
Pick-and-shovel work
Rowing
Swimming

© Strawn

ACTIVITIES AND HEARTBEATS —
CHOOSE THE ONE FOR YOU

Figure 9-6.

343

- **140-150:** playing tennis, walking at the rate of about four miles an hour, figure skating, playing badminton, or chopping and sawing wood.
- **150-160:** speed skating, playing handball, mountain climbing, downhill skiing, or vigorous dancing.
- **Over 160:** playing hockey, rowing a boat at peak effort, cross-country skiing, playing basketball, or running fast uphill.

Be consistent. It does not really matter how much you exercise at any one time or what kind of exercise you choose, but it is critical that you exercise consistently. Occasional bursts of strenuous activity are worse for your body than no activity at all. Do *something* every day, because the progress that you make will diminish rapidly if you become inactive for even a short time.

Do not exercise for at least two hours after you have finished eating a heavy meal.

When temperatures and humidity are extremely high, avoid exercising outdoors; instead, choose something like handball, swimming, basketball, bowling, or ballroom dancing that can be done indoors for days when weather conditions make exercising outdoors hazardous.

Do not be afraid to rest during exercise. No one says that you have to keep up a grueling pace for a solid hour with no breaks; in fact, it is not healthy. Sit on the bench for a few minutes in the middle of a fast-paced game of basketball; slow to a jog and then a walk, and stop to inspect some unique tree pods when you are out running near the park.

Be sure to choose exercise activities that can be done year-round, especially critical if you live in an area that experiences vast changes in climate. Running might be fine in the spring in the Colorado Rockies, but it is not fun or easy to plow through a few feet of snow around your old running course. If you live where there are changes in climate, plan for them. In Colorado, for instance, you might run in the spring, play handball or racquetball during the summer, swim indoors during the fall, and cross-country ski when the snow falls. Make sure that you have activities for all kinds of seasons, plus all kinds of weather — do not let a few days of rain or smog throw you off kilter. Have some alternatives up your sleeve.

If you smoke, stop. Smoking constricts the lung capillaries and restricts the ability of the heart and lungs to circulate oxygen through the body.

Make sure that all parts of your body are being worked. As

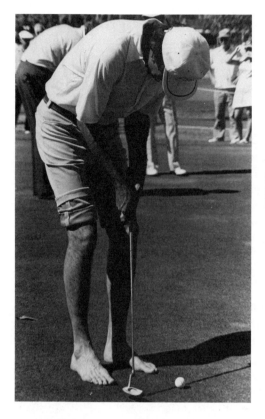

Golf may be popular and relaxing, but it does not promote cardiovascular fitness.

mentioned, you should choose an aerobic exercise that will strengthen your heart and lungs, but you should also choose isotonics or isometrics that will exercise the muscles of your neck, shoulders, chest, upper back, waist, lower back, abdomen, legs, and feet.

Learn to breathe deeply while you exercise. Draw as much air as you can into your lungs, and release it explosively. Do not try to hold the air in your lungs.

If you have an erratic schedule, plan your exercise activities in spurts throughout the day instead of all in one time block. If you are sitting in class all day, for example, you might run a mile in the morning before class, play a game of tennis during lunch, and bicycle for fifteen minutes before you settle down to study. Take a break from studying midevening to do some calisthenics or weight lifting.

Make sure that you are eating a well-balanced diet to provide you with the strength and nutrition that you need. Exercise requires energy, and you need to eat the foods that will give you strength and energy. Get plenty of fresh fruits and vegetables.

Do not make time commitments that are impossible. For instance, do not decide that you are going to exercise every Saturday morning if you have a part-time job on Saturdays that you need to juggle with your studying. Do not commit to a full-scale exercise program if all you can afford is fifteen minutes after your classes each night. Do what you can, but making commitments that you cannot keep causes discouragement and abandonment of the exercise plan.

Get some friends to join you. Exercising is always more fun, and you will stick to it better if you are in a group. Besides companionship, others in the group provide support and help.

Consider your body type when choosing exercises. If you have a round, soft body with little muscle development and relatively small bones, you will do best at activities like archery, bowling, cycling, swimming and golf. Those who have fragile, delicate bodies with thin muscles and thin bones should choose something like badminton, basketball, hiking, jogging, tennis, or running. Those with muscular bodies, big bones, and hard, rugged appearance can participate in any activity with reasonable success.

Wear the proper clothing for the exercise that you choose. Many like jogging, walking, or running, because the clothing is uncomplicated, and the only expense is a good pair of shoes. Dress so that your body is protected; use the proper equipment for exercise. Dress for the weather, and do not dress so much that perspiration is trapped next to your skin. Perpsiration should be absorbed by clothing or should be allowed to evaporate. Do not get overheated.

Make sure that you drink plenty of fluids. You should not fill your stomach with water during the course of exercise, but you should drink enough to keep your thirst quenched and to replace the fluids that you lose through perspiration.

EXERCISE PROBLEMS AND INJURIES ━━━━━━

Those who have been inactive for any length of time may, due to overexertion, develop some minor problems when they first begin to exercise.[5] If you begin slowly, and work up gradually, you will be able to

346

avoid most of these problems and injuries. Further protection can be obtained by careful warming up and cooling down just before and after exercise.

Blisters

Wearing good, properly fitted shoes can help you avoid blisters. At the first hint of discomfort, cover the area with some moleskin or with a large bandage. If you do get a blister, puncture the edge with a sterilized needle, drain the accumulated fluid (be careful not to brush off the skin), treat the blister with an antiseptic, cover the blister with sterile gauze, and circle the area with foam rubber (you can also get commercially made bandages for blisters).

Muscle Soreness

It is almost impossible to avoid some muscle soreness when you first start exercising, but exercise modestly at first, and do mild stretching exercises before you begin. When soreness does occur, repeat some of the mild stretching exercises; avoid putting too much strain on the sore muscles. Gentle massage and soaking in a warm tub can also help relieve the pain and stiffness.

Muscle Cramps

Cold muscles cramp more readily, and it is essential that you warm up before you exercise. Many times, cramping is due to salt and fluids lost through perspiration. If you suffer from cramps occasionally, stop exercising, stretch the muscle that is cramping, and rest while you drink fluids (a good idea is a drink like Gatorade which helps to replace lost potassium). If you get cramps often, see your doctor.

Bone Bruises

Hikers and joggers sometimes get painful bruises on the bottoms of the feet. These bruises can be avoided by careful foot placement and by using quality footwear. You can also try cushion innersoles if you suffer from bone bruises. There is no instant cure for a bone bruise; ice can help reduce pain and hasten healing slightly. Apply heat forty-eight to seventy-two hours after the injury to aid healing. If you pad your shoes carefully, you can continue exercising.

Knee Problems and Injuries

Pain and tenderness in the knee may be a sign of a knee injury, a problem that can affect your ability to exercise for the rest of your life. Knee injuries often lead to arthritis and can restrict your ability to participate in a number of activities. Because of their potential seriousness, you should see a doctor whenever you injure a knee. Before you get to the doctor, use ice packs to help reduce the inflammation and ease the pain.

You can prevent knee problems by striking your foot from heel to toe when running or jogging, wearing shoes that are in good condition (avoid worn shoes), and wearing shoes and other footgear that provide you with proper support.

Low Back Pain

Pain radiating down the buttocks and leg, and tightness or pain in the hamstring, can result from lack of physical activity, poor posture, inadequate flexibility, and weak abdominal or back muscles. Doing specific exercises designed to improve the strength of the back and the abdominal muscles and improving your posture can relieve most of these pains, which are generally not a result of exercise.

Ankle Problems

Wearing high-topped gym shoes helps prevent ankle sprains if you are playing basketball, tennis, or handball; if you have had weak ankles or previous ankle injuries, you should avoid low-cut shoes. A sprained ankle should be iced immediately; immerse your foot in a bucket of ice water as soon as possible after the sprain to reduce swelling and bruising. If the sprain is serious, you should see your doctor. Ankle wraps and taping allow for exercise after a sprain, but you should avoid putting stress on your ankle during exercise.

Achilles Tendon Injuries

When rubbed long enough, as in exercise of some kinds, the bursa located beneath the Achilles tendon becomes inflamed and incapable of lubricating the movements of the tendon. Other Achilles tendon injuries include rupture, inflammation, or partial rupture.

You can prevent Achilles tendon injuries by having ample warm up before exercise, by avoiding sudden start and spurts, and by avoiding sudden changes of direction during exercise.

Achilles tendon injuries are characterized by pain and tenderness behind the ankle when you stand or put weight on your foot. Minor injuries may indicate themselves by pain and stiffness in the back of the heel after a night's sleep.

Ice helps to relieve the pain. You should not exercise your ankles or do exercising that causes you to put weight down on your feet for several weeks. In severe cases, see your doctor.

Shin Splints

Tenderness in the lower third of the leg, inside the shin area, that is accompanied by pain with toe extension and pain with weight bearing is indicative of shin splints. Shin splints are caused by a lowered arch, irritated membranes, tearing of the muscle from the bone, a muscle spasm (due to swelling of the muscle), a hairline fracture of the bones of the lower leg, a muscle strength imbalance, or other factors.

Rest is the best cure; taping or using a sponge heel pad can help in some cases, but a physician can diagnose the cause of the shin splint and can prescribe specific treatment.

You can prevent shin splints by including exercises to strengthen your skin muscles, gradually adjusting to exercise, running on soft surfaces, occasionally reversing direction when running on a curved track, and using the heel-to-toe method of striking your foot on the ground when running or jogging.

Stressful Exercise

To avoid undue strains on your heart and body systems, you should avoid unfamiliar, exhaustive, or highly competitive exercise until you have gradually built your strength and endurance. Avoid sudden vigorous exercise until you have built endurance, and then make sure that you warm up properly.

EXERCISE WARNING SIGNS

Any of these warning signs can be indicative of danger. If any of these occur *even once,* stop exercising immediately and call your physician:[6]

1. **Abnormal heart action** — pulse irregular, fluttering, pumping, or palpitations in chest or throat; sudden burst of rapid heartbeats; very slow pulse when a moment earlier it had been high.
2. **Pain or pressure** in the middle chest or in the arm or throat, either during exercise or after exercise.
3. **Dizziness,** lightheadedness, sudden loss of coordination, confusion, cold sweat, glassy stare, pallor, blueness, or fainting. Stop exercise immediately, lie down with your legs and feet elevated, and rest until symptoms stop. Then call your doctor.

If any of the following occur, try the suggested remedy first; if, after a brief period of time, the symptom does not clear up, call your doctor.

1. **Persistent rapid heart action** five to ten minutes after you have stopped exercising. Keep your heart rate lower during exercise (monitor with pulse), and cool down after exercising.
2. **Flare-up of arthritis.** Rest, and do not resume exercising until the symptoms of arthritis have disappeared. If you cannot get relief with your usual remedies, call your doctor.

The following can usually be remedied without medical attention, but if they are a presistent problem, you should call your doctor.

1. **Nausea or vomiting after exercise.** Exercise less vigorously, and take a more gradual cool-down period.
2. **Extreme breathlessness** lasting more than ten minutes after you stop

exercising. Do not exercise so vigorously; never become so breathless during exercise that you cannot speak while exercising.

3. **Prolonged fatigue** even twenty-four hours after exercising or **insomnia** that was not present before starting the exercise program. Exercise less vigorously, and increase your level gradually.

4. **Side stitch.** A spasm in the diaphragm, the side stitch can be relieved by leaning forward while sitting, attempting to push the abdominal organs up against the diaphragm.

HEALTH CLUBS

The kind of exercise that you can get at health clubs is generally not the kind that improves lung and heart function; most cater to isotonic and isometric needs. There are a few exceptions: some offer swimming or cardiovascular exercise such as the exercycle or jogging on a treadmill. If your main exercise needs are for cardiovascular exercise, and if you are on a limited budget, you will probably not be wise to consider joining a health club. If you do, you should look for some factors that indicate the quality of the club.[7]

Ask for the qualifications of the staff. Former athletes or sportsmen who have little or no training are not qualified to run a health club, where staff members are catering to people who have usually been unfit for a period of time and now desire to get fit or lose weight. Good qualifications would include training as a physiotherapist, a remedial gymnast, or an academically qualified teacher of physical education.

The health club should have a variety of good-quality equipment, including leg-exercising machines, a selection of barbell and dumbbell weights, horizontal and sloping benches, wall pulleys, and, most important, a pulsometer.

The health club personnel should require that they check your pulse before they allow you to start exercising. Any health club whose staff gives you the go-ahead to start exercising without giving you any kind of a stress test or pulse test should be viewed with caution.

Good health clubs strictly monitor the progress of their patrons; a club whose staff members allow you to choose your own weights, program your own exercising, or pedal too long on the exercycle is not properly monitoring your progress, and you may not benefit from the gradual buildup of exercise.

You should not join a health club unless you are sure that you have the time to go at least once each week; any less, and you are missing the benefits besides losing money. If you have unused exercise books or equipment at home, you are probably a poor candidate for a health club, most of which require long-term contracts. The classified ads in newspapers in most major cities are full of ads pleading for buyers to relieve owners of their health club memberships.

Watch out for health clubs that try to lure members with special introductory offers; most of the time they are no bargain, and in some cases, the "special" price offered is actually higher than the membership cost.[8]

Ask a health club staff member if you can have two or three trial visits before signing a contract; that way, you can see if you can really utilize the equipment and if you have time to visit the club. If the staff refuses to let you try the facilities two or three times, steer clear!

Take the time to make exercise a regular part of your life — and you will reap the benefits of a longer, happier life that is free from many diseases and afflictions.

Notes

1. Lawrence E. Lamb, ed. *The Health Letter* (San Antonio, Texas: Communications, Inc., September 26, 1975), vol. 6, no. 6.
2. Adapted from Donald B. Ardell, *High Level Wellness* (Emmaus, Pennsylvania: Rodale Press, 1977), pp. 151-158.
3. List of tips compiled and adapted from Laurence E. Morehouse, "You and Your Heart," *Reader's Digest,* October 1971, p. 79; Charles T. Kuntzleman and the editors of *Consumer's Guide, Rating the Exercises* (New York: William Morrow and Company, 1978), pp. 65-77; "The Fitness Mania," *U.S. News and World Report,* February 27, 1978, p. 38; "Are You Getting the Right Kind of Exercise?" *Changing Times,* January 1978, p. 35; and the President's Council on Physical Fitness and Sports, *Cureton's Basic Principles of Physical Fitness Work,* 1973.
4. Morehouse, "You and Your Heart," p. 79.
5. Mary Carpenter, "See Dick Run! See Jane Run! Everybody's Doing It Now!" *SCI/DI,* August 1978, p. 12; and Brian J. Sharkey, *Fitness and Work Capacity* (U.S. Department of Agriculture, Forest Service, Washington, D.C.: U.S. Government Printing Office, May 1977), pp. 55-56.
6. Adapted from Lenore Zohman, *Exercise Your Way to Fitness and Health,* 1974, as reprinted in Sharkey, p. 57.
7. "What To Look for in a Health Club," pp. 152-153 in *Feel Younger, Live Longer* (New York: Rand McNally, 1976).
8. "Thinking of Joining a Health Club? Exercise Caution!" *Family Health,* February, pp. 34, 36.

Self-Evaluation

Assessing Your Fitness

Perform each of the activities below. Read the instructions carefully, and make sure that you follow them precisely. Then check the response that applies to you; be honest in your response. You should *not* take this test without medical permission if you are currently undergoing medical treatment for any problem or if you have a history of heart disease. Stop at once if you feel overstressed.

1. Standing straight, arms to your sides, take a deep breath. Can you hold it for forty-five seconds? (Time yourself with the second hand of a watch.)

   Yes _____   No _____

2. Standing straight, take any clothing off from around your waist. Pinch your body at the waist, holding the flesh between your thumb and forefinger. Can you grab less than one inch of flesh?

   Yes _____   No _____

   (Every quarter of an inch in excess of one inch indicates about ten pounds of body fat.)

3. Standing straight, exhale, letting all of the air out of your lungs. Using a tape measure, measure your chest around the widest part. Next, inhale as deeply as you can, hold the breath, and measure your chest again at the same place. Were there at least three and one-half inches in difference (two and one-half inches for women)?

   Yes _____   No _____

4. Lie down on the floor with your legs flat on the floor. Hook your feet under an immovable object (a heavy dresser, a bed, or a chair that someone is sitting on). Hold your arms straight out in front of you; keeping your arms held straight, sit up slowly until you are in a sitting position. You may bend your knees slightly. Can you repeat this exercise ten times?

   Yes _____   No _____

5. Lie facedown on the floor, and place your hands, palm down, on the floor directly under your shoulders. Keeping your body rigid, do a push-up by straightening both arms at the same time, and then lowering slowly to the original position. Can you, without undue stress, repeat the push-up five times?

   Yes _____   No _____

354

6. Stand with your back straight and flat against a wall; extend your arms straight out in front of you. Raise up to your tiptoes, slowly bend your legs, and move downward until you are in a squatting position; straighten back up again, keeping your arms extended, by sliding back up the wall. Can you repeat this exercise ten times? (If you have cartilage problems in either knee, skip this test.)

Yes _____   No _____

7. Place a strong chair in front of you that has a seat at a distance about eighteen inches from the floor. Face the chair; step up and down onto the seat of the chair, alternating legs. Can you repeat the exercise twenty times?

Yes _____   No _____

8. Run in place for three minutes. Time yourself with a stopwatch or a watch with a second hand. Lift your feet at least four inches off the ground as you run in place. At the end of three minutes, take your pulse, using the method described in this chapter (record for six seconds, multiply by ten). Is your pulse under 120 beats a minute at the end of the exercise?

Yes _____   No _____

9. Sit on the floor with your legs wide apart in front of you and your hands clasped behind your head. Lean forward and touch each elbow to the opposite knee. Can you touch each knee with an elbow without any undue strain?

Yes _____   No _____

Scoring: If you answered "no" to any of the above nine questions, you are not as physically fit as you should be. If you answered "no" to three or more, you are in poor physical condition. The tests included here are designed to measure suppleness, lung capacity, heart strength, endurance, stamina, muscular strength, and body fat. If you had to answer "no" to any question, you should improve the exercise program that you now have; if you do not now have an exercise program, you need to get one. If you were able to complete all of the tests as indicated, but if you suffered pain, discomfort, shortness of breath, or exhaustion due to the exercise test, you should answer "no" to that test.

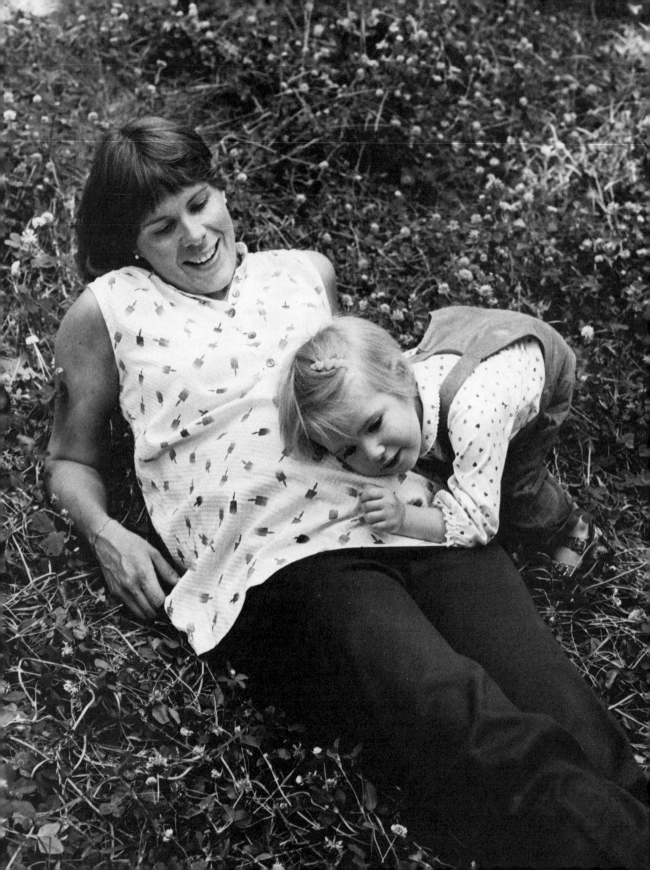

10
Reproduction and Childbirth: New Beginnings

Some of the greatest changes in attitude that have occurred in medicine in the last century are those concerning one of the most basic human functions: that of bearing children.

Many ancient cultures viewed reproduction as a mysterious ritual, little understood and often feared. Even half a century ago, sexuality — the feelings and social patterns that accompanied the physiological drives of sex — was not openly discussed. A woman about to give birth was given general anesthesia and was awarded with her newborn when she awakened. Her anxious husband kept company with a brood of other anxious husbands in a smoke-filled room down the hall.

All of that has changed. We are free — and encouraged — to discuss our sexuality; open forum has led us to a greater understanding of how we function together as men and women and how cultural roles have contributed to our feelings about ourselves. Expectant fathers participate much more actively in both the pregnancy and the birth. We are realizing that there *are* alternatives.

THE FEMALE REPRODUCTIVE SYSTEM ▬▬▬▬▬

   The external genitalia are known collectively as the vulva. A pad of
fatty tissue, the mons veneris is located over the pubic bone; extending
downward and backward from the mons are two folds of skin called the
labia majora — the outer lips of the vulva, sometimes referred to as the
major lips. They surround the inner lips, the labia minora, which are
sensitive and delicate folds of tissue that are not covered by pubic hair
and that swell and darken in response to sexual stimulation. The labia
minora vary greatly in size from woman to woman and sometimes
increase in size with sexual activity. The labia minora join at the upper
front of the vulva just above the clitoris, the seat of sexual sensation in
women.

Figure 10-1.

FEMALE REPRODUCTIVE SYSTEM

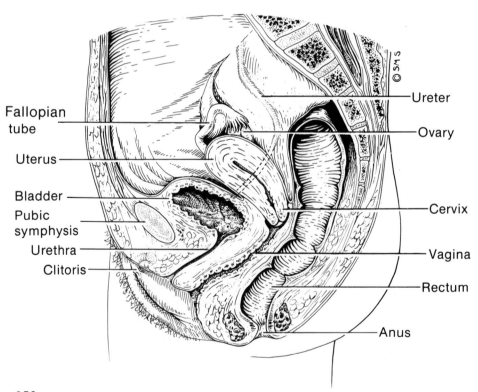

Protected by a soft hood of tissue, the clitoris is often considered the counterpart to the male penis. Composed mainly of erectile tissue and richly endowed with blood and nerves, the clitoris is the part of the genitalia that is most sensitive to touch, and it becomes erect during sexual excitement. It is much smaller than the penis, although it varies in size from woman to woman, and it does not, of course, have a passage for the elimination of urine.

Just below the clitoris is the urethra, the opening of the urinary passage; the labia help direct the flow of urine. Just behind the urethra is the opening to the vagina.

Surrounding the opening of the vagina is the hymen, a membrane that varies in thickness and toughness from woman to woman. In normal circumstances, an unbroken hymen has an opening large enough to permit unrestricted menstrual flow and the insertion of a small tampon. It usually remains intact until it is surgically broken or is ruptured through sexual intercourse. In some women, however, it is so thin and delicate that it is broken through exploration with a finger, the insertion of a tampon, or physical exercise. In other cases — usually extremely rare — the hymen is so thick and tough that it blocks the entire vaginal opening, blocking the menstrual flow; this condition must be surgically corrected. Even after a woman's hymen has been broken and stretched, small parts of the membrane remain.

Lying at an angle between the urinary bladder and the rectum is the vagina, the passageway that connects the outside of the body to the mouth of the uterus.

The inside lining of the vagina is soft, pliable, and moist; although there are no glands, the lining is covered with a mucous membrane. Moistening in the vagina comes mostly from the uterus, although some changes occur during pregnancy, when the vagina secretes a liquid substance that contains lactic acid.

The outer part of the vagina is composed of tough, fibrous tissue and is surrounded by strong muscles that permit the vagina to contract during sexual intercourse and to dilate enormously during childbirth, permitting passage of the baby through the vagina.

At the mouth of the vagina, just inside the vaginal opening, are the Bartholins glands, which secrete the thick lubricating substance essential to intercourse. The secretions of the Bartholins glands are activated in response to sexual stimulation.

Shaped like a flattened, hollow, inverted pear, the uterus is a muscular organ that receives the fertilized egg and houses the growing fetus until birth. The lower part of the uterus is sometimes called the neck of the uterus, or the cervix. The *os,* the opening in the cevix, leads from the uterus to the vagina. The cervix dilates during childbirth to enable the child to move from the uterus into the vagina. The upper part of the uterus is called the corpus. The interior walls of the uterus — so close together most of the time that there is barely a slit — are lined with a mucous membrane called the endometrium, which undergoes change in response to hormones.

The entire uterus is about the size of a small pear or a clenched fist. It is surrounded by a network of strong muscles that contract the uterus to expel the baby at birth.

About four or five inches long, the fallopian tubes (oviducts) extend outward from the top of the uterus, one on each side. Fingerlike projections at the ends of the fallopian tubes are extremely close to the two ovaries but are not actually joined; wavelike motions of the fimbria (the fingerlike projections) and slight suction created by the fallopian tubes draw the ovum into the tube. Tiny cilia, hairlike projections that line the fallopian tubes, continue a wavelike motion to move the ovum along toward the uterus. It is in the fallopian tubes that union of the ovum and sperm takes place.

Approximately the size of an almond and grayish-white in color, the ovaries produce the ova and act to secrete two ovarian hormones — estrogen and progesterone — that are essential to reproduction. While the male produces new sperm constantly, the female is born with all of the ova that she will ever have — a number that ranges from 40,000 to 400,000. Each month, one (or more) of these ova ripens and leaves one of the ovaries, but the female does not actually produce more eggs.

Menstruation

At the beginning of the menstrual cycle, the lining of the uterus is generally quite thin; as a Graafian follicle (which contains the developing ovum) matures and ripens in the ovary, it secretes estrogen, which causes the endometrium to thicken, grow, and become rich in blood and other nutrients capable of nourishing a fetus. This estrogen secretion and change of the endometrium continue for about ten days in the first phase of the menstrual cycle, the proliferative phase.

Just prior to ovulation, the second or secretory phase begins in which the embryo-nourishing substances are released from the endometrium.

THE MENSTRUAL CYCLE

Conception is possible on two or three days out of each month if an intricate set of hormone interactions properly prepare the reproductive organs.

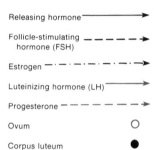

Releasing hormone ⟶

Follicle-stimulating hormone (FSH) ⟶ (dashed)

Estrogen ⟶ (dash-dot)

Luteinizing hormone (LH) ⟶

Progesterone ⟶ (long dash)

Ovum ○

Corpus luteum ●

From Day 1

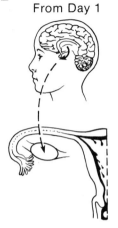

The first day of menstruation represents the beginning of a cycle. It lasts four or five days, during which the hypothalamus secretes a releasing hormone, which signals the pituitary to release follicle-stimulating hormone, FSH.

From Day 5

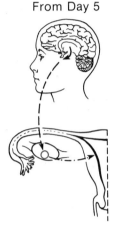

FSH causes the follicles in the ovaries to (1) produce ova and (2) begin estrogen secretion.

Days 5 to 14

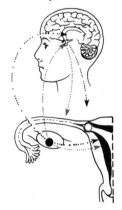

Estrogen (1) causes the lining of the uterus to thicken and (2) causes the hypothalamus to promote luteinizing hormone (LH) release from the pituitary.

Days 14 to 21

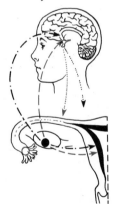

LH causes rupture of the follicle with release of the ovum. The follicle is changed into a corpus luteum which secretes progesterone, a hormone which (1) prepares the uterine lining for implantation and (2) stops the flow of FSH and LH.

Days 21 to 28

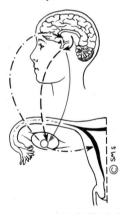

If the ovum is not fertilized, the corpus luteum ceases hormone production; the lining degenerates and is shed as menstrual bleeding. If fertilization does not occur, progesterone secretion stops and the menstrual flow begins.

Figure 10-2.

361

MAJOR CHANGES DURING THE MENSTRUAL CYCLE

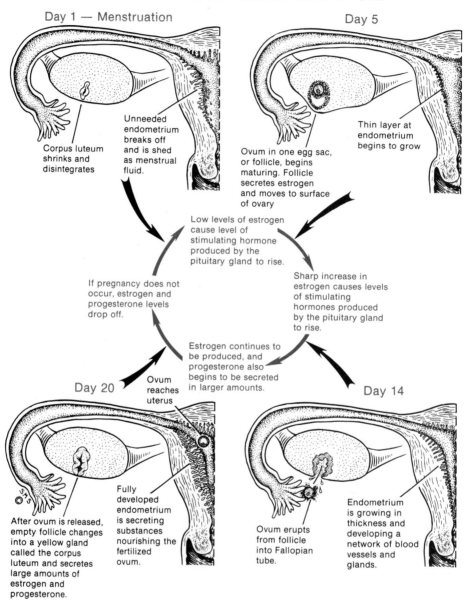

Day 1 — Menstruation

Corpus luteum shrinks and disintegrates

Unneeded endometrium breaks off and is shed as menstrual fluid.

Day 5

Ovum in one egg sac, or follicle, begins maturing. Follicle secretes estrogen and moves to surface of ovary

Thin layer at endometrium begins to grow

Low levels of estrogen cause level of stimulating hormone produced by the pituitary gland to rise.

If pregnancy does not occur, estrogen and progesterone levels drop off.

Sharp increase in estrogen causes levels of stimulating hormones produced by the pituitary gland to rise.

Estrogen continues to be produced, and progesterone also begins to be secreted in larger amounts.

Day 20

Ovum reaches uterus

Fully developed endometrium is secreting substances nourishing the fertilized ovum.

After ovum is released, empty follicle changes into a yellow gland called the corpus luteum and secretes large amounts of estrogen and progesterone.

Day 14

Ovum erupts from follicle into Fallopian tube.

Endometrium is growing in thickness and developing a network of blood vessels and glands.

Figure 10-3.

362

Table 10-1
PROBLEMS ASSOCIATED WITH MENSTRUATION

Problem	Symptoms	Cause	What to Do
Toxic Shock	Vomiting, diarrhea, fever, rash on palms and soles of feet.	Extended retention of tampons; prevents normal removal of staphylococcal toxin by menstrual flow.	1. Avoid highly absorbent tampons. 2. Change every 3-4 hrs. 3. Alternate tampons with sanitary pads. 4. Remove tampons and see a physician if symptoms appear.
Premenstrual Syndrome	Most common in middle-aged adults. Breast tenderness, bloated feeling, headache, tension, irritability, fatigue and depression. Flaring of other chronic problems.	Salt and fluid accumulation in all body tissues.	1. Decrease salt & fluid intake. 2. Mild analgesics aspirin. 3. If symptoms remain, see your doctor.
Dysmenorrhea	Cramping in lower abdomen during menstruation occasionally with nausea and vomiting, headache, pain in back and thighs.	*Simple* — poor posture, sedentary life style, fatigue. *Complex* — hormonal, cysts, tumors, pelvic inflammatory disease.	Usually treated with analgesics, heat to the abdomen, rest and exercise. Hormones, drugs or surgery if cause is more complex.
Endometriosis	Pelvic pain 2-7 days before menstruation until cessation of flow, abnormal uterine bleeding, painful intercourse and/or defecation, sterility.	Retrograde menstruation through fallopian tubes into abdominal cavity. Endometrial tissue outside of uterus.	Become pregnant if condition has just begun; hormone therapy, and/or surgery.

Then, in the third phase, ovulation occurs, and the Graafian follicle becomes a yellowish body called the corpus luteum, releasing the ovum and producing progesterone. The ovum is swept into the fallopian tubes, where it travels toward the uterus, a journey that takes about ten to twelve days. If fertilization does not occur, the corpus luteum gradually disintegrates, and about fourteen days after ovulation has occurred, the lining of the uterus is shed, leaving the body through the vagina in the fourth phase, menstruation. The menstrual flow or fluid is composed of blood, mucous, and cell fragments.

Female Hygiene

Some discharge from the vagina is normal. The healthy vagina cleanses itself daily, carrying out with the discharge the old cells, bacteria, and menstrual blood. Normal vaginal discharge is usually sticky, scant, and clear or white. There are changes during the cycle, however, and the discharge may change in character or appearance while remaining "normal." Normal, healthy vaginal discharge has a mild odor and dries to a yellowish color.

The best hygiene is soap and water. Wash the area of the vulva once each day with mild, nonperfumed soap, rinse thoroughly with warm water, and dry completely. Avoid clothing that is too tight, and avoid wearing synthetic underwear that retains the moisture of the vaginal secretions and perspiration. Cotton underwear is most absorbent and should be worn with loose-fitting clothing to minimize the risk of irritation. Itching or burning may be due to the laundering detergent.

Douching

For most women, douching is unnecessary. Douching removes the normal vaginal secretions and can lead to an imbalance of the vagina's

---

TABLE 10-2

COMMON REPRODUCTIVE TRACT INFECTIONS*

Problem	Symptoms	Treatment
Vaginitis — Bacterial infection, spread by sexual contact	Yellow or grey-green vaginal discharge, vaginal itching	Antibiotics, medicated douche
Trichomoniasis — protozoan; spread by sexual contact or contaminated objects	Itching; thick greyish-white discharge; foul odor. Painful and frequent urination	Medication, douche. Treatment somewhat difficult; risky during pregnancy
Manilia Candida — Yeast infection	Itching and redness of Labia. "Cottage cheese" discharge	Antibiotic vaginal cream, vinegar douching (1 Tblsp./ quart of water) may prevent reinfection
Pubic Lice (crabs) Sexual or other close contact	Mild to intense itching	Shampoo, cream, or lotion, called *Kwell*, applied after thorough cleansing
Veneral Warts Virus	Warts on the genitals	Various medications, surgical removal, freezing cauterization

*For other sexually transmitted diseases, see chapter on Infectious Diseases.

---

usually healthy environment, leading to vaginal infection. In addition, the force of douching can push contaminated fluid or material into the uterus or fallopian tubes, where it can lead to massive infection. In any case:

1. Do not douche more than once a week.
2. Use only plain warm water — it cleanses just about as well as anything else and is less irritating.
3. Use gentle pressure — *never* hang a bag douche from the shower head or curtain rod! A hanging bag should be hung no more than two or three feet above your body; if you use a bulb syringe, use gentle pressure.
4. Never douche in the presence of an infection — the pressure of the douche could force contaminated water into the uterus or fallopian tubes.

Menopause

Occurring anywhere between the ages of thirty-five and fifty-eight — and usually around the age of fifty — menopause marks the end of menstruation. Menopause is a significant event in a woman's life, because it marks the end of the reproductive period.

A number of physical changes take place in connection with the menopause. Most common are "hot flashes," flushes of the upper body and the face that are often followed by profuse perspiration and periods of chilliness. Occasionally, numbness, tingling of the hands, headaches, dizziness, and palpitations of the heart may accompany the hot flashes.

Other significant physical changes that may occur with menopause include thinning of hair on the head; thickening and darkening of hair on the upper lip; constipation; urinary frequency; softening of the bones or chemical changes in the bones that cause them to become brittle; pain in the joints; tenderness and pain in the muscles; loss of elasticity in the skin, resulting in flabbiness of the breasts, upper abdomen, and upper arms; overweight (the famous "middle-age spread"); tendency to high blood pressure; and nervousness that includes fatigue, irritability, apprehension, and, sometimes, crying spells. Depression often occurs with menopause as women who have married and established families watch their children leave home to marry and establish their own families — a condition known as the "empty nest syndrome".

Adjustment to menopause depends a great deal on how well the woman has adjusted to problems throughout her life. Those who are immature and emotionally unstable generally have a difficult time, but women who have learned to solve problems in a mature, calm way and who have learned to deal with their emotions generally adjust to menopause well.

Because the metabolism is slowed after menopause, a woman's dietary needs are reduced. Good nutrition is, as always, essential, but caloric intake should be substantially reduced. A woman who has gone through menopause needs to make sure that she has enough calcium and vitamin D in her diet. Exercise can improve muscle tone, improve circulation, help to reduce high blood pressure, and can prevent weight gain following menopause.

Hysterectomy

Hysterectomy — partial or total surgical removal of the female reproductive tract organs — is an operation that reached new highs in the late 1970s (more than 700,000 a year were being performed in the United States alone). In some cases, a hysterectomy can save a life; in others, the surgery is used as a corrective measure for what may be, in reality, a minor medical problem.

Reasons for Hysterectomy

There are four situations in which a hysterectomy may be performed to save a woman's life:

1. To remove a cancerous vagina, cervix, uterus, fallopian tubes, or ovaries.
2. As part of lifesaving surgery involving removal or correction of the bladder or intestine when it is technically impossible to avoid removing the uterus as well.
3. To stop severe, uncontrolled bleeding (hemorrhage) that threatens the life of the woman.

4. To correct severe and uncontrolled infection that could spread and threaten the life of the woman.

While hysterectomy has been used widely to correct a number of medical conditions, some medical situations do warrant the performance of a hysterectomy:

1. A woman's monthly menstrual flow is so heavy that it causes anemia, and it has resisted medication or hormone therapy.
2. Extensive endometriosis exists.
3. A woman has recurrent pelvic infections that are difficult to control with medication and that leave an extensive amount of scar tissue.
4. The woman has lost muscular support in the pelvis (usually as a result of childbirth), and this condition is interfering with normal bowel or bladder function.
5. The woman has large fibroid tumors or an extensive number of fibroid tumors — especially a problem if they cause disabling pain or interfere with bladder function.

▬▬▬▬▬ THE MALE REPRODUCTIVE SYSTEM

The male reproductive system consists of both external and internal organs of reproduction. The two external organs are the penis and the scrotum.

The penis, designed to conduct the sperm to the outside and to penetrate the vagina, is composed of erectile, spongy, cavernous tissue. The glans penis, located at the end of the penis, is highly sensitive and richly endowed with nerves — the counterpart to the female clitoris.

In an uncircumcised male, the glans penis is covered by a fold of skin called the foreskin. Elastic in nature, it stretches easily and can be pushed back to expose the glans penis. It is not attached to the glans penis directly but is attached about one inch below the glans.

As a result of stimulation by touch, sight, smell, or thought, the penis, normally flaccid, becomes large and stiff — necessary to prepare for penetration of the vagina in intercourse. However, an erection does not necessarily signal the need to have an ejaculation or to experience intercourse.

Erection is accomplished by messages from the spine that cause the arteries that feed blood to the corpus spongiosum, a bed of erectile tissue

MALE REPRODUCTIVE SYSTEM

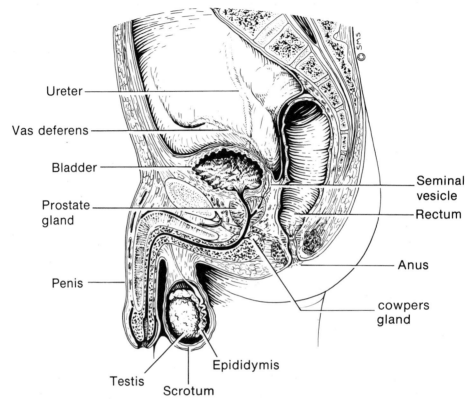

Ureter

Vas deferens

Bladder

Prostate
gland

Penis

Testis

Scrotum

Epididymis

Seminal
vesicle

Rectum

Anus

cowpers
gland

Figure 10-4.

that encloses and surrounds the urethra, to dilate, resulting in erection.
The muscles at the base of the penis contract, preventing the flow of the
blood out of the vessels; there is generally about six times the normal
amount of blood in the penis during erection.

The scrotum is the dark-colored pouch of skin below the penis that
holds the testicles. The scrotum varies in texture and color from male to
male but is generally darker in pigmentation than the skin on the rest of
the body and is usually wrinkly in appearance.

There are two testicles that descend from the abdominal cavity into
the scrotum about one month before birth. The descension into the
scrotum is essential to fertility, since a temperature about four degrees

368

lower than normal body temperature is required for the production of sperm. Occasionally, testicles do not descend, and sperm production fails to occur. If one descends, however, the man is usually fertile.

Each testis in the adult male is filled with about eight hundred tightly coiled tubes called *seminiferous tubules.* Sperm develop in these tubules, and testosterone (the male sex hormone) develops in the cells surrounding the tubules.

The epididymis is a long, coiled structure that rests on the testicles within the scrotum. As new sperm are produced in the seminiferous tubules, the old sperm are pushed into the epididymis, where the sperm mature in a fluid produced by the epididymis until they are either ejaculated or until they disintegrate.

As sperm leave the epididymis, they are carried by a long excretory duct called the vas deferens. There is one duct leading from each testicle; about eighteen inches long, each duct leads up into the pelvis, around the bladder, and down toward the urethra. The end of the vas deferens that is closest to the penis is wider, forming a small pouch called the ampullae, which stores sperm.

As the sperm pass through the vas deferens and eventually through the penis during ejaculation, secretions from several glands are added to make up the seminal fluid.

1. **The seminal vesticles,** located at the end of the vas deferens, produce a substance that gives the sperm cells energy for the movement required to reach the ovum.
2. **The prostate gland** secretes an alkaline substance that counteracts the acid environment of the vagina and aids in movement of the sperm. The prostate gland is located at the juncture of the vas deferens and the urethra below the urinary bladder.
3. **The Cowper's glands,** adjacent to the prostate gland, produce an alkaline fluid that neutralizes the acidity of the urethra and lubricates it for the passage of the seminal fluid through the urethra.

COMMON SEXUAL DISORDERS

Sexual problems occur in an estimated one-half of American marriages. While a few are the result of strictly physical causes (such as diabetes, injury, or birth defects), most are emotional or psychological in origin and result from other marital problems. Some are even due to simple ignorance about normal sexual functioning.

Male Sexual Dysfunction

Impotence is the inability of a man to achieve an erection or his inability to maintain it long enough to complete the act of intercourse. There are three kinds of impotence — organic, psychogenic, and functional.

Organic impotence, the least common of the three, occurs when there is something physically wrong with the structure of the penis, its blood supply, or with the nervous supply. In such a condition, the individual cannot achieve an erection even though emotionally and psychologically aroused.

More common is functional impotence — where the nervous system is temporarily not functioning due to fatigue, certain drugs, too much alcohol, inadequate hormone levels, circulatory problems, or physical exhaustion.

By far the most common type of impotence is psychogenic — emotional inhibitions or fears that affect approximately 85 percent of those men who are impotent. The fears or emotional inhibitions block the impulses that control the erection process. Such emotional inhibitions range from self-doubt on the job to fear of causing a pregnancy.

It should be remembered that a single failure to achieve erection on a given occasion does not indicate impotence. Almost all men are unable to achieve an erection or to maintain it long enough at some time. Impotence is indicated by a failure to achieve an erection in one-fourth of all attempts. A man who has had a successful and satisfying sex life may suddenly one day, for any number of reasons, be unable to achieve or maintain an erection. If this happens several times in a row, his own fear and apprehension about the situation may serve to compound the problem, causing the impotence to linger. This fear of failure literally becomes a type of self-fulfilling prophecy.

Premature ejaculation simply denotes a lack of voluntary control over the ejaculatory reflex. Like impotence, occasional loss of control is of no concern. Becoming anxious over the situation can turn it into a chronic problem.

Some men simply do not recognize the sensations that immediately precede ejaculation. Other men — especially those whose sexual life began early under situations of high anxiety (in parked cars, fear of being caught) — have been conditioned to ejaculate quickly. Premature ejaculation can also result from using withdrawal as a birth control practice, or from selfishness and disregard for his wife's pleasure. In only rare cases is there a physical cause for premature ejaculation.

Female Sexual Dysfunction

Frigidity. No connection has been established between a woman's lack of responsiveness toward sex and her partner's technique, her upbringing, her lack of sex education, her religious beliefs, traumatic sexual experiences, attitudes toward sex, general mental health, or premarital and extramarital sexual experience. The inability to be sexually responsive strikes women in any circumstance, any age group, and any range of experience. Some women simply find no physical enjoyment in the act of intercourse.

Orgasmic difficulty. There are three main complaints about orgasmic difficulty that are most common: the inability to achieve orgasm at all; the ability to achieve orgasm through means other than intercourse (such as masturbation), but not through intercourse; and the inability to achieve an orgasm quickly enough during the act of intercourse.

The causes of orgasmic difficulty are much the same as the causes of frigidity — a woman who has feelings of guilt or anxiety may not be able to "let herself go" enough to experience an orgasm through intercourse even when she is relaxed and happy.

Vaginismus is a powerful, painful contraction of the muscles that surround the vagina. The most severe cases make penetration completely impossible; more mild cases simply make penetration difficult, delaying it for a time. In a small percentage of the cases, vaginismus may be due to a physical abnormality — such as an infection that makes intercourse extremely painful. Most commonly, it is due to emotional trauma associated with early, traumatic sexual experiences (including rape) or with fear of intercourse. Strangely enough, vaginismus rarely afflicts women in lower socioeconomic strata; the phenomenon almost exclusively affects women in upper income groups. Treatment of vaginismus demands patience and understanding from the husband, who can cause considerable harm by trying to force the woman to have intercourse while she is suffering from the painful spasms.

PREGNANCY

The ovum remains alive for about forty-eight hours after it is released from the ovary, and fertilization occurs most of the time in the end of the fallopian tube farthest from the uterus. During intercourse, the semen is deposited in the upper end of the vagina. It contains millions of sperm cells that begin the journey through the cervix, the uterus, and the fallopian tube, a journey requiring about seven or eight hours.

Figure 10-5.

MENSTRUATION, OVULATION, PREGNANCY

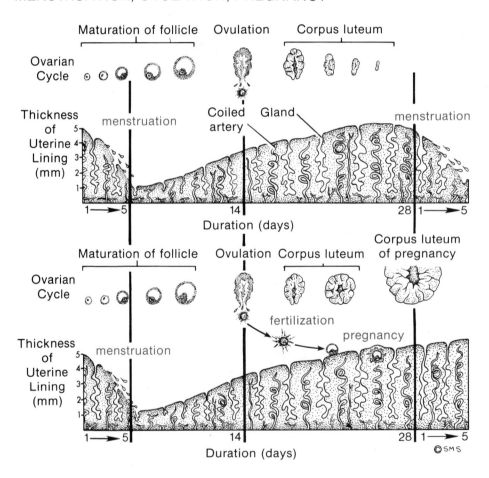

OVULATION, FERTILIZATION OF AN OVUM

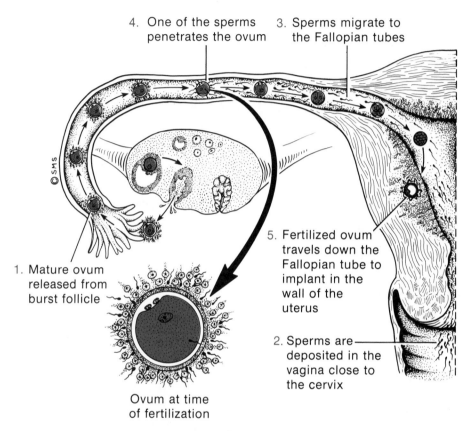

4. One of the sperms penetrates the ovum

3. Sperms migrate to the Fallopian tubes

1. Mature ovum released from burst follicle

5. Fertilized ovum travels down the Fallopian tube to implant in the wall of the uterus

2. Sperms are deposited in the vagina close to the cervix

Ovum at time of fertilization

Figure 10-6. During sexual intercourse, sperm cells are deposited in the vagina in the seminal fluid ejaculated by the man. They then travel up through the uterus to the Fallopian tubes to meet the ovum. Fertilization occurs when one of the sperms penetrates the ovum, after which the fertilized egg continues its journey to the uterus.

The sperm stay alive in the uterus and fallopian tubes about three days. The fertile days of the menstrual cycle are the three days preceding ovulation, the day of ovulation, and the day following ovulation.[1] By charting the menstrual cycle over a period of one to two years, the period of fertility can generally be accurately calculated.

When the sperm reach the ovum, they group around it in enormous numbers, but only one fertilizes it. The process of fertilization is completed when one sperm penetrates, the tail drops off, and the head

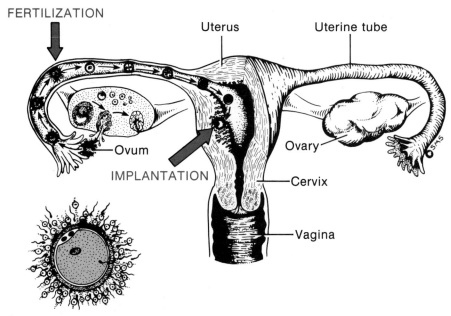

FERTILIZATION

Uterus

Uterine tube

Ovum

IMPLANTATION

Ovary

Cervix

Vagina

Ovum at Moment of Fertilization

Figure 10-7. In the uterus, the fertilized egg attaches itself to the uterine lining.

merges with the nucleus of the ovum. The fertilized ovum, or zygote, then moves to the uterus, where it becomes implanted in the endometrium and begins the growth process.

Pregnancy is diagnosed by means of a test usually administered by a physician. A number of in-home pregnancy tests available on the market have an accuracy of about 95 to 98 percent[2] if used correctly.

Changes During Pregnancy

A number of changes occur in the body during pregnancy, and these can be used to determine pregnancy even before a test confirms the condition.

374

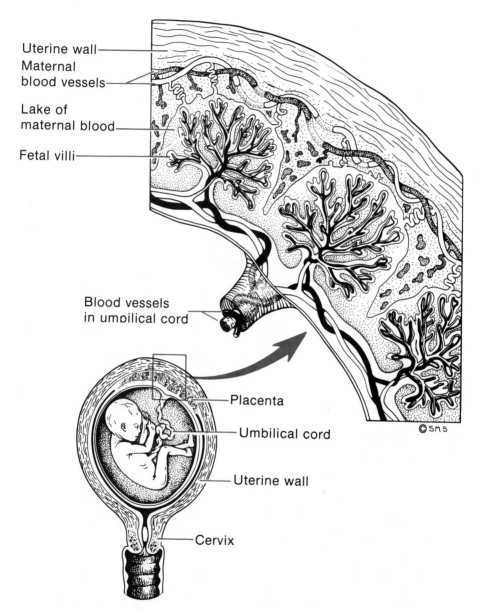

Figure 10-8. The placenta develops early in pregnancy and normally occupies an area high in the uterus. The maternal and fetal circulations do not mix, but are able to exchange nutrients and waste products across the placenta. Maternal blood is pumped into "lakes" which surround the villi containing delicate fetal blood vessels. The placenta now secretes hormones.

Labels in figure:
- Uterine wall
- Maternal blood vessels
- Lake of maternal blood
- Fetal villi
- Blood vessels in umbilical cord
- Placenta
- Umbilical cord
- Uterine wall
- Cervix

©SMS

The first, and most obvious, symptom of pregnancy is the cessation of menstruation. That is the only symptom that some women ever experience; most, however, suffer one or more of the following during pregnancy:[3]

1. Nausea and/or vomiting, especially during the first trimester of pregnancy, and usually during the morning (hence the term "morning sickness"). The nausea and vomiting may occur later in the day, and in some it is a special problem after meals.
2. A sensation of weight in the uterus due to the swelling of the growing embryo.
3. Abundant salivation *(ptyalism)*.
4. Pain and tenderness in the breasts; because of the development and growth of the mammary gland, the breast feels tight. Additional blood circulation to the breasts results in large blue veins appearing just beneath the skin. The breasts enlarge, and the skin around the areola darkens. The areola itself darkens and gets larger; the oil glands surrounding it become prominent and begin secreting sebum, an oily fluid. The nipples become larger, get darker, and are erectile.
5. Sudden dizziness; in some cases, women faint frequently, although such fainting is not common.
6. Bladder problems, especially the frequent, urgent need to urinate. As the uterus increases in size, it places pressure on the bladder. The problem decreases as the pregnancy advances, since the uterus rises in the abdomen; the problem recurs during the last month or two of pregnancy, when the uterus descends again.
7. Toothaches and headaches, especially a problem to those who are prone to them or who have frequent headaches and toothaches when not pregnant.
8. Changing moods, especially frequent irritability and depression.
9. Changing tastes in food; many women develop a craving for some foods and a loathing for others. This appears to be purely psychological. In many cases, cigarettes and coffee, which tend to increase nausea, are intolerable.
10. Hot flashes in the face and upper half of the body, accompanied at times by tingling in the hands.
11. Unjustified fatigue; inability to do simple tasks that ordinarily require little energy.
12. During the final months of pregnancy, breathing can become difficult due to the fetus crowding the diaphragm and lungs.

CHILD ABUSE & NEGLECT

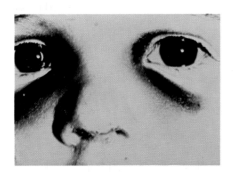

Child Abuse

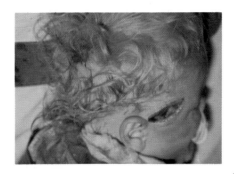

Physical Abuse

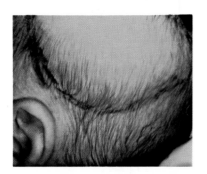

Child Neglect

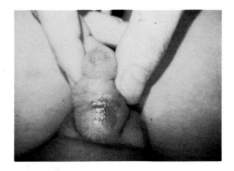

Sexual Abuse

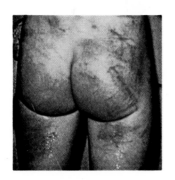

Physical Abuse

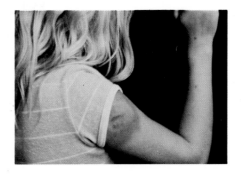

Physical Abuse

FETAL GROWTH & DEVELOPMENT

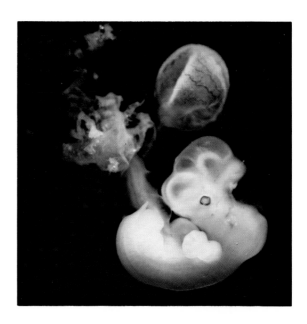

5 weeks old, two-fifths of an inch long.

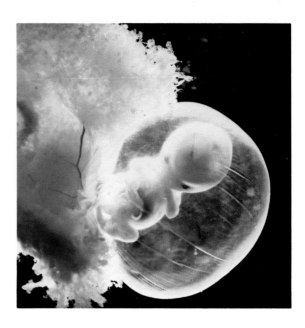

7 weeks old, nearly an inch long, and weighing about 2 grams.

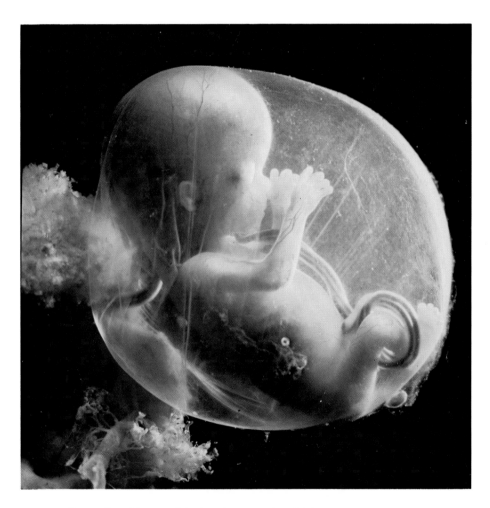

3 months old, over 3 inches long, and weighing almost an ounce.

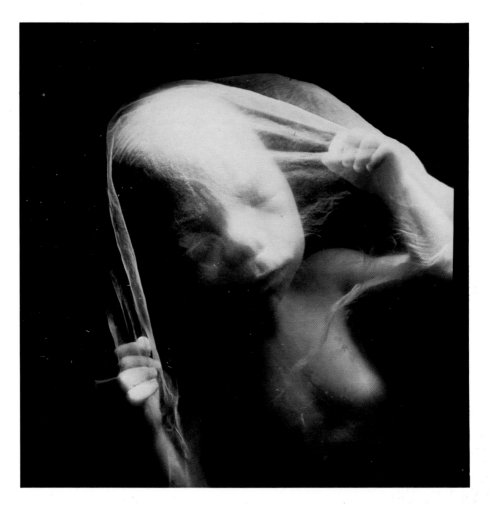

4 months old, more than 6 inches long, and weighing about 7 ounces.

FETAL GROWTH & DEVELOPMENT

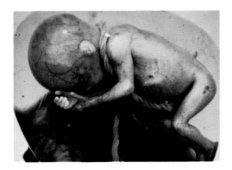

Fetus in Amniotic Sac

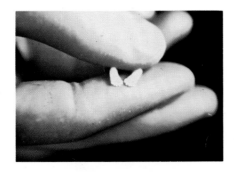

Feet of Ten Week Fetus

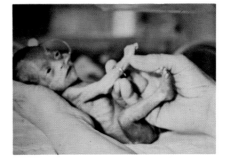

Premature Infant Approximately 5 months

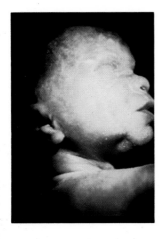

Premature Stillbirth

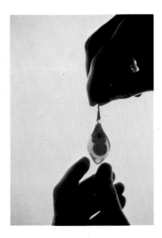

Early Fetus in Amnion

CHILDBIRTH

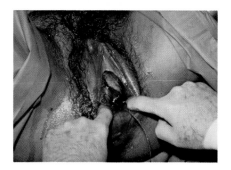

Early Crowning

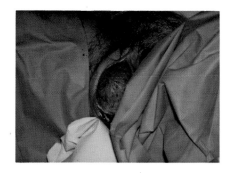

Late Crowning

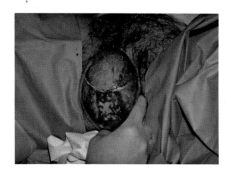

Head Delivering

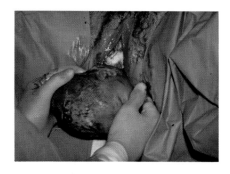

Head Delivers and Turns

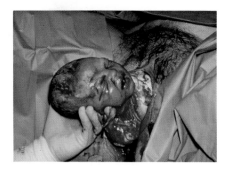

Shoulders Deliver

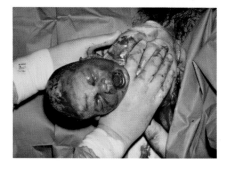

Chest Delivers

CHILDBIRTH

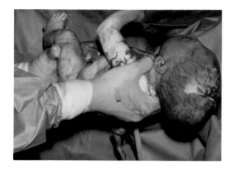

Infant Delivered

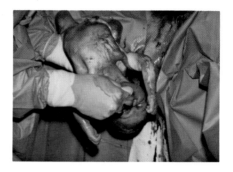

Suctioning Airway

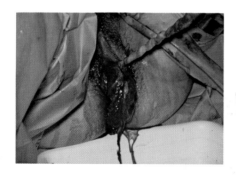

Placenta Begins Delivery

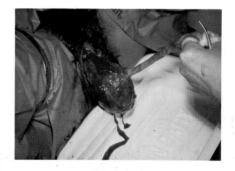

Placenta Delivers

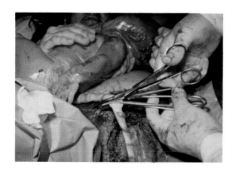

Cutting of Cord

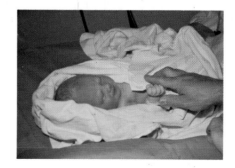

Wrap the Baby

CARDIOVASCULAR DISEASE

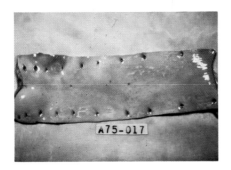

Inside Surface Normal Artery

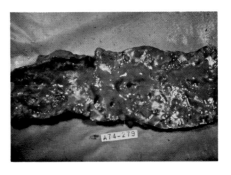

Inside Surface Severe Atherosclerosis

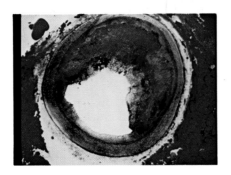

Artery Cross-Section Atherosclerosis

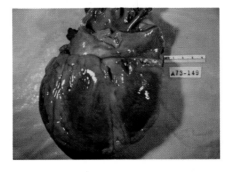

Myocardial Infarction

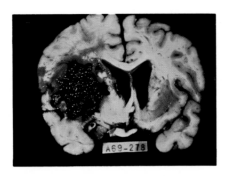

Cerebralvascular Accident (Stroke)

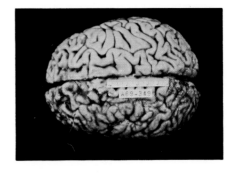

Stroke Damaged Brain

13. Pigmented brownish-pink striations appear on the breast, the skin of the abdomen, around the vulva, and on the thighs. The linea nigra, a brown pigmented line in the center of the abdomen, appears. Brownish-pink patches of pigmentation — often called "pregnancy mask" — appear on the face.

14. Alterations in the vagina include congestion with blood vessels, making it appear reddish or violet. The cervical canal becomes filled with a thick mucous plug that prevents infection from entering the uterine cavity; the mucous-forming glands around the cervix are so active, in fact, that many women experience heavy vaginal discharge during pregnancy.

Most of the above changes are temporary, and the body returns in most cases to normal within a few months following the pregnancy. Changes in the breasts usually last as long as the mother nurses the baby, and some of the pigmentation changes may be permanent.

Signs of Trouble in Early Pregnancy

Miscarriage

Miscarriage — spontaneous abortion — is much more common than many people think, occurring in about 15 percent of all pregnancies. Most miscarriages occur between the fourth and twelfth weeks of pregnancy. Something happens to alter the course of the pregnancy, and the pregnancy naturally ends before a hazardous situation develops.

Signs that indicate an impending miscarriage include:

1. Abdominal pain, with or without fever.
2. The last period was late; current bleeding is extremely heavy, containing blood clots and, possibly, small clumps of tissue; menstrual cramps are more severe than usual.
3. The period lasts longer and is heavier than usual, featuring five to seven days of bleeding characteristic of the usual "heavy" days.
4. Heavy bleeding (a good cue to a hemorrhage situation is soaking ten tampons or pads in a period of two hours).

Always seek medical attention for a miscarriage, even if it occurs

Figure 10-9.

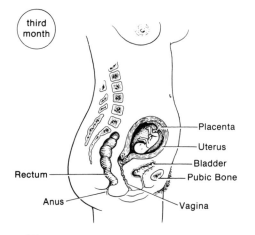

third month

The baby is now about 3 inches long and weighs about 1 ounce. It may continue to develop in the position shown or may turn or rotate frequently. The uterus begins to enlarge with the growing fetus and can now be felt extending about halfway up to the umbilicus.

Placenta

Uterus

Bladder

Pubic Bone

Rectum

Anus

Vagina

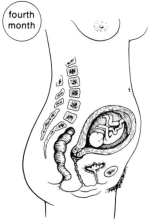

fourth month

The baby is now about 6½-7 inches long and weighs about 4 ounces. It has a strong heartbeat, fair digestion, and active muscles. Its skin is bright pink and transparent and is covered with a fine, downlike hair. Most bones are distinctly indicated throughout the body.

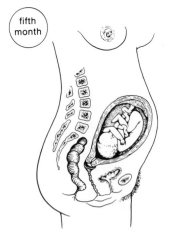

fifth month

The baby measures about 10-12 inches long and weighs from ½ to 1 pound. It is still bright red. Its increased size now brings the dome of the uterus to the level of the umbilicus. The internal organs are maturing at astonishing speed, but the lungs are insufficiently developed to cope with the conditions outside of the uterus.

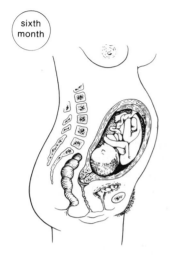

sixth month

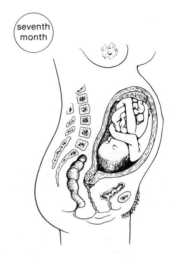

seventh month

At the end of the 6th month, the baby measures 11-14 inches and may weigh from 1¼-1½ pounds.

At 7 months, the premature baby has a fair chance for survival in nurseries cared for by skilled physicians and nurses.

In the absence of premature labor, the growth and maturation of the baby in the last 2 months are extremely valuable. From 1½ to 3 pounds at the beginning of the month, it will add from 2-2½ more pounds and will lengthen to 16½-18 inches by the end of the eighth month.

At birth or full term, the baby weighs on an average about 7 pounds if a girl and 7½ if a boy. Its length is about 20 inches.

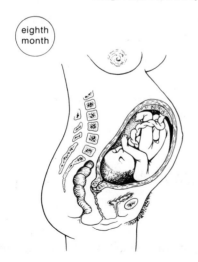

eighth month

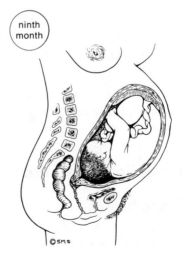

ninth month

©SMS

early in the pregnancy — the miscarriage may be incomplete, leaving behind pieces of tissue that will cling to the uterine wall and cause infection or hemorrhage.

Ectopic Pregnancy

Ectopic pregnancy — implantation of the zygote outside the uterine cavity, usually in a fallopian tube — can be life-threatening if it is not diagnosed and corrected early. The developing fetus increases in size, stretching the tissue of the tube and eventually (usually about the seventh or eighth week of pregnancy) causing the tube to rupture. This complication can result in severe hemorrhage.

Indicators of ectopic pregnancy include the following:

1. Irregular or light bleeding after a late period or after an abnormally light period; this light bleeding or spotting is accompanied by abdominal pain.
2. Fainting or dizziness (a sign of internal bleeding).
3. Sudden, intense pain in the lower abdomen, usually localized on one side; the pain may be accompanied by cramping or may become persistent. Do not look for bleeding from the vagina as a sign of tubal rupture: internal bleeding will not show through the vagina.
4. A history of gonorrhea or pelvic infection. Scar tissue may block the fallopian tubes, causing the zygote to implant there.
5. Conception occurred with an IUD in place.

A physician or emergency room should be contacted in the event of any symptoms suggestive of ectopic pregnancy.

Complications Later in Pregnancy

Toxemia

Usually occurring late in pregnancy or just after delivery, toxemia is

380

divided into two phases — preeclampsia and eclampsia. Preeclampsia, occurring during pregnancy, is characterized by high blood pressure, swelling of body tissue (especially the ankles and feet), and the presence of protein in the urine. The earliest and most dependable sign of toxemia is high blood pressure. Eclampsia is characterized by convulsions and, in some cases, coma.

While it is not certain what causes toxemia, women who are at risk for developing the disease have been identified: those who (a) have their first baby at a young age, (b) are diabetic, (c) have a family history of eclampsia, (d) have high blood pressure, (e) are suffering from malnutrition, or (f) have vascular or kidney disease.

Treatment for preeclampsia involves getting bed rest, drinking plenty of fluids, and being observed closely by a physician. Eclampsia requires medication.

Hemorrhage

During the first half of pregnancy, hemorrhage is usually a result of miscarriage or ectopic pregnancy. During the second half of pregnancy, hemorrhage can be a sign of abnormal placental location, chronic high blood pressure, dietary deficiencies, toxemia, injury, or premature separation of the placenta. The most serious hemorrhage occurs just after birth in cases where the placenta is torn. External massage of the uterus, external ice bag application to the uterine area, and medication are usually helpful in controlling postpartum hemorrhage. When other attempts fail, placing the baby at the mother's breast usually causes the uterus to contract enough to stop the bleeding.

Determining the Due Date

The due date of a baby is usually calculated from the first day of the menstrual period: (1) Subtract three months from the date of the first day of the last menstrual period; then add seven days. For instance, if the last menstrual period started on August 10, go back three months to May 10, and add seven days: May 17; (2) Count 280 days from the first day of the last menstrual period.

While these are only estimates, they are generally quite accurate; a physician can determine the due date more closely as the pregnancy advances by assessing various signs and symptoms and by monitoring the fetal growth.

TWINS

IDENTICAL TWINS

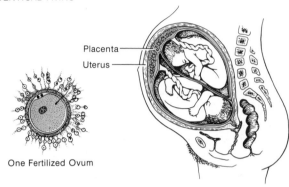

Placenta
Uterus

One Fertilized Ovum

NONIDENTICAL TWINS

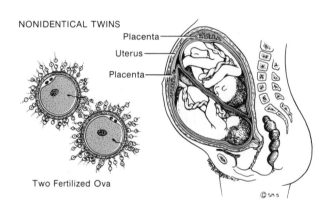

Placenta
Uterus
Placenta

Two Fertilized Ova

Figure 10-10. Identical twins are the result of a fertilized egg dividing into two identical cells which then separate and develop independently. Since both twins are derived from one sperm and one egg, they are genetically identical. Nonidentical twins are no more genetically similar than ordinary brothers and sisters; they develop from two different ova (each fertilized by separate sperms) and have separate placentas.

Ultrasound

With ultrasound — echoes of sound waves translated into visual images — it is possible to follow the development of the fetus without the use of x-rays. No pain is involved, and no instruments intrude into the baby's sheltered world. Ultrasound is usually used to answer some clinical question about whether the pregnancy is progressing normally. By far the most common use of ultrasound is to determine true fetal age when the date of conception is unknown due to a miscalculation or mistake. Ultrasound is also used to confirm the suspicion of a multiple pregnancy.

382

In a sonogram (or ultrasound picture), the bones — the densest tissue — show up as white areas, while the less dense tissues, such as muscles show up as gray. The fluid-filled areas are reflected as black areas on the pictures. Ultrasound can detect a fetus as early as the seventh week of pregnancy and can follow the fetal development throughout the pregnancy.

Labor and Childbirth

Stages of Childbirth

Childbirth is divided into three stages, the first one being labor. In labor, the cervix effaces (thins) and dilates. In early labor, the cervix dilates two or three centimeters. The woman may experience abdominal cramping and mild, regular contractions. In the second, or active phase of labor, dilatation progresses from three to seven centimeters. Uterine contractions will be longer, lasting between forty and sixty seconds. They will be more intense and will occur more frequently (every three to five minutes). In the third or transition phase of labor, the cervix dilates from seven to ten centimeters. When the cervix is fully dilated, the baby's head can pass through. Contractions during this phase become very frequent (every two or three minutes) and are intense and long-lasting (fifty to ninety seconds). This is generally considered the most difficult phase of labor, but it is soon followed by the next stage of childbirth — expulsion.

During expulsion, the baby moves down the birth canal and is born. The mother must add her own bearing-down efforts to the uterine contractions in order to push the baby out of the birth canal. The miraculous process of birth involves flexion, then extension of the baby's head, and internal rotation in order for the baby to deliver.

In the third stage of childbirth, delivery of the placenta, the woman will experience quite mild contractions — perhaps as few as one or two. A shot is administered in the arm or hip following delivery of the placenta to help keep the uterus contacted and prevent bleeding.

The final phase is called postpartum, and during this period, the mother's vital signs stabilize. She is carefully monitored during this recovery phase.

MECHANISMS OF NORMAL LABOR

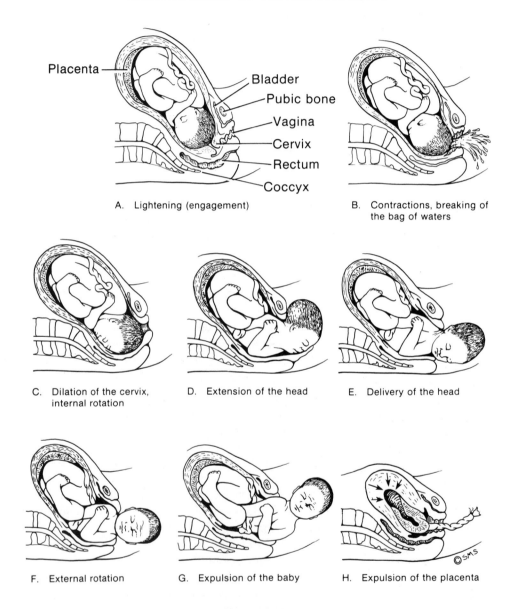

A. Lightening (engagement)

Placenta
Bladder
Pubic bone
Vagina
Cervix
Rectum
Coccyx

B. Contractions, breaking of the bag of waters

C. Dilation of the cervix, internal rotation

D. Extension of the head

E. Delivery of the head

F. External rotation

G. Expulsion of the baby

H. Expulsion of the placenta

Figure 10-11.

384

Kinds of Delivery

Once women were put under general anesthesia during birth; now, a wide range of options is available to women. The following methods are in general use in the United States.

Natural Childbirth

In its strictest sense, natural childbirth describes birth that occurs with the benefit of no painkillers and with the parents having no training in breathing techniques, relaxation techniques, or other such education in prenatal classes. In many areas, it means that the mother does not even go to the hospital to have the baby. Natural childbirth is often used to describe the condition that allows the mother to be awake, aware, and undrugged during delivery — usually in a hospital. Some women experience intense pain during natural childbirth, and others feel little pain or no pain at all.

Prepared Childbirth

A recently coined term, prepared childbirth refers to the situation where the parents are given the best possible preparation for the childbirth — including classes, lectures, exercise instruction, explanation of theories on labor management, display and demonstration of infant care, and tours of maternity and obstetrics departments in the hospital where the birth will occur. The theory behind prepared childbirth is to educate the parents to the fullest extent possible so that myths will dissolve and education will alleviate fear and apprehension concerning the birth process.

LeBoyer Method

Concerned with the trauma that birth imposes on the baby, a French doctor devised a method of delivery that is designed to reduce such trauma. The lights in the delivery room are dimmed, there is little noise

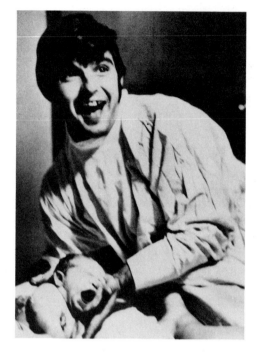

In the Lamaze method, the husband is trained to be an active part of the delivery team and is critical in coaching his wife in the breathing techniques.

(the doctors and nurses are encouraged to speak with soothing voices), the room temperature is kept higher than usual, and the baby is given a soothing, warm bath as soon as it is born. Many doctors disagree with this method, and if you desire to use it, you will need to discuss it with your doctor in advance.

Lamaze Method

Named after another French doctor, the Lamaze method centers on breathing techniques that are designed to reduce the pain of labor and delivery. Relaxation techniques are taught, and the woman is trained to almost hypnotize herself by staring fixatedly at some object of her own choosing. The husband is trained to be an active part of the delivery team and is critical in coaching his wife in the breathing techniques. The Lamaze technique requires extensive training in prenatal classes; Lamaze classes are currently the most popular prenatal classes in the nation.

Dick-Read Method

A British doctor designed the classes that teach a method of slow abdominal breathing that are supposed to allow the mother to concentrate on the signals that her body sends during labor and delivery. The Dick-Read method is reputedly harder to learn and master than some of the other relaxation techniques; there are no assistants or props used in the Dick-Read method — the woman operates with only the help of the doctor in the actual delivery.

Bradley Method

An approach that is more than thirty years old, the Bradley method combines breathing exercises, relaxation exercises, emphasis on proper nutrition, and coaching by the husband. The emphasis of the Bradley method is on the woman and her husband being able to do what comes naturally for them during pregnancy, labor, and delivery.

Cesarian Section

A number of factors may make it necessary for the baby to be taken through a surgical incision in the uterine wall rather than passing through the vagina. Some of these include venereal disease (the baby passing through the birth canal can be infected from contact with chancres or herpes sores); vaginal injuries that could be aggravated by normal delivery; certain disease conditions (including diabetes, which in many cases results in stillbirths if the baby is allowed to go full term); excessive birth weight (that may cause pelvic fracture); obstruction of the birth canal; or prolonged labor that endangers the life of the baby. In some cases, the baby does not present itself for birth in the normal head-down position; instead, the buttocks may appear in the birth canal first, or an arm and leg may be presented. Unless the physician can quickly turn the baby to the proper position without injury to the baby or the mother, emergency cesarian is performed.

The surgical incision leaves a scar on the uterine wall, and, although this is controversial, subsequent babies may also have to be delivered cesarian. The concern is that allowing the baby to go full term and allowing the uterus to contract as in normal labor can result in rupture of the uterine wall at the scar site.

Midwives

In forty-eight of the fifty states, a woman can legally choose to have her baby delivered by a midwife instead of a physician. In order to qualify, the midwife has to be trained by an accredited institution and must be licensed as a certified nurse-midwife. In twenty states, lay midwives — women who have some training in the procedures of childbirth but who are not certified — can deliver a baby.

Women generally choose midwives because of their preference for a female practitioner (and their inability to find a woman obstetrician), their preference for less technical birth surroundings, or the economic factors involved (a midwife charges much less than an obstetrician in most cases, and since many midwives deliver at home, the costs are further reduced).

Birthing Rooms

A number of hospitals across the nation have adopted the concept of providing a birthing room for women who desire it. Under most conditions, the birthing room is decorated like a bedroom — with carpeting, wallpaper, and occasional furniture. Instead of being moved from a labor room to a delivery room, the couple comes first to the birthing

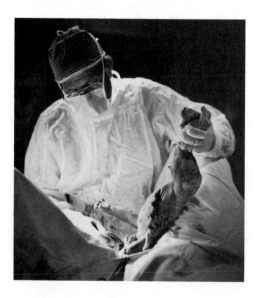

A variety of birthing options are now available.

388

room and stays there during the entire birth process. The husband is allowed to be present, and in most hospitals, the woman may choose to have one or two other adults present for the labor and birth. The baby is not taken from the mother following birth; the mother and father are allowed to bathe and dress the baby, and the mother is given the baby immediately to feed or cradle. If there are no complications, the couple is free to take the baby home within twelve to twenty-four hours.

While the birthing room is similar to a home, it has benefits that home delivery lacks. Some technical procedures — such as the enema, the episiotomy (a small incision at the vaginal opening to aid in birth), and the perineal shave — are left up to the woman's preference, as at home. But, unlike a home birth, a hospital team and full lifesaving equipment wait just around the corner in case of complications.

Home Birth

During the late 1970s and early 1980s, the home birth movement gained great momentum, with thousands of mothers opting to give birth at home with the aid of a midwife and husband and family members. While some women choose home birth because of financial reasons, many choose it because of their dislike of what they describe as the sterile, antiseptic atmosphere of the hospital and their inability to enjoy the birth experience because of the commotion, the glaring lights, and the bevy of equipment. Others object to rigid rules set up by the hospital, to not being able to dress and bathe the baby, and to the enforced separation of baby and mother after birth.

The one danger that exists in home delivery is the possibility of complications. Even a woman who has successfully and without problem given birth to several children may suddenly develop complications that may endanger her or her baby. Too often, the home is located far enough from the hospital to prevent transportation in the few minutes that it takes for a baby to die from lack of oxygen, insufficient circulation, or a host of other complications. In addition, a mother may develop sudden problems (such as hemorrhage or skyrocketing blood pressure) that may cause her death if immediate help is not available. While midwives are trained in normal birth procedures, few have the knowledge and the equipment on hand to deal with life-threatening emergencies.

Breast or Bottle Feed?

Physicians now encourage breast feeding because of its benefits to both mother and child, but there are several reasons why you should not breast feed:

1. Certain disease conditions make it impossible for a woman to breast feed because of the effect on her (such as diabetes) or because of the possibility of passing the disease on to the infant (tuberculosis).
2. Women who take regular medication should not breast feed, since the medication may be passed to the infant in the mother's milk.
3. Women who do not want to breast feed should not force themselves to do so; the emotional upset involved often interferes with the flow of milk and disturbs both the mother and the baby. Women who do not have the support of family members may have trouble breast feeding for the same reasons.

On the positive side, breast milk seems to offer immunity to the infant; newborns and babies who breast feed are generally able to resist colds, pneumonia, gastrointestinal disorders, and measles. Infants are rarely allergic to mother's milk, while many develop severe allergic reactions to cow's milk. And infants who drink cow's milk tend to get a much higher caloric intake (because the infant is encouraged to drink the whole bottle), resulting in overweight and obesity among infants.

Special Demands of Pregnancy

Of primary concern to many couples is the ability to continue sexual relations during pregnancy. Under normal conditions and in a pregnancy without complications, sexual intercourse is not harmful to the mother or baby and can be continued until shortly before birth. Intercourse should not occur after the amniotic sac has ruptured because of the danger of introducing infection into the uterus, and intercourse should be avoided if the woman has vaginal bleeding or abdominal cramps during pregnancy.

Some women do not want to have sex during pregnancy; for some it is out of a desire not to harm the baby, and for others it is a result of diminished sex drive (a common occurrence). In some cases, it is the husband who does not want to have sex during pregnancy. Most physicians advise couples to do what is most comfortable for them if there are no complications that would contraindicate sexual intercourse. As the pregnancy advances, it is generally thought wise to prevent excessive pressure from being exerted on the abdomen.

While you should concentrate on eating a well-balanced, nutritious diet that will provide all of the essential nutrients needed during pregnancy, you should avoid overeating — it leads to excessive weight gain, dangerous for you and the baby. A reasonable weight gain is about twenty-four pounds, or two and one-half to three pounds per month. Dieting should be avoided during pregnancy because of possible harm to the fetus.

Toxic substances including coffee, cigarettes, alcohol, and caffeine (found in high concentrations in chocolate and some soda drinks) should be avoided. No drugs should be used without the physician's approval — including aspirin. If you visit a general practitioner while you are pregnant or go to a dentist or any other doctor who is not aware of your pregnancy, you should make him or her aware so that you can avoid exposure to x-ray and so that prescriptions can be written accordingly.

If the woman feels well and can handle the demands, she is encouraged to keep working until the baby is due. Quit working if the job entails exposure to risks (such as lead) or excessive fatigue. Avoid work that strains your back or abdomen.

Exercise and mild sports are appropriate at the time of pregnancy. Swimming is particularly beneficial, as are biking, playing tennis, or playing golf, although you will have to slow your pace somewhat. Sports that require a fine sense of balance — such as hiking — may become increasingly difficult as the center of gravity changes.

Long travel may be uncomfortable toward the end of pregnancy due to swelling in the ankles and pain in the legs. The wearing of both a shoulder strap and lap seat belt when traveling in a car helps to decrease risk of injury. Near the end of pregnancy, when delivery is imminent, stay close to the hospital and obstetrician, or the baby may be delivered in unfamiliar surroundings.

Rh Incompatibility

About 85 percent of all adults have in their red blood cells a protein agent termed an Rh factor (and are thus termed "Rh positive"), while 15 percent lack this agent (and so are "Rh negative"). A serious condition

Rh INCOMPATABILITY

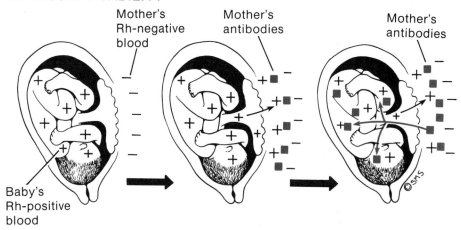

Figure 10-12. As shown, some of the Rh-positive blood of the child leaks through the placenta to the Rh-negative blood of the mother. The mother's body reacts by developing antibodies that return to the baby's bloodstream and destroy some of the red blood cells. If enough antibodies reach the child, anemia of varying severity will result. Adapted from Rene Dubos, *Health and Disease*, Life Science Library, 1965.

results only when the mother is Rh negative and the fetus is Rh positive. If fetal Rh-positive red blood cells leak into an Rh-negative mother's circulatory system, the Rh-negative mother develops antibodies against the foreign Rh-positive antigens from the fetus. This occurs most commonly during delivery of her first Rh-positive child. With succeeding Rh-positive pregnancies, and during those pregnancies, the mother's Rh antibodies rise sharply.

The antibodies pass from the Rh-negative mother through the placental barrier to the Rh-positive fetus. The antibodies agglutinate and destroy the red blood cells of the fetus as fast as they are formed. This hemolytic disease is known as erythroblastosis fetalis. It may result in stillbirth, or the newborn may develop jaundice, a severe anemia, and edema. Death may ensue.

Prevention is accomplished by injecting the mother with serum containing antibodies (the drug is called Rhogam) to Rh-positive red blood cells. As a result, Rh-positive cells that she receives from her infant are destroyed, and she never develops her own antibodies. The injection must be given within seventy-two hours of birth, miscarriage, or abortion to be effective. With this treatment, most instances of Rh incompatibility can be prevented.

Many couples find it desirable or necessary to postpone childbearing and space their children. A variety of factors should be considered by the couple such as religious values, health factors, economic circumstances, and various pressures and stresses which may adversely affect the couple or their offspring.

If a couple decide to postpone pregnancy, they must choose among a variety of alternative methods which vary considerably in their effectiveness, risks, and side effects. Some methods are only available with a physician's prescription and should be used after medical consultation to assure safety. The more commonly used methods, their effectiveness, advantages, disadvantages, and risks are reviewed in the appendix.

ABORTION

Abortion refers to the interruption of pregnancy sometimes within the first twenty weeks before the fetus can survive outside the womb. There are several kinds of abortion:

1. **Spontaneous.** Also called miscarriage, spontaneous abortion is usually due to some condition in the mother that would have prevented normal fetal growth. About one in ten to fifteen pregnancies end in miscarriage, and about 75 percent of all miscarriages occur during the first three months of pregnancy. Common causes of miscarriage include disease in the mother, abnormalities in the placenta, or abnormalities in the developing fetus.
2. **Psychogenic.** Psychogenic abortions are miscarriages that are emotionally produced.
3. **Self-Induced.** Probably the most commonly attempted form, self-induced abortion refers to "home remedy" methods used by the mother to terminate the pregnancy. Most such crude methods are insufficient to end the pregnancy, and unfortunately, most result in serious damage to the mother instead.
4. **Selective.** A selective abortion is performed in the same way as a

I feel I should end on a personal note. For my own part, I favor making abortion available on an unrestricted basis. My reasons are those customarily given, and I have no new arguments to add. At the same time, I am far from happy finding myself in this position.

Abortion is taking of human life. No legal or scientific theorizing can change that basic fact. My fear is that sanctioning abortion will direct our sensibilities from moral principles to pragmatic matters of cost and inconvenience. That aspect of abortion concerns me as much as anything else.

Moreover, I find I have sympathy for those on the other side. Far from being fanatics, they conceive of a social and moral order where citizenship has its duties and passions are held in check. They believe strongly in the family. Theirs may be a stern, even punitive, ethic, but they are people who have contributed their share to society, at no small cost to themselves.

I am not convinced that those supporting abortion have a parallel vision. Theirs is a highly personal outlook, stressing freedom and choice and pleasure. What is lacking is any sign of concern over the society we will have, and the people we will be once their ends are attained. A fully active sexual life may be fine. But we should consider where it can take us. Opponents of abortion have done just that. Its supporters prefer to avoid such questions.

Hacker, Andrew. "Of Two Minds About Abortion," *Harpers Magazine*, Queens College, September 1979.

therapeutic abortion after the mother discovers (as a result of amniocentesis) that her baby is abnormal. Selective abortion is sometimes used to prevent the birth of children with serious genetic defects, such as Down's Syndrome.

5. **Therapeutic.** Performed under a surgeon's care, a therapeutic abortion is elective and utilizes medical and clinical techniques. Therapeutic abortions are a matter of considerable controversy at present. The justifications for therapuetic abortion may be divided into "hard" and "soft" reasons according to Granberg:[4]

The "hard" reasons are:

1. If the woman's health is seriously endangered by the pregnancy.
2. If she became pregnant as a result of rape.
3. If there is a strong chance of a serious defect in the baby.

The "soft" reasons are:

1. If the family has a very low income and cannot afford any more children.

2. If she is not married and does not want to marry the man.
3. If she is married and does not want any more children.

Surveys show that the acceptability of these reasons varies considerably in our population, an observation which suggests that attitudes with regard to pregnancy and abortion are highly diversified. Some of the concerns are exemplified by the following questions:

1. Is abortion physically and psychologically safe?
2. What are the alternatives to abortion in unwanted pregnancy?
3. What ethical, spiritual, and religious considerations are involved?
4. Is abortion a responsible method of birth control?
5. How will abortion affect future fertility and family planning?
6. How will abortion affect a couple's existing relationship?
7. What are the long-range implications of this decision?
8. How, when, by whom, and where is it best to get an abortion?
9. How much does an abortion cost in time and in money?
10. What are the legal aspects of getting an abortion?
11. Is parental or spouse consent needed? Is financial aid available, etc.?
12. What happens during the abortion procedure?
13. How will I feel after the abortion?

And on the more emotional side, particularly with regard to "soft" reasons:

1. Does abortion betray an increasing calousness to life?
2. Is abortion a responsible solution to irresponsible sexual intercourse?
3. Is abortion a personal or a social issue — or both?

Counseling is particularly important so that the ramifications can be explored completely by all persons involved. In general, counselors explain procedures and alternatives rather than give advice, broadening the perspective so that decision making is more closely related to the facts of the issue.

INFERTILITY

The dilemma faced by millions of couples was brought into the spotlight by the birth of Louise Brown on July 27, 1978 — the first "test-tube baby," conceived outside the womb and implanted with normal uterine development until birth. A number of factors can lead to infertility, and they can develop in the male or the female (or, in some difficult cases, both).

Male Factors of Infertility

The male is the cause of the infertility in 30 to 40 percent of the cases, due to abnormalities in:

1. **Sperm production.** In order for conception to occur, the sperm must be plentiful, normal, and mobile enough to swim to the ovum as it travels down the fallopian tube. When sperm are abnormal in number or quality, the viability for conception is poor. When the problem is mild, the condition may respond to treatment that consists of abstaining from tobacco and alcohol, eating a sufficient amount of nutritionally balanced food, and getting good exercise and adequate rest. In some cases, hormone therapy may be effective. Rarely the cause of low sperm production is varicose veins in the scrotum; the condition can be surgically corrected with return to normal sperm production.

2. **Sperm blockage.** While problems with sperm production are the most common, in some cases the sperm are not able to be discharged through the penis, even though they are produced in normal numbers. The blockage generally occurs in the network of tubes that carry the sperm from the testicles to the penis; new methods of microsurgery have been successful in locating and correcting such blockages.

Female Factors of Infertility

Generally, infertility that originates with the female accounts for 60 to 70 percent of the infertility problems and is more difficult to discover and more complex to treat.

1. **Egg production.** About one-fifth of the women complaining of

396

infertility suffer from lack of hormones sufficient to cause the ovaries to release mature ova. Fortunately, drug therapy with clomiphene (Clomid), which acts to release the egg from the ovary, has been successful in treating a number of these women. In more difficult cases, Pergonal or HCG (a powerful hormone) may be used. Multiple births are more common when these substances are used to promote ovulation.

2. **Ovum transport.** The most common problem in female infertility is one of getting the ovum from the ovary to the uterus. Scar tissue in the fallopian tubes (a result of gonorrhea or other infections) or malformations in the tubes prevent the ovum from passing toward the uterus, and, in extreme cases, prevent the sperm from reaching the ovum. As with the male, microsurgery has been successful in correcting some of these defects.

3. **Cervical environment.** This is the most diffcult of all infertility problems to solve — the sperm are incompatible with the environment at the cervix. Sometimes it is due to the mucous secreted in the vagina (some women actually secrete a spermicide that destroys sperm before they even reach the cervix); other times, the mucous renders the sperm immobile. While this situation is difficult to treat, some cases have responded to therapy to improve the character of the cervical and vaginal environment.

GENETIC AND BIRTH DEFECTS

The National Foundation — March of Dimes defines a birth defect as an abnormality of body structure or function, whether genetically determined or the result of environmental influence on the unborn baby, or both.[5]

Hereditary influences are difficult to control. Individuals who have a history of a particular defect in their family line should realize that they may possibly pass the characteristic to their children. The likelihood that the trait will show up in the offspring varies considerably, depending on the manner of its inheritance.

There are three main divisions of environmental influences that may affect the baby.

ELEMENTARY PRINCIPLES OF INHERITANCE

How Dominant Inheritance Works

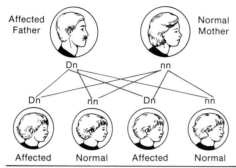

How X-Linked Inheritance Works

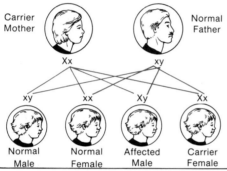

How Recessive Inheritance Works

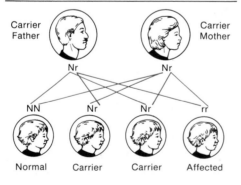

Figure 10-13.

One affected parent has a single faulty gene (D) which dominates its normal counterpart (n). Each child's chances of inheriting either the D or the n from the affected parent are 50%.

In the most common form, the female sex chromosome of an unaffected mother carries one faulty gene (X) and one normal one (x). The father has normal male x and y chromosomes. The odds for each male child are 50-50: (1) 50% risk of inheriting the faulty X and a normal y; (2) 50% chance of inheriting normal x and y chromosomes. For each female child, the odds are: (1) 50% risk of inheriting one faulty X to be a carrier like mother; (2) 50% chance of inheriting no faulty gene.

Both parents usually unaffected carry a normal gene (N) which takes precedence over its faulty recessive counterpart (r). The odds for each child are: (1) a 25% risk of inheriting a double dose of r genes which may cause a serious birth defect; (2) a 25% chance of inheriting two Ns, thus being unaffected; (3) a 50% chance of being a carrier.

1. **Direct maternal factors.** The mother's general physical characteristics and her history of physical and mental health can be related to fetal health. Among the factors are: (1) **Metabolic disorders.** Diabetic women, for example, more often have miscarriages, stillbirths, and children with many different kinds of defects without necessarily passing the disease on to the child. Other examples include maternal phenylketonuria (PKU) and thyroid disorders, which may cause mental retardation in offspring; and (2) **Maternal age.** Stillbirths are more frequent among teenage mothers. Miscarriages and mongoloid babies occur more among women thirty-five years and older. In the first case, it is thought that the girl's reproductive system may not have fully matured; in the latter, the system may have begun to break down with environmental influences affecting later developing ova cells.

2. **Environmental causes acting on the mother during pregnancy.** These include influences brought to bear upon the unborn child as a result of the mother's getting sick, eating poorly, or taking harmful

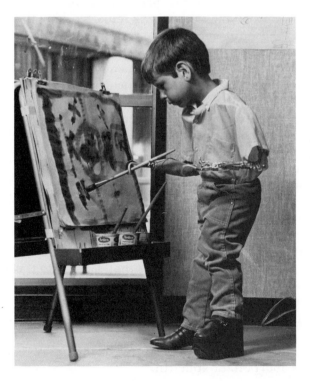

The risk of many birth defects can be reduced through genetic counseling, screening, and appropriate prenatal care.

drugs, especially during the first trimester. They include: (1) **viral disease and infections;** (2) **venereal disease;** (3) **drug use;** (4) **smoking;** and (5) **diet.**

3. **Effects of the larger environment.** These include elements in the mother's general environment to which she may or may not know that she has been exposed. Three common examples are: (1) **radiation;** (2) **pollutants;** and (3) **some pesticides.**

DRUGS AND PREGNANCY

Pregnant women should keep in mind continually the fact that they and the fetus are inseparable. If you are pregnant, you need to remember that anything you take into your body affects your baby. Particularly consequential are drugs — medication that may benefit you may harm your unborn baby.

Until recently, doctors thought that the placenta served as an effective barrier between the mother and the growing fetus, blocking the passage of drugs and other harmful substances while permitting an exchange of life-giving elements, like food and oxygen. We know now, however, that the placenta is like all other human membranes — it is capable of being penetrated by chemical substances, including drugs.[6]

The biggest problem concerning ingestion of drugs during pregnancy is the fact that the greatest and most critical period of fetal development takes place in many cases before a woman even knows that she is pregnant: during the first three months (first trimester) of pregnancy. The most critical developmental period for the fetus — and the period during which it is particularly susceptible to damage from drugs — begins on the thirteenth day of pregnancy. Few women know for sure that they are pregnant that early.

The higher the dose and the more frequently the drug is taken, the more likely it is that the fetus will be exposed to the drug — and the more the fetus is exposed to the drug, the more likely it is that damage to the fetus may occur.[7]

The most common defects associated with a mother's drug use during pregnancy include the following:[8]

- Congenital malformation, often of the facial features or the limbs.
- Miscarriage, spontaneous abortion, or stillbirth.

400

- Abnormal physical growth, especially stunted growth.
- Inability of the infant to adjust to life outside the uterus.
- Abnormal metabolism.
- Alteration of vital physiologic function.
- Long-term mental or neurologic damage.
- Development of cancer in the child years after delivery.

In some cases, drugs *must* be taken during pregnancy. A woman who develops an infection or who has cardiac disease, high blood pressure, thyroid disease, diabetes, or a seizure disorder must be treated.[9] Even in these cases, you should be sure that you take only *necessary* medication — not medication just to relieve symptoms. In all cases, you should weigh the risks of taking the drug versus the risks of not taking the drug. Remember, you can cause damage to your fetus before you even receive confirmation that you are pregnant, so avoid using any unnecessary drugs if you even *suspect* that you might be pregnant.

Drugs During Breast Feeding

Just as a number of drugs can be harmful if taken while a woman is pregnant, some drugs can cause danger to an infant if his mother ingests them while she is breast feeding him. Mother's milk is generally considered to be the perfect food, unable to be improved; it becomes less than perfect when contaminated, especially by drugs.[10]

Chemicals enter mother's milk from the mother's bloodstream. Many — if not all — drugs are detectable in some amount in the mother's milk, but most of these drugs are not harmful to the infant. Because an infant's enzyme and metabolic systems are not fully developed, he cannot tolerate some drugs in even minute doses, even though those drugs would not normally be harmful to the infant. The use of any substances during pregnancy should be cleared with a physician.

Effects of Smoking During Pregnancy

A woman who smokes while she is pregnant can damage the fetus in a number of ways; the more the woman smokes, the more damage the fetus is likely to sustain.[11] Stopping smoking at any time during the pregnancy will help and can reduce the chances of permanent damage.

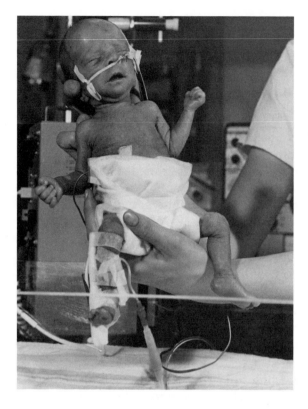

Medical technology greatly increases survival rates of premature infants.

Recent studies indicate that no smoking during the forty-eight hours preceding birth can help increase the available oxygen supply to the fetus and can reduce the damage at birth.[12]

A number of effects have been repeatedly observed and definitely linked to maternal smoking:

1. Premature delivery.
2. Low birth weight. Women who smoke are twice as likely to deliver a low birth weight baby as women who do not smoke.
3. Stillbirths. The risk of having a stillborn infant is 30 percent higher for those who smoke.
4. Infant mortality. Infant mortality is about one-third higher in cases where the mother smoked during pregnancy.
5. Congenital malformations. Because of the toxins contained in cigarette smoke, a fetus can develop congenital malformations so serious

that miscarriage often results; in cases where miscarriage does not occur, the infant often dies shortly after birth.

6. Sudden Infant Death Syndrome. Seven of the eight suspected contributors to SIDS are related to conditions during pregnancy; five of those are directly attributable to cigarette smoking during pregnancy.

7. Health during the first year of life. Children born to mothers who smoked during pregnancy have much more likelihood of developing health problems during the first year of life.

Alcohol and Pregnancy

If you are pregnant, do not drink — you run a good chance of inflicting defects on your unborn baby that will last all of its life. Delivered under the auspices of the Department of Health, Education, and Welfare, that warning was prompted by research conducted and released by the National Institute on Alcohol Abuse and Alcoholism — research findings that link maternal alcohol intake with a defect known as fetal alcohol syndrome. The scope is broad: fetal alcohol syndrome is one of three leading causes of birth defects.[13]

Fetal alcohol syndrome apparently occurs only in cases of heavy maternal drinking. Moderate or occasional drinking, however, can produce symptoms similar to fetal alcohol syndrome and can result in infants who manifest the following:

1. Central nervous system dysfunctions — mental retardation, small head size, poor sucking and swallowing reflexes, and problems with eating.

2. Growth deficiencies — weight deficiencies, failure to thrive.

3. Facial malformations — narrow, flat head; cleft palate; flat midface; short, upturned nose; low nasal bridge; a broad space between nose and upper lip; a wide mouth with an extremely thin upper lip; slant-like eyes with heavily folded eyelids; a small jaw; smaller than normal eyes; eyes set wide apart; and large, protruding ears.

4. Skeletal malformations — joint malformations.

5. Heart malformations — heart murmurs, defects in the septum, and abnormal muscular formation of the heart.

6. Other abnormalities — abnormally pigmented skin, excessive hair growth, deformities of the external genitals, kidney defects, clubfoot, dislocated hip joints at birth, deformities of the toes, poor eye-hand coordination, and abnormal liver structure and function.

Caffeine and Pregnancy

Caffeine readily crosses the placenta and is absorbed by the fetus; unlike an adult, the fetus during development and the baby following birth lack the enzymes required to metabolize caffeine. Instead of being metabolized and eliminated from the body, then, the caffeine is absorbed and retained, where it causes developmental defects and some cases of spontaneous abortion, stillbirth, and miscarriage. Premature birth is much more common among caffeine users, and the babies born prematurely are much more likely to suffer complications.

CAUTION LIGHT ON CAFFEINE

For many people the consumption of caffeine starts at an early age — before birth even — and continues for much of a lifetime. Caffeine is taken up by the bloodstream of the mother and crosses the placenta to reach the fetus. It appears in the milk of mothers who breast-feed their newborns while regularly consuming foods, drinks, and drugs that contain caffeine.

Most people probably know there is caffeine in a cup of coffee or tea. Perhaps not as many realize it is also in some soft drinks, and even fewer may know they are taking in caffeine when they sip a cup of cocoa, munch on a chocolate bar, or take some pills for a headache or cold. It is even used in some foods.

The implications for health of caffeine consumption have been matters of concern and debate for years. This concern has now been heightened by new evidence from animal tests confirming earlier findings that caffeine causes irreversible bith defects and other abnormalities in the fetuses of pregnant rats — adverse effects that also have occurred in experiments with mice and rabbits. But the critical question — still unanswered — is whether this commonly ingested substance poses the same hazards and dangers to unborn children as it does to animals.

Caffeine is a drug, and it acts as a stimulant to the central nervous system, although it does not affect all the people the same way. If consumed in large enough doses, it can cause insomnia, nervousness, irritability, anxiety, and disturbances in the heart rate and rhythm. It also seems to have an effect on coronary circulation, blood pressure, the diameter of the blood vessels and secretion of gastric acids. There is also recent concern about the possible behavioral effects of caffeine on children and on their brain growth and development.

So while further evidence is being gathered on the possible relationship between caffeine and birth defects, a prudent and protective mother-to-be will want to put caffeine on her list of unncessary substances which she should avoid.

Among babies born to caffeine users, low birth weight is common, and in some cases, the birth weight is so low that the baby's health is endangered. Some children suffer physical and mental impairment directly connected to low birth weight as a result of excessive caffeine use on the part of the mother.

Excessive caffeine use by mothers (in excess of eight cups of coffee a day or the equivalent ingestion of caffeine) also results in a lowering of the baby's muscle tone and functional abilities. Children whose mothers used caffeine regularly during pregnancy are generally retarded in physical activity development and in functional abilities (such as walking, sitting, crawling, or holding their head up).[14] Excessive caffeine use during pregnancy also apparently contributes to a significantly higher percentage and incidence of breech birth.[15]

Current legislation is requesting that the Food and Drug Administration require warning labels on over-the-counter drugs and on coffee, tea, and other foods that contain caffeine, warning users that the caffeine contained in the products causes birth defects.[16]

Notes

1. L. M. DelBo, *A Guide for the Future Mother* (Englewood Cliffs, New Jersey: Prentice-Hall, Inc., 1977), p. 29.
2. Jacqueline Maio, "Pregnancy Tests: No Sure Thing, But Sometimes Helpful," *FDA Consumer*, June 1979, p. 4.
3. DelBo, p. 42.
4. Donald Granberg and Beth William Granberg, "Abortion Attitudes, 1969-1980: Trends and Determinants," *Family Planning Perspectives*, September/October 1980, p. 252.
5. Excerpted from *National Foundation — March of Dimes, Birth Defects*, (White Plains, New York: National Foundation — March of Dimes, 1977), and National Institute of General Medical Sciences, "What are the Facts About Genetic Diseases?" (Bethesda, Maryland: National Institues of Health, 1974).
6. Thomas E. O'Brien and Carol E. McManus, "Drugs and the Human Fetus," *Grassroots* (March 1978 Supplement), March 1978, p. 3.
7. Molly J. Brog, "Birth Defects and Drugs," *Life and Health*, June 1980, p. 3.
8. John F. Henahan, "What to Tell Your Pregnant Patients About Drinking: 'Don't,'" *Modern Medicine*, Apirl 15, 1977, pp. 29-33; and Reba Michels Hill, "Drugs that an Unborn Baby Can't Tolerate," *RN*, August 1977, pp. 35-39.
9. Peter E. Fehr, "Guidelines for Prescribing in Pregnancy," *Modern Medicine*, June 15, 1976, p. 41.
10. Annabel Hecht, "Advice on Breast Feeding and Drugs," *FDA Consumer*, November 1979, p. 21.
11. "Smoking and Pregnancy," *Family Health*, May 1979, p. 8; Sadja Goldsmith Greenwood, "Warning: Cigarette Smoking is Dangerous to Reproductive Health," *Family Planning Perspectives*, vol. 11 (no. 3), May/June 1979, pp. 168-172; Butler, pp. 43-49; American Academy of Pediatrics, "Effects of Cigarette Smoking on the Fetus and Child," *Pediatrics*, vol. 57 (no. 3), March 1976, pp. 411-413; and "When a Mother Smokes During Pregnancy, Will It Affect Her Baby?" *Clinical Pediatrics*, June 1974, pp. 485-486.
12. "Even a Late Break From Smoking Could Help Fetus," *Medical World News*, September 17, 1979, p. 48.
13. "Fetal Alcohol Syndrome: New Perspectives," *Alcohol Health and Research World*, Summer 1978, p. 2.
14. "Coffee May Perk Up Pregnant Mom But Not Her Baby," *Medical World News*, April 17, 1978, p. 8.
15. "Coffee May Perk Up Pregnant Mom," p. 13.
16. "Birth Defect Warning Asked on Caffeine," *FDA Consumer*, November 1978, p. 22.

Self-Evaluation

Section 1
Chance of Having a Healthy Baby

Consider carefully your own plans for children, if you have decided to have children. Read each of the following questions thoroughly, and circle the response that most closely resembles your preferences and decisions.

1. I plan on having my first baby when I am (or when my wife is):
   a. under the age of twenty
   b. between twenty and thirty-five
   c. over the age of thirty-five

2. I plan on having my first baby when my husband is (or when I am):
   a. under the age of twenty
   b. between twenty and forty-five
   c. over the age of forty-five

3. I plan on spacing my children:
   a. one year or less apart
   b. two years and nine months or more apart
   c. between one and two years apart

4. I plan on having:
   a. more than three children
   b. three or fewer children

5. I plan on receiving:
   a. care from my doctor during the last half of my pregnancy
   b. care from my doctor throughout my pregnancy
   c. care from my doctor during my early pregnancy, but after that the baby is just growing so I will not receive as much medical care

6. I plan on having:
   a. no genetic counseling
   b. genetic counseling if it is needed

7. As a woman, I plan on:
   a. dieting while I am pregnant so I will not gain too much weight
   b. eating a well-balanced diet that is adequate in calories
   c. eating whatever I feel I need to keep up my strength and satisfy my cravings

8. As a woman, I plan on:
   a. smoking during pregnancy
   b. abstaining from alcohol and tobacco during pregnancy
   c. drinking alcohol during pregnancy
   d. both smoking and drinking during pregnancy

9. As a woman, I plan on:
    a. using only basic over-the-counter drugs (like aspirin) when I am pregnant, but refraining from unusual drugs
    b. using no drugs during pregnancy unless my doctor specifically approves them
    c. using over-the-counter remedies and old prescription drugs that I know are safe

10. As a woman, I plan on:
    a. getting involved in some new sports activities to get some exercise during pregnancy
    b. continuing in those sports and exercises I have already participated in during pregnancy
    c. taking it easy and refraining from exercise during pregnancy

Scoring: The "b" response to each question is the factor that is most likely to insure the health and well-being of you and your baby. If you checked more than two of the questions with responses other than "b", you should be prepared to examine your thinking concerning the important subject of childbearing.

**Section 2
Reproductive Tract Infection**

Examine the appropriate list below, and circle any symptom that you now have or have had in the last two weeks.

Women	**Men**
yellowish vaginal discharge	genital itching
grayish-green vaginal discharge	itching during urination
thick discharge with foul odor	small bumps along shafts of pubic hair
vaginal itching	
painful intercourse	visible lice in pubic hair
painful urination	painful intercourse
frothy, thin, gray vaginal discharge	dry, painless warts on penis, scrotum, or anus
frothy, greenish-white vaginal discharge	
	small, painful blisters on penis
reddened vulva	ulcerated sores on penis
frequent urination	swollen penis

itching and redness of vulva that spreads to thighs

thick, white, lumpy vaginal discharge

itching of area under pubic hair

tiny lice visible in pubic hair

dry, painless warts around anus or vulva

vulvar pain

tender, hot, swollen lump at entrance to vagina

small, painful blisters on vulva or buttocks

ulcerated sores on vulva or buttocks

genital swelling

fever

enlarged lymph nodes in the abdomen

fever

enlarged lymph glands in the abdomen

Scoring: The above lists represent the signs and symptoms common to reproductive tract infections. If you circled one or two, you may have an infection; if you circled more than two, it is extremely likely that you have contracted a reproductive tract infection. You should make an appointment with your doctor, and you should avoid sexual intimacy until you are examined for such an infection.

Section 3
Birthing and Birth Defects

It is essential for prospective mothers to prepare for their babies before they are born. What she does to her body before conception often makes a difference in the success of the birth process. Females, assess your preparations for childbearing by answering the following questions. Males, answer according to your wife or prospective wife.

Yes   **No**

_____ _____ 1. Pelvic examination by a qualified doctor shows tipped uterus, small frame, endometriosis, or organic disorders.

Yes	No		
———	———	2.	Had a recent abortion.
———	———	3.	A current history of anemia.
———	———	4.	Under the age of eighteen years.
———	———	5.	Under five feet, two inches in height.
———	———	6.	Have a chronic heart problem.
———	———	7.	Is obese (weight is 20 percent greater than indicated by standard age, sex, height charts).
———	———	8.	Rh negative blood factor.
———	———	9.	No history of rubella (german measles) or vaccine.
———	———	10.	Close relatives who are mongoloid, diabetic, or have other genetic-based diseases.
———	———	11.	Have a history of sexually transmitted diseases.
———	———	12.	Have diabetes.
———	———	13.	Have lived in an area of high radiation exposure.
———	———	14.	Prolonged, high-concentration exposure to pesticide of all types.
———	———	15.	Had x-ray treatment or x-ray examination in the past year without pelvic shielding.
———	———	16.	Smoke less than half a pack of cigarettes per day.
———	———	17.	Drink less than five ounces of alcohol per week.
———	———	18.	Smoke more than half a pack of cigarettes per day.
———	———	19.	Drink more than five ounces of alcohol per week.
———	———	20.	Take stimulant, hallucinogenic, sedative and opiate drugs, or smoke marijuana or hashish daily.

If you answered yes to any items from 1-7, there is a slight risk involved; items 8-12 indicate a moderate risk; items 13-17 indicate high risk; and items 18-20 indicate extreme risk to child development and health of the mother.

This assessment is not a conclusive test instrument. The purpose is only to give an indication to possible degrees of risk. If you fall into any of the categories and are pregnant or expect to be pregnant in the next several months, you are advised to consult your physician and change your life-style where appropriate.

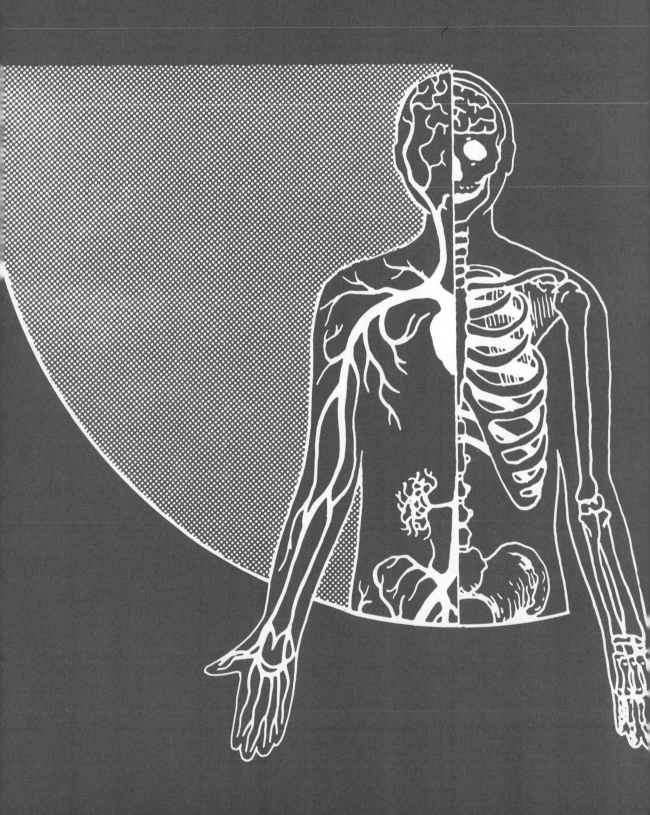

Part IV
Reducing Risks

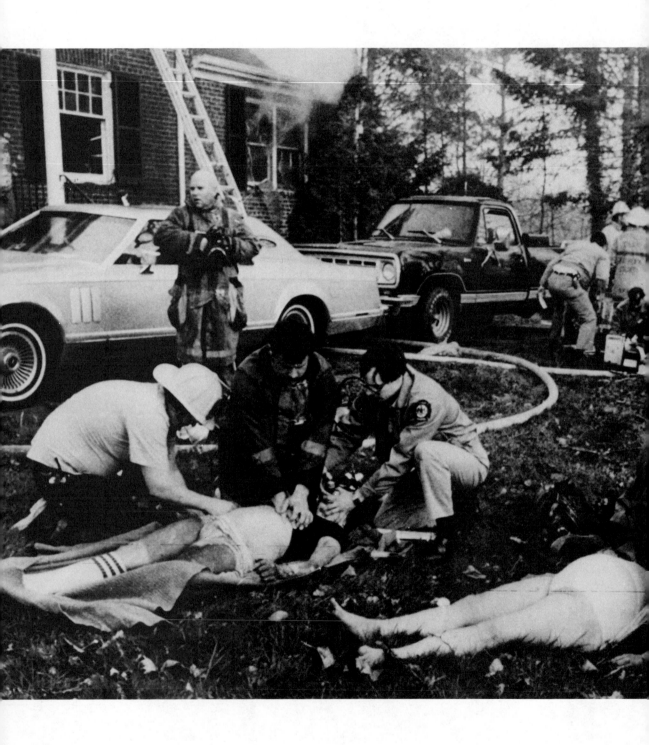

11
Cardiovascular Disease: Have A Heart

Pass the salt, please.

No, I'm too tired this morning — let's *drive* over to campus.

I piled on twenty pounds during my freshman year!

I tried to cut down on my smoking once, but final exams make me so nervous. . . .

Heart disease is the number one killer in the United States today.[1] And, ironically, you can do more to prevent your chances of being affected by heart disease than you can to combat any other major cause of death. By the way — heart disease is not just a disease of the middle-aged executive with gray hair sprinkled around his temples and a paunch tucked under his belt. Heart disease is claiming its victims from college campuses, too.

But heart disease, for the most part, is preventable. All it takes is a basic understanding of what factors affect your heart's performance, what life-styles present a risk for your heart, and how you can overcome those risks.

DISEASES OF THE CIRCULATORY SYSTEM ━━━━

Seven major diseases affect the heart and its system: hypertension (high blood pressure), heart attack, congestive heart failure, stroke, atherosclerosis (sometimes called arteriosclerosis), rheumatic heart disease, and congenital heart disease.

HYPERTENSION ━━━━━━━━━━━━━━━━

One in every four adults in the United States has high blood pressure.[2] It is a major killer, leading to congestive heart failure, stroke, and kidney failure. And it is a mysterious, silent killer: 90 percent of those who have high blood pressure manifest no symptoms.[3]

There are two forms of hypertension, essential and secondary. Both are serious, but the essential type is by far the most common. Secondary hypertension is, as the term implies, hypertension secondary to some other disorder. Two common disorders giving rise to secondary hypertension are kidney disease and some malfunctioning of the endocrine system. Essential hypertension has no underlying disorder. The hypertension is itself the disorder. Its cause is not known, and, though treatment is available, there is no cure.

Measuring Blood Pressure

You have probably had a test for blood pressure. An inflatable rubber cuff (called a sphygmomanometer) is wrapped around the upper arm; a sufficient amount of air to cut off the circulation is pumped into the cuff. As the air is gradually let out of the cuff, the technician listens with a stethoscope as the first blood rushes through the artery; he notes the pressure on the gauge as he hears the first sound of rushing blood. Pressure at that point is called *systolic:* it is the amount of pressure exerted when the heart contracts. A systolic pressure of about 120 is considered normal (if you are older than forty-five, a slightly higher reading is still considered normal).[4]

416

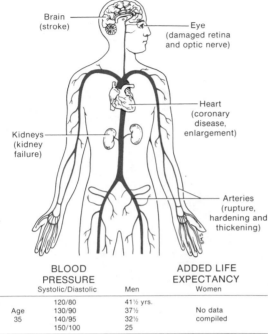

Figure 11-1. Hypertension target areas.

Brain (stroke)

Eye (damaged retina and optic nerve)

Heart (coronary disease, enlargement)

Kidneys (kidney failure)

Arteries (rupture, hardening and thickening)

	BLOOD PRESSURE Systolic/Diastolic	ADDED LIFE EXPECTANCY Men	Women
Age 35	120/80	41½ yrs.	
	130/90	37½	No data
	140/95	32½	compiled
	150/100	25	
Age 45	120/80	32 yrs.	37 yrs.
	130/90	29	35½
	140/95	26	32
	150/100	20½	28½
Age 55	120/80	23½ yrs.	27½ yrs.
	130/90	22½	27
	140/95	19½	24½
	150/110	17½	23½

Source: Metropolitan Life Ins. Co.

The technician continues to release air from the cuff until the sounds of the blood become muffled or disappear; the technician again checks the gauge. This number is a measurement of the *diastolic* pressure: the lowest level of pressure exerted, between beats, when the heart is at rest. A diastolic pressure of about 80 is considered normal (again, normal is slightly higher for those over forty-five).[5]

From the two numbers noted at your systolic and diastolic pressures, you get your blood pressure — 120/80. Those with hypertension, whose systolic blood pressure is over 150mm Hg, have more than twice the chance of suffering an MI (myocardial infarction or heart attack) than a man whose systolic blood pressure is under 120mm Hg.[6] At any age, a

417

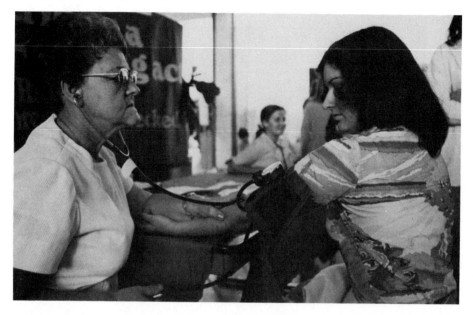

Early detection of hypertension can greatly reduce the risk of cardiovascular disease.

systolic pressure of 160 or more and a diastolic pressure of 95 or more is considered dangerous.[7]

Causes

Contributing factors that seem to lead to the development of high blood pressure include:

1. **Heredity.** Hypertension often runs in families;[8] this may be due either to strict genetic factors or to the fact that family members usually lead the same general life-style.
2. **Race.** Black people are 50 percent more likely to develop high blood pressure.[9]
3. **Age.** The prevalence of hypertension increases with age.
4. **Emotional stress.** Blood pressure naturally goes up during periods of emotional crisis, because the body is preparing itself for an emergency. Some people, however, react to life as if it is a series of

FOODS WITH HIGH SALT CONTENT
(those with highest salt content are in color)
Asparagus (canned)
Bacon
Beets (canned)
Boullion
Broth
Butter (salted)
Calf's liver
Carrots (canned)
Catsup
Cheese (including cottage)
Chili sauce
Corned beef (canned)
Corn (canned)
Corn chips
Frankfurters
Green beans (canned)
Ham (especially cured)
Lima beans (canned and frozen)
Lobster
Luncheon meats
Margarine (salted)
Milk (more than 2 glasses a day)
Milk chocolate
Mustard
Olives (green and ripe)
Oysters (frozen)
Peanuts (salted
Peas (canned)
Pickles
Pizza
Popcorn (salted or buttered)
Potato chips
Pretzels
Relish
Sardines (canned in oil)
Salmon (canned pink)
Soy sauce
Sausage
Sauerkraut
Tomatoes (canned)
Tuna fish (canned in oil)
Worcestershire sauce
Waffles (enriched)
TUNA
SOY SAUCE
HAM
Olives
SMS

Figure 11-2.

emergencies, and their bodies never have a chance to calm down and return to normal.[10]

5. **Smoking.** Nicotine is known to raise blood pressure chemically; heavy cigarette smoking is known to be a factor in the development of hypertension.[11]

6. **Body chemistry.** For an unknown reason, some people secrete into the blood stream chemicals that cause high blood pressure; these secretions generally originate in the kidneys or the adrenal glands.[12]

7. **Diet high in fats and salt.** Chemically, fats and salt act together to accelerate the development of atherosclerosis, which, in turn, leads to heart attacks and stroke and the development of high blood pressure.[13] According to some researchers, too much salt ingested at an early age (especially in baby food) can cause a predisposition toward high blood pressure later in life.

8. **Kidney defects.**[14]

9. **Adrenal cortex defects.**[15] Defects of the adrenal cortex cause it to secrete aldosterone (or some other similar hormone), which causes the body to retain sodium, resulting in the same condition as would occur by eating too much salt.

10. **Diseases of the pituitary, thyroid, or parathyroid glands.**[16]

11. **Toxemia.**[17]

12. **Blood and blood vessel defects** (generally due to birth defects).[18]

13. **Obesity.**[19]

Symptoms

Unfortunately, hypertension rarely exhibits any symptoms at all — 90 percent of those who have high blood pressure are unaware that anything at all is wrong.[20] There is usually no pain. If symptoms do occur, they generally include nagging headaches in the back of the head and upper part of the neck, dizziness, shortness of breath, excessive flushing of the face, fatigue, and insomnia.

What Can You Do

1. **Cut down on salt.** This is probably one of the most important ways in which you can fight the development of high blood pressure. We

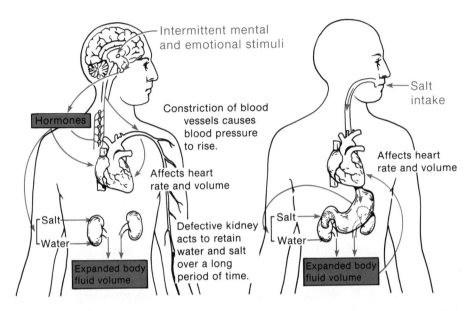

Intermittent mental and emotional stimuli

Salt intake

Hormones

Constriction of blood vessels causes blood pressure to rise.

Affects heart rate and volume

Affects heart rate and volume

Salt
Water

Defective kidney acts to retain water and salt over a long period of time.

Salt
Water

Expanded body fluid volume

Expanded body fluid volume

Figure 11-3. What causes the most common type of high blood pressure known as essential hypertension? There are hundreds of different causes that research scientists are looking at in an effort to discover the underlying mechanism. However, the two most prevalent factors appear to involve salt and stress.

need about 230 milligrams of sodium (found in ordinary table salt) every day — but some estimates cite that Americans consume about *twenty times* that amount. Because we get so much salt in the foods that we eat, watch your intake of table salt.

2. **Stop smoking.**

3. **Lose weight if you need to.** Every pound of fat places an added burden on the heart. If you are overweight for your height and frame, your heart is forced to pump more blood through a larger network of blood vessels — and the added work is a major cause of high blood pressure.

4. **Exercise.** Before you embark on any program of exercise, you should check with your doctor. If you dive in too quickly and try to do too much too soon you could end up overworking your heart and creating worse problems than you are trying to prevent. *Mild* exercise, like walking or light jogging, can be beneficial in lowering high

blood pressure; rigorous exercise, however, can be dangerous. If you are in the clear and the doctor gives you the go-ahead, work out an exercise program that gives you *some* kind of physical activity every day and some kind of vigorous exercise at least once a week.

5. **Calm down.** Stress is a highly suspicious culprit in the development of high blood pressure.

Treatment

The most effective therapeutic approach is use of antihypertensive drugs, with diuretics being the mainstay of therapy. Drugs working through the nervous system to dilate the arteries are employed if the diuretic does not adequately control the hypertension. These drugs have varying side effects ranging from a stuffy nose to impotence. Drowsiness, nausea, and depression are other side effects commonly seen.

HEART ATTACK

Almost 700,000 Americans each year succumb to heart attacks; many more suffer heart attacks each year and live.[21] About three out of five survive their initial episode. The chances of surviving subsequent heart attacks decrease dramatically; very few live through a third "attack."

Heart attack refers to a situation in which an artery of the heart becomes blocked either by fatty deposits (atherosclerosis), by a blood clot (thrombosis), or by vessel spasms. When an artery becomes obstructed, the heart muscle tissue beyond that artery dies; death of heart tissue is referred to as *myocardial infarction*. As a result, the heart muscle may suddenly quiver, a condition referred to as *fibrillation*. Fibrillation, unless corrected immediately (within seconds), leads to death.[22]

Causes

Some factors that contribute to heart attack include:

422

WHAT YOU SHOULD KNOW
ABOUT HEART ATTACK AND STROKE

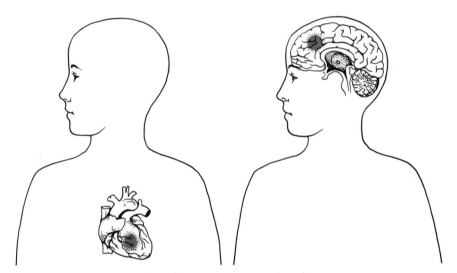

Figure 11-4. Heart attack and stroke.

Heart Attack: An estimated 3,990,000 have coronary heart disease. More than 684,000 die of heart attack each year — 350,000 before they reach the hospital. Many thousands of these might have been saved if the victims had heeded the warning signs.

Stroke: An estimated 1,700,000 persons are afflicted by stroke. More than 214,000 suffer fatal strokes annually. Many fatal strokes could be prevented if hypertension (high blood pressure), a leading cause of stroke, is diagnosed and controlled.

The warning signs of heart attack: Prolonged, oppressive pain or unusual discomfort in center of chest; Pain may radiate to shoulder, arm, neck, or jaw; Sweating may accompany pain or discomfort; Nausea, vomiting, and shortness of breath may also occur.

The warning signs of stroke: Sudden, temporary weakness or numbness of face, arm, or leg; Temporary loss of speech or trouble in speaking or understanding speech; Temporary dimness or loss of vision, particularly in one eye; An episode of double vision; Unexplained dizziness or unsteadiness; Change in personality, mental ability, or the pattern of headaches.

Act immediately. Sometimes these symptoms subside, then return. When you experience one or more warning signs, call your doctor and describe these symptoms in detail. If he's not immediately available, get to a hospital emergency room at once. Be prepared to act. Instruct others to act if you cannot. Keep a list of numbers — doctor, hospital, ambulance or other emergency services, and police — next to your telephone, and in a prominent place in your pocket, wallet, or purse. Adapted from American Heart Association.

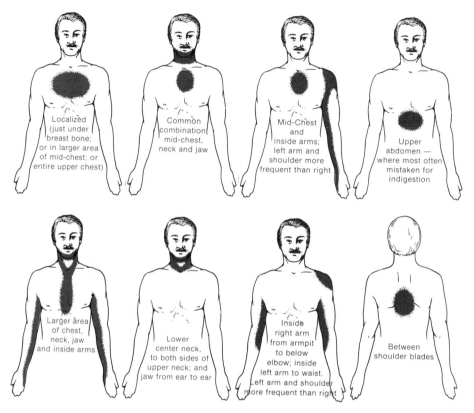

Figure 11-5 labels:

Localized (just under breast bone; or in larger area of mid-chest; or entire upper chest)

Common combination; mid-chest, neck and jaw

Mid-Chest and inside arms; left arm and shoulder more frequent than right

Upper abdomen — where most often mistaken for indigestion

Larger area of chest, neck, jaw and inside arms

Lower center neck, to both sides of upper neck; and jaw from ear to ear

Inside right arm from armpit to below elbow; inside left arm to waist. Left arm and shoulder more frequent than right

Between shoulder blades

Figure 11-5. Early signs of a heart attack. Pain, in one form or another, almost always accompanies a heart attack. Ranges from a mild ache to one of unbearable severity. When severe, pain is often felt as constricting, like vise on chest. Pain also often includes the burning and bloated sensations that usually accompany indigestion. Pain may be continuous and then might subside — but don't ignore it if it does. Could be in any one or combination of locations shown here. Courtesy Metropolitan Life Insurance Company ©.

1. **Overweight,** especially extreme overweight (thirty or more pounds exceeding ideal weight for height and frame).
2. **High blood pressure.**
3. **Smoking.**
4. **Lack of exercise and general sedentary life-style.**
5. **Diabetes** (including a family history of diabetes).
6. **Family history of heart attack** among immediate family members (parents, brothers, sisters).
7. **High blood cholesterol level** (generally over 200 mg percent).
8. **Age.** The chances of suffering a myocardial infarction rise dramatically with the passing years.[23]

424

Figure 11-6. Risk factors in coronary heart disease.

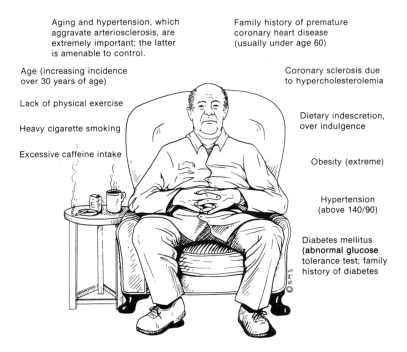

Aging and hypertension, which aggravate arteriosclerosis, are extremely important; the latter is amenable to control.

Age (increasing incidence over 30 years of age)

Lack of physical exercise

Heavy cigarette smoking

Excessive caffeine intake

Family history of premature coronary heart disease (usually under age 60)

Coronary sclerosis due to hypercholesterolemia

Dietary indescretion, over indulgence

Obesity (extreme)

Hypertension (above 140/90)

Diabetes mellitus **(abnormal glucose** tolerance test; family history of diabetes

Figure 11-7. Causes of heart pain and heart attack.

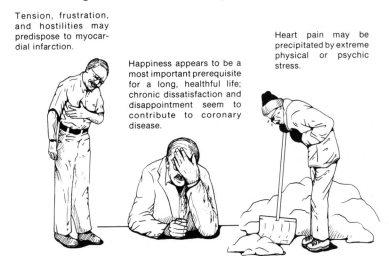

Tension, frustration, and hostilities may predispose to myocardial infarction.

Happiness appears to be a most important prerequisite for a long, healthful life; chronic dissatisfaction and disappointment seem to contribute to coronary disease.

Heart pain may be precipitated by extreme physical or psychic stress.

9. **Personality.** In recent years, claims have been made about a certain personality type being more susceptible to a "coronary." The person who becomes impatient at delay, who feels compelled to challenge a competitive or aggressive person, or who attempts to do more and more in less and less time, to specify a few factors, was reportedly more prone to a heart attack than the easygoing individual.

Warning Signs

Pain, in one form or another, almost always accompanies heart attack.[24] Besides pain, early warning signs include difficulty in breathing, heart palpitations, nausea, vomiting, cold sweats, paleness, weakness, and a sense of anxiety or impending doom.

CONGESTIVE HEART FAILURE ━━━━━━━━━━

Congestive heart failure is *not* a heart attack — but a heart attack is one of the conditions that can cause congestive heart failure. Congestive heart failure results when the heart muscle has been damaged by heart attack, rheumatic fever, atherosclerosis, high blood pressure, or birth defects. As a result, the heart's pumping capacity is reduced well below normal, and fluids begin to accumulate in the extremities and in the lungs.[25] If the heart is not strong enough to empty the ventricles at each contraction, congestive heart failure results. This failure can involve either the right, or left, or both sides of the heart. In-flowing blood flows into the heart faster than the heart can move it out.

Left side failure means that the blood entering the left ventricle flows in from the lungs faster than the weakened ventricle can move it out through the aorta. Blood backs up into the lungs, producing pulmonary congestion. Shortness of breath, especially upon exertion, is an obvious sign. Lying flat on the back may also bring on shortness of breath. This can be alleviated by sleeping on a pillow or two so that the head and shoulders are slightly elevated.

Since blood collects in the vessels in the lungs, plasma leaks out of the capillaries and into the air sacs of the lungs. This produces the cough accompanying shortness of breath. Dizziness, weakness, or fatigue are common symptoms, these being the result of the inability of the heart to meet the oxygen needs of the body.[26]

Right side failure means that the incoming blood from the systemic circulation cannot be moved to the lungs by the heart fast enough, causing the blood to back up in the tissues of the body. In time, fluid seeps out of the capillaries and into the tissues of the body, similar to what occurs in the lung with left side failure.

The legs and feet become swollen as a consequence. An individual may observe that the shoes fit normally in the morning but are tight by the end of the day. Sometimes the complaint is of increasing belt size or dress size. This is evidence of fluid accumulating in the abdominal cavity. Another sign is distended neck veins.[27]

If a patient suffers from both right and left side failure, he will have two sets of symptoms.

The key to prevention is to prevent damage to the heart muscle — in other words, take measures to prevent high blood pressure, heart attack, and atherosclerosis; get prompt treatment for rheumatic fever; and follow a therapeutic program to help deal with congenital heart disease.

STROKE

A stroke is an "accident" involving a blood vessel in the brain. For some reason, the blood supply is cut off to the brain because the artery can no longer carry the blood normally, and brain cells begin to die. Several factors may produce stroke:

1. **Hemorrhage.** Due to high blood pressure or some forms of disease (including infection of the arteries), a wall of the artery may burst, causing blood to spill into the surrounding tissue.
2. **Thrombosis.** A clot in a blood vessel in the brain may obstruct blood flow, and the tissue that is normally supplied by that artery is damaged or killed.
3. **Compression.** An object in the brain — usually a tumor, a section of swollen tissue, or a blood clot from another vessel — can press on a blood vessel, exerting sufficient pressure to cut off the blood supply and restrict the flow of blood to outlying tissue.
4. **Spasm.** As a result of some diseases of the arteries, a blood vessel may briefly spasm, tightening and closing sufficiently to reduce or shut off blood flow. Some spasms are mild and of brief duration;

427

RISK FACTORS IN HEART ATTACK AND STROKE

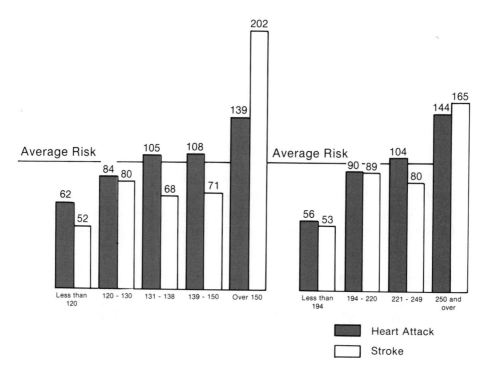

Figure 11-8. Risk factors in heart attack and stroke. A man whose blood pressure at systole (the moment the heart contracts) is over 150 has more than 2 times the risk of heart attack and nearly 4 times the risk of stroke of a man with systolic blood pressure under 120. A man with blood cholesterol measurement of 250 or above has about 3 times the risk of heart attacks and stroke of a man with cholesterol below 194.

permanent damage generally does not accompany a brief spasm. Others may be severe enough to cause a stroke.[28]

It should be kept in mind that once a brain cell is lost, it is not replaced. The disruption caused by loss of brain cells can be slight or severe. The disruption can be gone in a few days, or last for weeks and months, or may even be permanent. Brief episodes are in truth "mini" strokes and serve as warnings that a more serious stroke may occur.

THE DANGER OF HEART ATTACK
AND STROKE INCREASES WITH THE
NUMBER OF RISK FACTORS PRESENT

CIGARETTE SMOKING

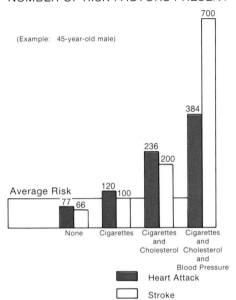

(Example: 45-year-old male)

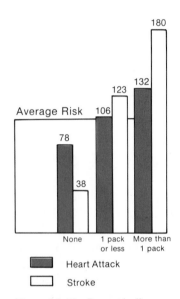

Figure 11-9. This chart shows how a combination of 3 major risk factors can increase the likelihood of heart attack and stroke. Source: The Framingham Massachusetts Heart Study.

Figure 11-10. For each disease (heart attack and stroke), columns below the horizontal line indicate lower than average risk, while columns above the line represent higher than average risk.

Other warning signs are experiencing transient episodes of dizziness or staring blankly into space.

Symptoms of a stroke include:[29] difficulty in speaking, jumbled speech, or loss of the ability to speak; inability to understand the speech of others; sudden weakness or numbness in an arm or leg, in the face, or on one side of the body; loss of vision in one eye; dimming of eyesight in one or both eyes; brief episodes of double vision; dizziness or unsteadiness that cannot be attributed to another cause; a change in mental capacities, such as the sudden inability to remember the past or a sudden inability to calculate math; a change in personality; a pattern of headaches significantly different than the headaches normally experienced; difficulty in completing simple thought processes; or paralysis of some extremity (arm or leg) or of the face or one side of the body (such paralysis is generally permanent).

You run a risk of developing a stroke if you have high blood pressure, have had fleeting symptoms of minor strokes or have had a stroke before; have diabetes; are overweight; eat foods that are high in animal fats; have heart diseases of any kind; have arteriosclerosis; or smoke.[30]

ATHEROSCLEROSIS

By far the most common chronic disease affecting Americans,[31] atherosclerosis is a slow, progressive disease that begins early in life and generally goes undetected until middle or old age or until it causes a major medical problem.

Atherosclerosis deposits begin on the inside wall of a blood vessel — generally at a spot where the artery was abnormal or injured previously in some way.[32] Cholesterol, fats, and other fatty substances begin to accumulate in the arterial wall, and the deposit, or plaque (atheroma), begins to build. The interiors of the arteries are normally smooth and spacious. Plaque will narrow the arteries and cause the lining of the artery to become roughened, limiting the ability of the vessel to conduct the flow of blood and promoting the formation of clots. As the size of the plaque increases, the artery loses its flexibility, adding to the possibility that even more plaque will accumulate. If the plaque is allowed to continue increasing in size, the flow of blood is shut off due to blockage.

Any artery in the body can be affected by plaque buildup.[33] The ones that are most often affected, however, are the major arteries leading to the heart, lungs, brain, legs, and kidneys.

Plaque formation varies from person to person — and sometimes from artery to artery in the same person. In some instances the formation is rapid and is accompanied by a great deal of damage to the artery; in other cases, plaque formation and buildup are slow and gradual and little damage takes place.

RHEUMATIC FEVER

Rheumatic fever most usually strikes children between the ages of five and fifteen and is always preceded by a streptococcal infection (strep throat). Not *all* strep infections lead to rheumatic fever, but those that go untreated or undetected are apt to progress to rheumatic fever in susceptible people.

While the death rate from rheumatic fever used to be high due to the inability to conquer infection, the discovery of penicillin and its widespread use has greatly reduced the mortality rate. The main concern is damage to the heart valves — damage that may be permanent and that may shorten life.

The best prevention consists of prompt treatment of streptococcal infections. *Any* sore throat that lasts longer than three days should be seen by a doctor and tested. If strep throat is confirmed, proper treatment — including vigorous therapy with penicillin or another antibiotic — should be undertaken.

CONGENITAL HEART DEFECTS

Congenital heart defects — those defects found in the heart at birth — result from abnormal development of the heart in the fetus.

Researchers have not yet isolated all of the factors that lead to congenital heart defects.[34] One cause is disease or illness suffered by the mother during the first trimester of pregnancy — German measles is a particularly grim culprit. Other viral diseases are currently suspected, but medical confirmation is as yet unavailable. Heredity seems to be a factor in the likelihood of developing congenital heart defects, and other factors such as drugs or medications and radiation have been implicated.

The most common defects of the heart manifest at birth include holes in the wall that divides the lower chambers of the heart, holes in the wall dividing the upper chambers of the heart, lack of closure between the artery delivering blood to the body and the artery delivering blood to the lungs, constriction or narrowing of the largest artery in the body (the aorta), and transposition of the arteries delivering blood to the

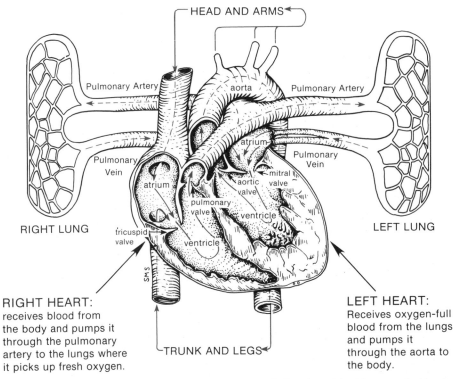

HEAD AND ARMS

Pulmonary Artery

aorta

Pulmonary Artery

atrium

Pulmonary Vein

Pulmonary Vein

atrium

mitral valve

aortic valve

pulmonary valve

ventricle

RIGHT LUNG

tricuspid valve

ventricle

LEFT LUNG

SMS

RIGHT HEART:
receives blood from the body and pumps it through the pulmonary artery to the lungs where it picks up fresh oxygen.

TRUNK AND LEGS

LEFT HEART:
Receives oxygen-full blood from the lungs and pumps it through the aorta to the body.

Figure 11-11. The heart and how it works. The heart is a 4-chambered double pump that beats 100,000 times a day while moving 4,300 gallons of oxygen-rich blood through the circulatory system to the entire body. As the heart beats, contractions of thick muscle wall (myocardium) pump blood from the heart through 60,000 miles of blood vessels. The heart rests only a fraction of a second between beats. The normal adult circulatory system contains about 8 pints of blood, recirculating continuously throughout the body. The heart has 2 pumping stations. The right heart pump receives the blood after it has delivered nutrients and oxygen to the body tissues, then starts on its journey to the lungs. The lungs cleanse the blood of waste gas (carbon dioxide) and provide it with a fresh supply of oxygen. The left heart receives this recycled blood from the lungs and pumps it through the circulatory system to its eventual return to the right heart. This recycling process is activated by a small node in the upper right chamber of the heart — actually an electrical impulse center — that normally regulates the heart to 60 to 80 beats a minute. The node sends out electrical impulses which travel through the heart's own intricate nervous system. This is the power source, the heart's own "pacemaker."

lungs and to the body (resulting in "blue babies," unable to get oxygenated blood).[35]

Death generally results if serious defects are not corrected; deaths in this case are usually due to the heart's inability to get an adequate blood

432

supply or to the baby's inability to deliver oxygenated blood to his organs and body tissues. Presently, only 12 percent of congenital heart disease cases die in the first year.[36] This is in stark contrast to a 90 percent fatality rate in the first year only a few short years ago.[37]

Recent advances in microsurgery have enabled doctors to perform heart surgery on infants who are only hours old, thus enabling medical teams to reverse the errors in an improperly formed heart. In some cases, the defects are not correctable but do not result in death. In these cases, the child generally has to exercise caution throughout his life in the kinds of activities in which he participates and in the kind of food that he eats.

DIAGNOSING HEART DISEASE

A number of tests and diagnostic tools have been developed that help determine the presence — and degree of involvement — of heart disease.

Blood Test

One important determinant of heart disease is the amount of lipid fats — particularly triglycerides and cholesterol — in the blood; the only way to determine that level is to examine a sample of blood.

Electrocardiogram

Commonly referred to as an ECG or EKG, the electrocardiogram gives a graphic representation of the electrical activity of the heart and can reveal irregularities in the heart rhythm thereby disclosing which portion of the heart muscle sustained injury as a result of a heart attack or other heart disorder.

Exercise Electrocardiogram

An exercise electrocardiogram is taken while the patient is exercising, most often while the patient walks or runs on a treadmill. It is designed to detect problems which surface only when the heart is placed under stress.

Flouroscopy

Fluoroscopy, a type of x-ray examination, allows the doctor to watch the heart in motion. It is useful in diagnosing irregularities in heart function and structure.

Echocardiography

Similar in technique to sonar, echocardiography can reveal the size of the heart chambers and great vessels, the motion of the heart valves, and the shape of the heart chambers and vessels without radiation.

Vectorcardiography

This advancement over the EKG features a three dimensional representation of the electrical impulses involved in initiating heart beats. Subtle aberrations in the electrical pattern that would be missed with the EKG are detected with this procedure.

Cardiac Catheterization

A thin, flexible tube made of material to which blood will not adhere (such as woven plastic) is threaded into the heart through a vein or artery (usually of the arm or leg). A cardiac catheter makes it possible to draw blood samples from the heart itself and to measure blood pressure in the individual heart chambers, across the heart valves, or across the great vessels.

COMMON SURGICAL PROCEDURES FOR HEART DISEASE PROBLEMS

Pacemakers

A pacemaker is an auxilliary artificial nerve center of batteries and transistors designed to take over the function of regulating the heart

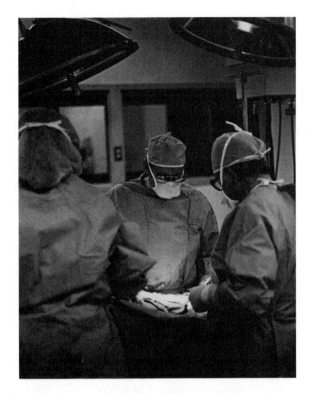

Surgical intervention has considerably decreased disability from heart disease.

beat. The device is usually implanted just under the skin near the shoulder or abdomen. Although the batteries require charging periodically, this is a non-surgical procedure, and pacemakers may go 10-15 years with no need for further surgical involvement.

Coronary Bypass

If some severe obstruction of coronary arteries exist, surgery may be performed to remove veins from some other part of the body and implant them in the heart in such a way as to bypass the obstructed arteries. This operation is common today and the survival rate is close to 99%.

Valve Replacement

Congenital defects, rheumatic fever, and occasionally infections of the heart may cause damage to the heart valves. If the damage is such that the valves simply will not allow adequate heart function, the valves will need to be replaced. Although valves from pigs have been used in the past, man-made valves are preferred presently. The operation has become rather routine and survival rates are high.

Notes

1. American Heart Association, *Heart Facts 1980* (American Heart Association, Inc., 55-005-D, 1977), p. 2.
2. Ibid., p. 2.
3. Ibid.
4. Theodore Irwin, *Watch Your Blood Pressure,* rev. ed. (Bethesda, Maryland: Public Affairs Commission, National Institute of Health, 1976), p. 3.
5. Ibid.
6. Weldon J. Walker, "Curbing Risk Factors *Has* Helped Reduce U. S. Coronary Deaths," *Modern Medicine,* vol. 44, June 1, 1976, p. 33.
7. Irwin, *Watch Your Blood Pressure,* p. 4.
8. *What Every Woman Should Know About High Blood Pressure* (Bethsda, Maryland: U.S. Department of Health, Education, and Welfare, National Institute of Health, 1974), DHEW Publication No. (NIH) 75-733, p. 1; and Irwin, *Watch Your Blood Pressure,* p. 12.
9. American Heart Association, *Heart Facts,* p. 10.
10. Irwin, *Watch Your Blood Pressure,* p. 13.
11. Ibid., p. 14.
12. Ibid.
13. Ibid.
14. Milton G. Crane, "High Blood Pressure," *Life and Health,* July 1976, p. 14.
15. Ibid.
16. Ibid., p. 15.
17. Ibid.
18. Ibid.
19. J. A. Scharffenberg, "What You Need to Know About High Blood Pressure," *Life and Health,* December 1978, p. 5.
20. Ibid.
21. John Ross, Jr., and Robert A. O'Rourke, *Understanding the Heart and Its Diseases* (New York: McGraw-Hill, 1976), p. 88.
22. "What Is a Heart Attack?" *Life and Health,* October 1976, p. 12.
23. *The Merck Manual,* 13th ed. (Rahway, New Jersey: Merck and Co. Inc., 1977), p. 382.
24. "Early Warning Signs of a Heart Attack," Card t.15135, Metropolitan Life Insurance Company.
25. *Congestive Heart Failure Fact Sheet,* Public Health Service, U.S. Department of Health, Education and Welfare, National Institute of Health, 1976, p. 1.

26. "Questions and Answers About Congestive Heart Failure — Patient Education Aid," *Patient Care,* vol. 14, October 15, 1980, p. 44.
27. "Diagnosing Congestive Heart Failure," *Patient Care,* vol. 14, October 15, 1980, p. 16.
28. Public Health Service, U.S. Department of Health, Education, and Welfare, National Institute of Health, Cerebral Vascular Disease and Strokes (Washington, D.C.: U.S. Government Printing Office, 1972), pp. 5-6.
29. *Cerebral Vascular Disease and Strokes,* p. 7; and "Stroke," p. 43.
30. *Cerebral Vascular Disease and Strokes,* p. 9.
31. Public Health Service, U.S. Department of Health, Education, and Welfare, National Institute of Health, *Arteriosclerosis Fact Sheet* (Washington, D.C.: U.S. Government Printing Office, 1978), p. 1.
32. *Arteriosclerosis Fact Sheet,* p. 2.
33. Ibid.
34. Public Health Service, U.S. Department of Health, Education, and Welfare, National Institute of Health, *Inborn (Congenital) Heart Defects* (Washington, D.C.: U.S. Government Printing Office, 1976), DHEW Publication No. (NIH) 76-1085, pp. 2-3.
35. *Inborn (Congenital) Heart Defects,* pp. 1-2.
36. Thomas W. Rowland, "The Pediatrician and Congenital Heart Disease — 1979," *Pediatrics,* vol. 64, August 1979, pp. 180-186.
37. Ibid.

Self-Evaluation

The purpose of this self-evaluation is to give you an estimate of your chances of suffering a heart attack. The Risk Factors are medical conditions and habits associated with an increased danger of heart attack. Not all risk factors are measurable enough to be included in this self-evaluation. See the end of the evaluation for other Risk Factors.

Study each Risk Factor and its score. Find the number applicable to you, and circle the number to which it corresponds. For example, if you are 37, circle the number 3. Then add all of the circled numbers. This total — your score — is an estimate of your risk.

If You Score:
6-11 — Risk well below average
12-17 — Risk below average
18-24 — Risk generally average
25-31 — Risk moderate
32-40 — Risk at a dangerous level
41-62 — Danger urgent. See your doctor now.

Heredity
Count parents, grandparents, brothers, and sisters who have had heart attack and/or stroke.

Tobacco Smoking
If you inhale deeply and smoke a cigarette way down, add one to your classification. Do NOT subtract because you think you do not inhale or smoke only a half inch on a cigarette.

Exercise
Lower your score one point if you exercise regularly and frequently.

Cholesterol or Saturated Fat Intake Level
A cholesterol blood level is best. If you can't get one from your doctor, then estimate honestly the percentage of solid fats you eat. These are usually of animal origin — lard, cream, butter, and beef and lamb fat. If you eat much of this, your cholesterol level probably will be high. The U.S. average, 40%, is too high for good health.

Blood Pressure
If you have no recent reading but have passed an insurance or industrial examination, chances are you are 140 or less.

Sex
This takes into account the fact that men have from 6 to 10 times more heart attacks than women of child-bearing age.

438

Test

Age	Score
10-20	1
21-30	2
31-40	3
41-50	4
51-60	6
61-70	
(& over)	8

Heredity	**Score**
No known history of heart disease	1
1 relative with cardiovascular disease — Over 60	2
2 relatives with cardiovascular disease — Over 60	3
1 relative with cardiovascular disease — Under 60	4
2 relatives with cardiovascular disease — Under 60	6
3 relatives with cardiovascular disease — Under 60	7

Weight	**Score**
More than 5 lbs. below standard weight	0
-5 to +5 lbs. standard weight	1
6-20 lbs. overweight	2
21-35 lbs. overweight	3
36-50 lbs. overweight	5
51-65 lbs. overweight	7

Tobacco Smoking	**Score**
Non-user	0
Cigar and/or pipe	1
10 cigarettes or less per day	2
20 cigarettes per day	4
30 cigarettes per day	6
40+ cigarettes per day	10

Exercise	**Score**
Intensive occupational and recreational exertion	1
Moderate occupational and recreational exertion	2
Sedentary work and intense recreational exertion	3
Sedentary occupational and moderate recreational activity	5
Sedentary work and light recreational exertion	6
Complete lack of all exercise	8

Cholesterol or Fat % in Diet   Score

	Score
Cholesterol below 180 mg.%. Diet contains no animal or solid fats	1
Cholesterol 181-205 mg.%. Diet contains 10% animal or solid fats	2
Cholesterol 206-230 mg.%. Diet contains 20% animal or solid fats	3
Cholesterol 231-255 mg.%. Diet contains 30% animal or solid fats	4
Cholesterol 256-280 mg.%. Diet contains 40% animal or solid fats	5
Cholesterol 281-300 mg.%. Diet contains 50% animal or solid fats	7

Blood Pressure   Score

	Score
100 upper reading	1
120 upper reading	2
140 upper reading	3
160 upper reading	4
180 upper reading	6
200+ upper reading	8

Sex   Score

	Score
Female under 40	1
Female 40-50	2
Female over 50	3
Male	5
Stocky Male	6
Bald stocky male	7

Because of the difficulty of measuring them, these Risk Factors are not included in the scoring:

Diabetes, particularly when present for many years.

Your character or personality, and the stress under which you live.

Vital capacity — determined by measuring the amount of air you can take into your lungs in proportion to the size of your lungs. The less air you can breathe, the higher your risk.

Electrocardiogram — if certain abnormalities are present in the record of the electrical currents generated by your heart, you have a higher risk.

Gout — is caused by a higher than normal amount of uric acid in the blood. Patients have an increased risk.

NOTE: If you have a number of Risk Factors, for the sake of your health, ask your doctor to check your medical conditions and quit your Risk Factor habits. The fact that various habits or conditions may be rated similarly in this evaluation does not mean that these are of equal risk. The reaction of individual human beings to Risk Factors — as to many other things — is so varied that it is impossible to draw valid conclusions for any individual. This evaluation has been developed only to highlight what the Risk Factors are and what can be done about them. It is NOT designed to be a medical diagnosis.

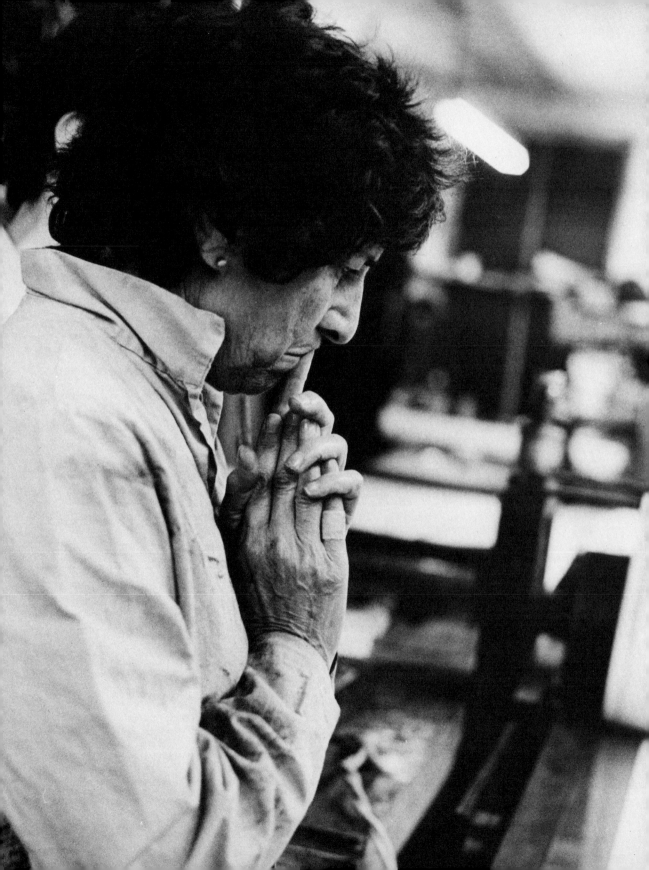

12
Cancer:
Beating the Odds

According to recent statistics, cancer will strike approximately two out of three American families. The tragedy lies in the fact that over 100,000 of those who die of cancer yearly could have been saved by earlier treatment — and that treatment can only result from earlier detection.

Cancer falls under a broader category of growths called neoplasms or tumors. Tumors fall into two major groups. One group, called benign tumors, are rather common. They grow slowly, never spread, contain cells that resemble the normal cells in the adjacent tissue, and are contained in a fibrous capsule. Generally speaking, they are harmless unless they cause pain, obstruct bodily functions, or are unsightly. These are sufficient reasons for surgical removal.

Cancer is the second type of tumor. Its main characteristic is abnormal, seemingly unrestricted growth of body cells. Unlike benign tumors, the resultant mass invades and destroys adjacent normal tissues. Sometimes cancer cells break off and leave the original mass to be carried by the blood or lymph to distant sites of the body, where they set up

A. Tumors can spread through direct extension
   and by the lymphatic and blood systems.

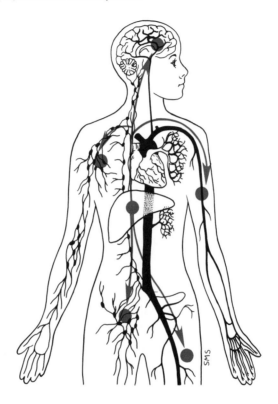

B. The steps of metastasis:

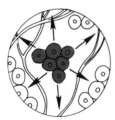 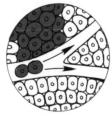 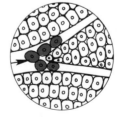 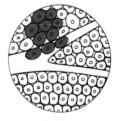

Tumor cells invade
surrounding tissue.

Tumor cell clumps,
called emboli, are
released into the
circulation.

Circulating emboli
are trapped in
small blood vessels.

Tumors penetrate
vessel walls into
adjacent tissue and
begin to multiply.
The process may
begin again.

444

secondary growths (mestatases), further attacking and destroying the organs involved.

Four factors tend to signal high risk for cancer, in general: overweight, smoking, drinking alcoholic beverages, and development of cancer in an immediate member of one's family. According to the American Cancer Society, certain factors indicate high risk for certain kinds of cancer.[1]

CAUSES OF CANCER

No one knows exactly what causes cancer, or whether the same factor is responsible for causing different kinds of cancer. If we knew exactly what caused cancer, of course, we would be much closer to

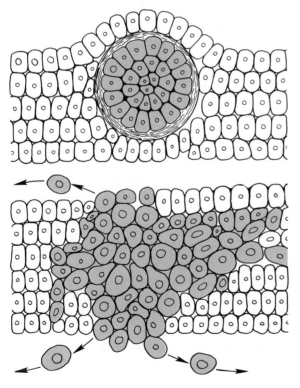

Figure 12-2. Benign tumors grow slowly, never spread, are encapsulated, and contain cells resembling normal precursors. Malignant tumors grow rapidly, are invasive, are rarely encapsulated, and contain many abnormal appearing cells. Source: *Chemistry*, Vol. 50, no. 1.

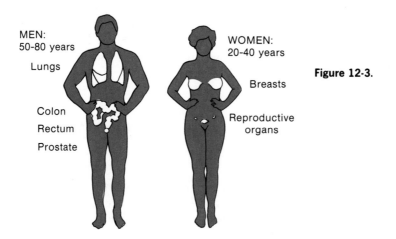

AGES AND TYPES OF CANCER
COMMON IN MALE AND FEMALE

MEN:
50-80 years

Lungs

Colon
Rectum
Prostate

WOMEN:
20-40 years

Breasts

Reproductive
organs

Figure 12-3.

finding an effective cure. But the causes appear to be as varied as the kinds of cancer. There are several factors that seem highly related:

1. **Condition of long-term irritation.** This includes extensive and frequent exposure to sunlight, which is believed to be a primary cause of skin cancer.
2. **Exposure to specific agents (carcinogens).** Many carcinogens originate in our environment. Federal agencies such as the Environmental Protection Agency (EPA) and the Food and Drug Administration (FDA) are currently embroiled in controversies, trying to establish a definition for "acceptable levels" of all kinds of environmental pollutants, from industrial waste to pesticides.
3. **Benign tumors that become malignant.** A prime example is that of leukoplakia, white patches on the mouth (benign) that eventually become malignant. Those tumors or conditions that may lead to cancer are termed *precancerous* or *premalignant.* Inroads have been made in treating such conditions (and identifying them early) before they become malignant.
4. **Hormones.** Evidence currently suggests that hormones are in some way involved in the development of certain cancers.

446

5. **Heredity.** Heredity, in terms of an influence toward or a predisposition to, a certain cancer is known as a familial influence. There is no single gene responsible. Only a few cancers exhibit familial tendencies, such as cancer of the breast, stomach, colon, prostate, and endometrium. The fact that an individual has at one time had cancer does not increase the possibility of a second episode.[2]
6. **Viruses.** There is some suspicion that cancer is caused by viruses in humans.

Figure 12-4. Source: Progress Against Cancer 1970, U.S. National Cancer Institute.

TYPES OF CANCER

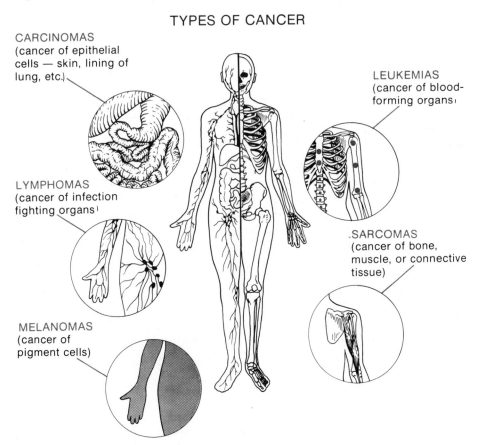

CARCINOMAS
(cancer of epithelial cells — skin, lining of lung, etc.)

LEUKEMIAS
(cancer of blood-forming organs)

LYMPHOMAS
(cancer of infection fighting organs)

SARCOMAS
(cancer of bone, muscle, or connective tissue)

MELANOMAS
(cancer of pigment cells)

Chemicals

One important chemical carcinogen is PCB — polychlorinated biphenyl. It has been on the market for almost forty years and is used in electrical transformers, capacitors, paints, inks, paper, plastics, adhesives, sealants, and hydraulic fluid. Traces of PCBs have been found in mothers' milk, in almost all human tissue samples collected in this country, in the flesh of fish from fresh water lakes and streams, in penguin eggs collected in Antarctica, and in animals captured in such remote spots as Greenland.

PCB produces cancer, mental retardation, reproductive disorders, skin lesions, liver problems, hair loss, and metabolic disorders. The average breast-fed baby is getting ten times more PCBs through its mother's milk than the FDA considers to be safe.

General Pollutants

Air pollution, which obliterates the skylines in many American cities, may also be linked to lung cancer.[3] Air pollutants come from industrial waste and from automobile exhaust — both of which contain carcinogenic elements.

Contamination of the water supplies can also cause cancer. One glass of tap water taken from a New Orleans household contained sixty-six organic chemicals; of those, eight were highly toxic potential carcinogens. There may be dangers in addition to pollutants; recent studies have raised concerns that the chemical used to *purify* culinary water, chlorine, may interact with other substances to produce carcinogens.[4] Fluoride has been recently investigated as a possible carcinogen.[5]

Radiation

Although radiation can damage the DNA and provoke mutations, it is a weak carcinogen. Radiation can cause leukemia. Radioactive strontium and iodine cause, respectively, bone and thyroid cancer.[6]

Foods

Complex chemical interactions in the foods that we eat may produce carcinogens.[7] Two of the most controversial food additives are sodium

448

nitrate and sodium nitrite — used in bacon, ham, and smoked foods and naturally present in some water supplies. The worst risk from foods is an indirect — but important — one: diets high in fat have been definitely linked to cancer. Those people with diets high in fat and low in fiber have a higher risk of developing several kinds of cancer, including cancer of the bowel, colon, stomach, breast, ovary, uterus, and prostate.[8] Heavy alcohol consumption is related to a higher risk of mouth, throat, esophageal, laryngeal, and liver cancer. The risk is even worse for heavy drinkers who smoke.

Drugs

Because drugs are taken in relatively large doses, researchers are more concerned with them than with the environmental or chemical additives to which we are exposed. Two examples are the increased risk of cancer related to the use of DES (diethylstilbesterol) and estrogen in treating pregnancy-related problems. Even the birth control pill — currently taken by millions of American women — has been implicated in certain kinds of cancer, especially cancer of the breast.

Drugs used to prevent rejection of human transplanted organs have also been shown to cause cancer, as have the drugs used in the treatment of psoriasis, acne, and sore throats.

DIAGNOSING CANCER

Diagnosing cancer often involves a complex network of laboratory tests designed to give physicians a clear picture of cellular activity in any suspected cancer area. But before those diagnostic tests take place, you may recognize that you may have cancer (either because you have recognized one or more of cancer's seven warning signals or because you know that you are a high-risk individual), and your doctor may perform a thorough physical examination to confirm that there may be a problem and that you need further testing.

The danger signs of cancer have been neatly organized by the American Cancer Society to facilitate memorization. The word "caution" is the skeleton upon which the danger signs are organized.

C = Change in bowel or bladder habits
A = A sore that does not heal
U = Unusual bleeding or discharge
T = Thickening or lump in the breast or elsewhere
I = Indigestion or difficulty in swallowing
O = Obvious change in wart or mole
N = Nagging cough or hoarseness[9]

Even if you do not exhibit one of cancer's seven warning signals, your doctor can detect early signs of cancer by checking the following:

1. Skin
2. Head and neck
3. Breast (whether you are male or female)
4. Pelvic area
5. Colon and rectum
6. Laboratory analysis of body secretions (i.e., urine, blood, etc.)

Further tests that your physician may recommend include:[10]

1. **Biopsy** — the surgical removal of a tiny piece of the tissue that might be cancerous. The tissue is examined carefully under a microscope for the presence of abnormal cells.

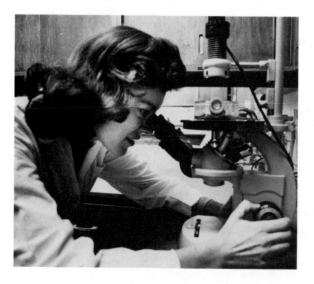

A biopsy analysis is used to determine the presence of cancer.

2. **Pap Smear** — the collecting of some cells from the cervix of the uterus with a cotton swab. These are further examined as in the biopsy and may suggest the need for further tests.
3. **Washings** from the stomach.
4. **Smears,** including smears from the nose and mouth, sputum samples, blood tests, and urine specimens.

MAJOR TYPES OF CANCER

Breast Cancer

Although the leading cancer killer in women, this malady is not unknown in men. In women, the malignancy occurs incident to or after

Figure 12-5. Self-Examination of Breasts (Looking).

Stand in front of a mirror with the upper body unclothed. Look for changes in the shape and size of the breast and for dimpling of the skin or "pulling in" of the nipples. Any changes in the breast may be made more noticeable by a change in position of the body and arms.

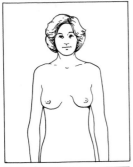
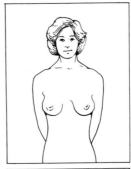

1. Stand with arms down.

2. Lean forward.

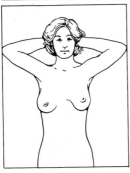
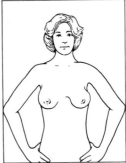

3. Raise arms overhead and press hands behind your head.

4. Place hands on hips and tighten chest and arm muscles by pressing firmly inward.

Figure 12-6. Self-Examination of Breasts (Feeling).

Lie flat on your back with a pillow or folded towel under your shoulders and feel each breast with the opposite hand in sequence. With the hand slightly cupped, feel with flattened finger tips for lumps or any change in the texture of the breast or skin; also, note any discharge from nipples or scaling of the skin of the nipples. Feel gently, firmly, carefully and thoroughly. Do not pinch your breast between thumb and fingers. This may give the impression of a lump that is not actually there.

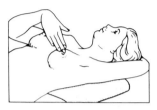

1. Place a pillow or folded towel under your left shoulder. This raises the breast and makes examination easier. Place your left arm over your head. With your right hand, feel the inner half of your left breast from top to bottom and from nipple to breastbone.

2. Feel the outer half from bottom to top and from the nipple to the side of the chest. Begin at outermost top of your right breast for 12 o'clock, then move to 1 o'clock, and so on around the circle back to 12. A ridge of firm tissue in the lower curve of each breast is normal. Then move in an inch, toward the nipple, keep circling to examine *every part of your breast,* including nipple. This requires at least three more circles. Now slowly repeat procedure on your left breast with a pillow under your left shoulder and left hand behind head. Notice how your breast structure feels.

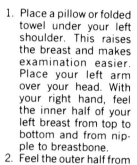

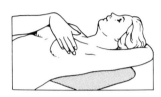

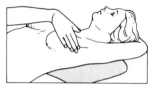

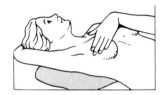

Finally, squeeze the nipple of each breast gently between thumb and index finger. Any discharge, clear or bloody, should be reported to your doctor immediately.

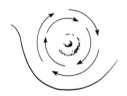

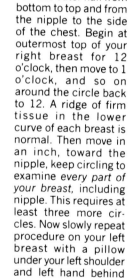

Pay special attention to the area between the breast and armpit itself.

Now, place the pillow or folded towel under your right shoulder. Repeat this same process for your right breast using the fingers of your left hand to feel.

452

menopause. Unmarried women, women who have married late, and those whose mother or sister have had the disease have a risk of breast cancer three times greater than the general population.[11]

Breast nodules occurring during the menstrual cycle must not be confused with suspicious lumps. To avoid this confusion, breast examination should be conducted after menstruation ceases. Suspicious lumps, usually detected by the woman herself, are most often found in the upper, outer quadrant of the breast. When manipulated, it seems to be fixed to breast structures and to be immovable. Other signs are an indrawing of the nipple, a dimpling of some part of the breast, unequal appearance of the two breasts when viewed in front of a mirror with the arms at the side or overhead, or a watery or bloody discharge from the nipple.[12]

Treatment usually involves surgical removal of the breast, associated lymph nodes and muscles. This procedure, known as a radical mastectomy, appears to be yielding to less radical procedures. The woman should be aware that there are alternative therapies. Her choice will influence survivability.[13]

Colon-Rectum Cancer

The hereditary presence of polyps (Familial polyposie), low fiber diet, and long standing ulcerative colitis are correlated with the malignancy. The most common symptom is a persistent change in bowel habits; often a pattern of alternating diarrhea and constipation. Other symptoms include intestinal bleeding, quite often inapparent.[14]

Hodgkin's Disease

This malignancy of the lymphatic system is much more common in men than in women. Early symptoms are usually fever and a nonspecific malaise accompanying the swollen cervical lymph gland. Cures for almost all patients are now possible through chemotherapy or radiation.

Leukemia

Leukemia comes in two forms, chronic and acute. Acute leukemia, usually found in children, is of shorter duration and generally runs a fatal course. It often starts out with symptoms of an acute illness. The patient is often dead within a few weeks or months. Chronic leukemia, which usually afflicts adults, takes a more sedate pace, allowing the individual years of life.

In most patients, leukemia begins silently. Sometimes it is not detected until the physician takes a routine blood count for a life insurance physical examination, for monitoring the course of an infection, or while preparing for surgery.[15] Eventually, the latent leukemia will rear its head and the disease will run its course.

Bleeding gums, internal hemorrhage, weakness, anemia, difficulty in warding off infections, and swollen glands are frequent symptoms.[16]

Treatment is by radiation or chemotherapy, and some long-standing remissions have been achieved, some as long as nineteen years. One type of leukemia in children now appears to be curable with chemotherapy.

Lung Cancer

This cancer is strongly linked to smoking cigarettes. The incidence for a nonsmoker is 3.4 per 100,000, whereas for a two pack or more a day smoker, it is 217 per 100,000.[17]

Coughing and wheezing are the usual symptoms. Coughing up blood will usually send the patient scurrying to see the doctor. By then it is often too late. Pneumonia or an abcess of the lung are complications that in themselves may cause death.[18] Chest x-rays will reveal a "shadow" in the lung, which in men who have been smoking for years is often regarded as malignant unless proven otherwise.

Oral/Facial Cancer

Most people — women, at least — realize that they can examine their own breasts to detect possible cancers, but few know that they can also examine their faces and mouths for cancer. Yet, oral/facial examination is perhaps even more critical: orofacial cancers occur at about four times the rate as breast cancers.[19]

All you need to perform the examination are a mirror, a gauze pad or handkerchief (clean, of course), and your own index finger — well-washed. Then examine these areas in these ways:

454

CANCER INCIDENCE BY SITE AND SEX*

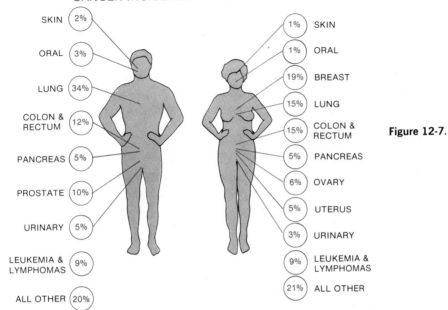

	Male	Female	
SKIN	2%	1%	SKIN
ORAL	3%	1%	ORAL
		19%	BREAST
LUNG	34%	15%	LUNG
COLON & RECTUM	12%	15%	COLON & RECTUM
PANCREAS	5%	5%	PANCREAS
		6%	OVARY
PROSTATE	10%	5%	UTERUS
URINARY	5%	3%	URINARY
LEUKEMIA & LYMPHOMAS	9%	9%	LEUKEMIA & LYMPHOMAS
ALL OTHER	20%	21%	ALL OTHER

Figure 12-7.

*Excluding non-melanoma skin cancer and carcinoma in situ.

CANCER DEATHS BY SITE AND SEX

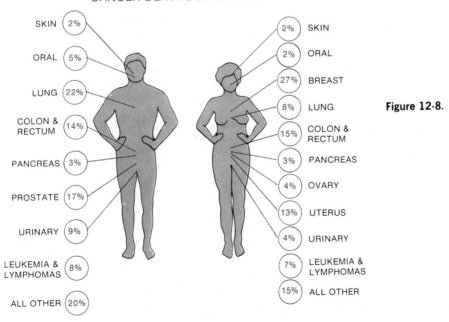

	Male	Female	
SKIN	2%	2%	SKIN
ORAL	5%	2%	ORAL
		27%	BREAST
LUNG	22%	8%	LUNG
COLON & RECTUM	14%	15%	COLON & RECTUM
PANCREAS	3%	3%	PANCREAS
		4%	OVARY
PROSTATE	17%	13%	UTERUS
URINARY	9%	4%	URINARY
LEUKEMIA & LYMPHOMAS	8%	7%	LEUKEMIA & LYMPHOMAS
ALL OTHER	20%	15%	ALL OTHER

Figure 12-8.

*Excluding non-melanoma skin cancer and carcinoma in situ.

455

1. Face: Look at the skin of your face, neck, and lips. See if any of the skin has changed color (without explanation) and if you have any lumps or sores. Make sure that you look at the area that is usually covered by your eyeglasses if you wear them.
2. Outer cheeks: Feel your outer cheeks carefully. Are there any lumps or swellings? Do you feel tenderness? Feel them all the way back to your ears and all the way down to your jaw.
3. Neck: Feel your neck closely, all the way around, paying special attention to the sides (where the lymph glands lie) and to your Adam's apple area. Is there tenderness, or do you feel lumps?
4. Roof of the mouth: Tilt your head back, and use your well-lighted mirror to look at both your hard and soft palate. Note any abnormalities — coloring, growths, tenderness, etc.
5. Tongue: You need to look at both the top side and under side of your tongue, again with the well-lighted mirror. Grasp your tongue with the gauze or handkerchief, and pull it out; extend it in all directions so that you get a good look at it from all sides. Note any growths, sores, or ulcerated areas.
6. Inner cheek: Use your index finger on the inside (and your thumb on the outside) to expose the lining of your cheek. Look for any ulcerations, growths, or white, red, or dark patches.
7. Lips: Evert your upper lip, and look for any possible white, red, or dark patches. Do the same with your lower lip. Also check for growths or sores.
8. Floor of the mouth. Lift up your tongue, and examine the floor of your mouth that is located underneath your tongue. If you have never looked under your tongue, you will find a rainbow of colors and a whole bevy of lumps. It is a good idea to have your doctor or dentist point out during your next examination what is normal.

Prostate Cancer

This common cancer, fortunately, is slow growing and slow to spread. The disease is also late starting, which explains why so many men who have it do not die of it. They die of other causes, and the cancer is not detected unless a postmortem examination is performed.[20] An estimated incidence of 70 percent of men over the age of seventy[21] gives an indication of how common this cancer is in aged men.

Due to the location of the prostate gland at the base of the bladder, a frequent symptom is difficulty in urinating, including a weak flow, difficulty in initiating urination, or frequent urination. Later, low back, thigh, or pelvic pain[22] is particularly suspicious.

Skin Cancer

Even though skin cancer is one of the more common cancers, it is generally curable. Skin cancer grows slowly and is usually readily visible. It is now known that exposure to ultraviolet light (ultraviolet light is present in sunlight) increases the risk of developing skin cancer. Skin cancer has increased twofold in the last twenty-five years primarily

SOLAR RADIATION AND SKIN CANCER.

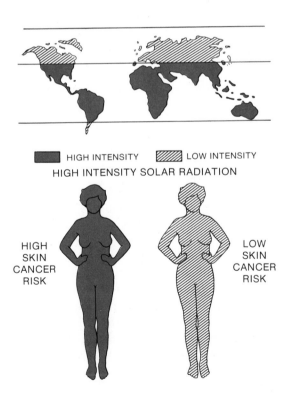

HIGH INTENSITY   LOW INTENSITY

HIGH INTENSITY SOLAR RADIATION

HIGH SKIN CANCER RISK

LOW SKIN CANCER RISK

Figure 12-9. Fair-skinned people exposed to intense ultraviolet radiation from the sun are at a higher risk of skin cancer than are others. Skin cancer occurs most frequently in the southern belt of the United States from New Mexico to the Atlantic Coast and in Australia, where solar radiation is more intense than in most areas of the United States. Source: Progress Against Cancer 1970, U.S. National Cancer Institute.

457

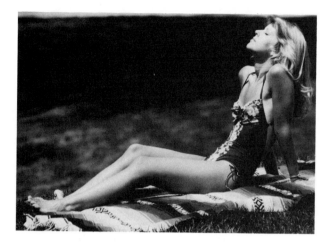

The "healthy" tan may promote cancer and premature aging of the skin.

because of the increase in sunbathing. The sunlamps used in many tanning booths produce ultraviolet light of the type that has been associated with skin cancer.

Testicular Cancer

Testicular cancer is the most common kind of cancer in men of ages twenty-nine to thirty-five. In fact, about 80 percent of testicular cancers occur in men of age forty and under.[23]

If testicular cancer is diagnosed early, it tends to be one of the most curable of cancers. But if it is not caught early, it is one of the most deadly. Because masses or enlargement of a testicle can be detected with relative ease, it is wise for men to practice self-examination once a month. This should be done after a warm bath or shower when the muscles of the scrotum are most relaxed and the contents can be most easily felt. Using the thumbs and fingers of both hands, you should probe the scrotum for hard lumps by rolling each testicle between the thumbs and fingers. Under normal conditions, the testicles are neither hard nor soft, but they have a sort of rubbery consistency. You should also feel for the epididymus and the spermatic cord to make sure that they are normal. The epididymus is on top of and behind each testicle. It should be a soft and slightly tender structure. The spermatic cord, which ascends from the epididymus and is behind the testicle, is a tubular structure that should feel firm and smooth to the touch.[24]

Uterine Cancer

There is more than one type of uterine cancer. The most common form is squamous cell carcinoma, which develops in women most frequently between the ages of forty and sixty. It begins with what is known as carcinoma-in-situ. Carcinoma-in-situ is confined to the cervix and is completely curable by surgery. Adenocarcinoma of the endometrium is the second most common form of uterine cancer. This cancer is associated with not having children. This is why its incidence is higher among nuns or women who have one or two children as opposed to women who have more children. Bleeding between periods, after intercourse, or after menopause is the most common symptom.[25]

TREATMENT

Surgery is by far the most effective method of treating cancer. It accounts for well over three-fourths of the cancers cured annually. If every cancer cell is removed, obviously the individual is cured. Achieving this desirable result often requires the removal of the lymphatics draining the area of the body in which the cancer was located in addition to removing the cancer. This necessitates the removal of large amounts of tissue and is known as radical surgery. On occasion it is disabling, sometimes disfiguring. Artificial limbs and reconstructive surgery are sometimes required in follow-up care. Less radical surgical procedures are available, but the evidence suggests lower cure rates.

Some cancers are inoperable. Some are due to the location of the tumor, i.e., cranial tumors. Some are due to the nature of the cancer, i.e., leukemia.

When surgery cannot be employed, the method of treatment is radiation or chemotherapy or both. These two are sometimes used in conjunction with surgery, the theory being to overwhelm the cancer by first cutting it out, then launching a two-pronged attack on any remaining cancer cells. Radiation seems to be most effective against cancers of the lymphatic system and rapidly dividing tumors. Conversely, slower dividing cancers are less susceptible; some are even resistant. This is why radiation can cure only a few cancers.

The medical profession has devised various ways of administering

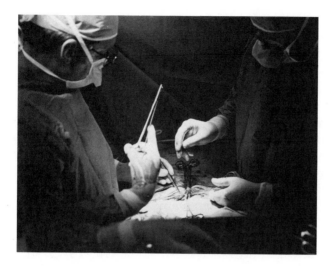

Surgery is the most successful treatment approach for cancer.

the radiation to the target tumor. Radioactive particles are surgically implanted in some tumors; radioactive isotopes that collect in certain tumors are used in other cases. Then there is the traditional mode of administering radiation: x-ray, radium, or radioactive cobalt. In these cases, radiation burns can occur where the emissions entered the body. Often the individual will go bald, lose his eyebrows, and become nauseated. The radiation patient can be quite ill for a while.

Chemotherapy can produce similar side effects, because the chemicals used are very toxic. The major advances involve Hodgkin's disease and acute lymphatic leukemia in children. Interferon, a hoped for potent treatment originating from within the body, has not materialized.

CANCER QUACKERY

Unfortunately, cancer victims are increasingly becoming victims of cancer quacks: doctors who prescribe unorthodox — and ineffective — methods of treatment at skyrocketing costs. An unproven therapy of recent fame is laetrile; presently one of the most highly promoted "cures" for cancer. Laetrile is an extract of apricot pits. Laetrile contains cyanide, and it is thought that cancer cells are more susceptible to the toxic effects of laetrile than are normal cells. This means that the cyanide element in

460

laetrile kills tumor cells, leaving healthy cells supposedly untouched. However, several people on laetrile therapy have died from cyanide poisoning, thus showing that cyanide does harm healthy cells.

PREVENTING AND REDUCING CANCER RISKS

The first line of defense against cancer is knowledge. Listen to your body and be aware of its function. Also, note some of these suggestions:[26]

1. Eat less high-fat beef, lamb, and pork; instead, eat more fish and poultry.
2. When you do decide to eat meat, select lean cuts; trim off all the visible fat before you cook and eat it.
3. Do not deep-fry food; bake, broil, roast, or stew it instead.
4. When you cook a soup or stew, make it ahead of time and refrigerate it overnight. The next day, remove all the fat that has congealed before you rewarm it.
5. Subsitute skimmed and low-fat milk and cheese for whole milk and cheese.

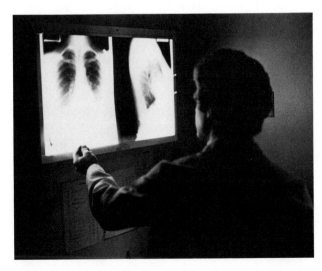

Early detection is the most important factor in preventing cancer death.

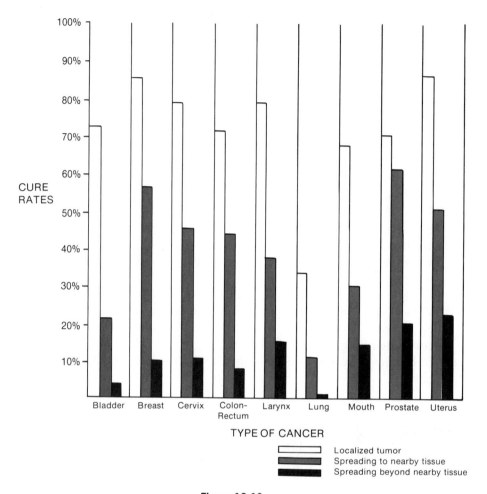

100%

90%

80%

CURE
RATES

60%

50%

40%

30%

20%

10%

Bladder　Breast　Cervix　Colon-　Larynx　Lung　Mouth　Prostate　Uterus
Rectum

TYPE OF CANCER

Localized tumor
Spreading to nearby tissue
Spreading beyond nearby tissue

Figure 12-10.

6. Eat only two to three eggs a week.
7. Substitute soft margarine for butter.
8. Use only liquid vegetable oil, never solid shortening (corn or soybean oil is best).
9. Avoid sugar-sweetened foods.
10. Eat more vegetables, beans, whole grains, and fruits.
11. Do not smoke.
12. Avoid smoke-filled rooms.

462

13. Avoid contact with car fumes and factory exhaust.
14. Do not get x-rays unless you really need them; refuse to let your doctor x-ray you as a routine.
15. Limit your exposure to the sun.
16. Use strong sunscreens when you are in the sun; reapply them after swimming or showering or if you are perspiring heavily.
17. Avoid long exposure to household solvent cleaners, cleaning fluids, and paint thinners.
18. Avoid eating many smoked or pickled foods.
19. Take great caution when you use pesticides, fungicides, and other garden and lawn chemicals.
20. Avoid ingestion of artificial sweeteners, like saccharin.
21. Do not drink alcohol.
22. Choose your occupation carefully.
23. Be careful about contraception; if possible, do not use oral contraceptives.
24. Avoid chronic irritation (including repeated infection).
25. Do not take any kind of medication needlessly.
26. When you buy bread, make sure that it contains whole grain *and* yeast.
27. Avoid eating prepared foods — especially anything that is "instant."
28. When you bake with flour, use whole wheat and whole grain as often as you can.
29. Examine your breasts once a month.
30. Perform any other self-examination that your doctor recommends.
31. Have regular physical checkups.
32. Learn the seven warning signals of cancer, and report to your doctor immediately if one persists longer than two weeks.

Notes

1. American Cancer Society, *1978 Cancer Facts and Figures*, pp. 4-5.
2. Cairns, *Cancer: Science and Society*, pp. 52-53.
3. "Cancer Hazards in the Modern Environment," *Progress Against Cancer*, the National Advisory Council, the U.S. Department of Health, Education, and Welfare, Public Health Service, and the National Institute of Health.
4. "Scare Over Cancer in Water — What Research Shows," *U.S. News and World Report*, December 2, 1974, p. 61.
5. "Fluoridation: The Cancer Scare," *Consumer Reports*, July 1978, pp. 392-396.
6. Cairns, *Cancer: Science and Society*, pp. 105-107.
7. "What Causes Cancer?" *Newsweek*, January 26, 1976, pp. 62-67.
8. "Can Diet Cause Cancer?" *Current Prescribing*, January 1977, p. 35.
9. American Cancer Society, *1981 Cancer Facts and Figures*, p. 20.
10. Department of Health, Education, and Welfare, *The Cancer Story*, p. 6.
11. William Boyd and Huntington Sheldon, *An Introduction to the Study of Disease*, 7th ed., Philadelphia: Lea and Febiger, 1977, p. 358.
12. Clara Gene Young and James D. Barger, *Introduction to Medical Science*, 3rd ed., St. Louis: C.V. Mosby Company, 1977, p. 50.
13. Benjamin F. Byrd, Jr., "Mastectomy Calls for More Than Surgery," *Consultant*, Vol. 15, August 1975, pp.48-49.
14. Boyd and Sheldon, p. 291.
15. Young and Barger, p. 359.
16. Boyd and Sheldon, p. 405.
17. Boyd and Sheldon, p. 257.
18. Young and Barger, p. 58.
19. "Self-exam for Orofacial Cancer," *Medical World News*, May 3, 1976, p. 23.
20. Young and Barger, p. 61.
21. Young and Barger, p. 343.
22. Young and Barger, p. 62; Boyd and Sheldon, p. 343.
23. Margaret Conklin, et al., "Should Health Teaching Include Self-Examination of the Testes?" *American Journal of Nursing*, December 1978, pp. 2073-2075.
24. *Ibid.*
25. Young and Barger, p. 49.
26. Jane E. Brody, "A Way to Reduce Your Chances of Getting Cancer," *Reader's Digest*, November 1977, pp. 131-134; Ruth Winter, "10 Ways You Can Avoid Cancer," *Science Digest*, May 1973, pp. 33-37; Guy R. Newell and Norma Golumbic, "What You Can Do to Protect Yourself Against Cancer," *AORN Journal*, Vol. 25, No. 5, April 1977, pp. 909-922; and Nicholas Gonzalez, "Preventing Cancer," *Family Health/Today's Health*, May 1976, pp. 30-34, 69-74.

Self-Evaluation

Section 1

An individual could conceivably rank himself in a Likelihood of Cancer Quotient to determine relative risk of developing cancer. Assuming all exposures to potential carcinogens, and all factors are of equal magnitude, a theoretical Likelihood of Cancer Quotient might look something like this:

Answer the following questions with a Yes or No. Score one point for every Yes and nothing for every No.

1. Do I smoke cigarettes?   Yes_____   No_____

2. Do I acquire more than ten hours of exposure to sunlight each week over one half of my body during the summer?   Yes_____   No_____

3. Am I light-skinned or a redhead?   Yes_____   No_____

4. Do I have more than one serving of meat each day for four or more days in a week?   Yes_____   No_____

5. Does my diet *not* include two slices of whole wheat bread or four servings of fruits and vegetables daily?   Yes_____   No_____

6. Have I had five x-rays of my body trunk in the past year?   Yes_____   No_____

7. Do I eat unrefrigerated left-overs that are more than eighteen hours old?   Yes_____   No_____

8. Do I *not* know the seven danger signs of cancer?   Yes_____   No_____

9. Do I have hypertension?   Yes_____   No_____

10. Does my job expose me to known carcinogens, i.e., asbestos?   Yes_____   No_____

11. Am I undergoing immunosuppressive therapy for any reason?   Yes_____   No_____

12. Has anyone in my family had stomach or colon cancer?   Yes_____   No_____

For women, answer and score these additional questions in the same manner.

1. Have I participated in pre-marital sex with more than one partner since the age of sixteen?   Yes _____ No _____

2. Have I given birth to *no* more than two children? (or, intend to do this?)   Yes _____ No _____

3. Have I waited until the late twenties or early thirties to give birth to my children? (or, intend to do this?)   Yes _____ No _____

4. Has a sister or has my mother developed breast cancer?   Yes _____ No _____

5. Do I have a diet high in fats?   Yes _____ No _____

Total your score. Double the score if you are fifty, and triple the score if you are sixty. Divide the score by your age for your Likelihood of Cancer Quotient. The higher the quotient, the greater the likelihood of developing cancer.

This little exercise, while interesting, is not scientific. It can only crudely estimate greater or lesser risk. There is no way of quantifying the risk, because norms have not been established. Further, there is no way of weighting different risk factors. Cigarette smoking probably deserves such a weighting, but how much is not known.

Not all cancers are touched by this little exercise. There is nothing for pancreatic, bladder, or prostate cancer, and all of these are leading cancer killers.

Section 2
Cancer Risk

Directions: Respond to each statement by answering yes or no.

Yes	No	Do you have extremely fair skin?
Yes	No	Do you have an outdoor occupation (i.e., farmer)?
Yes	No	Are you exposed to the sun (more than four hours per day for four months each year?)
Yes	No	Do you have a history of skin cancer or malignant moles?
Yes	No	Do you have moles on the soles of your feet or in areas irritated by tight clothing or shaving?

Yes	No	Do you have scars from severe burns?
Yes	No	Do you have a non-healing scaling sore on your skin?
Yes	No	You do not wear protective clothing (hats, long-sleeve shirts) when out in the sun for long periods.
Yes	No	You do not avoid excessive sunbathing.
Yes	No	You do not apply sunscreening ointment (different from regular suntan lotion).
Yes	No	You do not avoid contact with arsenic (found in some insecticides) and coal tar derivatives.
Yes	No	Has a member of your family ever had skin cancer or Hodgkin's disease?
Yes	No	You have had a mole removed.
Yes	No	You have had x-ray treatment (radiation therapy).
Yes	No	Do you smoke cigarettes, cigars, or a pipe?
Yes	No	Do you smoke more than one pack of cigarettes a day?
Yes	No	Do you drink beer, wine, or hard liquor daily?
Yes	No	Do you drink more than five beers, five glasses of wine, or three hard liquor drinks per day?
Yes	No	You do not have regular dental checkups.
Yes	No	Do you have a broken or crooked tooth that irritates the inside of your mouth?
Yes	No	Has a member of your family ever had cancer of the head and neck?
Yes	No	Have you ever had an x-ray treatment to the neck in youth?
Yes	No	Have you ever had a thyroid disorder?
Yes	No	Have you ever had a tumor in the throat or neck?
Yes	No	Do you work with or have you ever worked with: radioactive materials, asbestos, coal dust, stone or other minerals, nickel or chromates?
Yes	No	Have you ever had a respiratory disease? (i.e., tuberculosis, chronic bronchitis, emphysema, etc.)
Yes	No	Do you work daily with cleaning fluids, paints, dyes?
Yes	No	Have you ever had any urinary tract problems (i.e., infections, kidney stones, blood in the urine, etc.)?
Yes	No	Has a member of your family ever had cancer of the kidney or bladder?

Yes	No	Have you ever had stomach or duodenal ulcer, gall bladder disorder, pernicious anemia, hepatitis, cirrhosis of the liver, polyps of the stomach or colon, colitis?
Yes	No	Has a member of your family ever had stomach cancer, stomach ulcer, colon polyps, cancer of the colon or rectum?

For Men Only —

Yes	No	Have you ever had a prostate inflammation, venereal disease, or cancer of the prostate or testicles?
Yes	No	Are you over 50 years of age?
Yes	No	A physician has not examined your prostate regularly.

For Women Only —

Yes	No	Do you use female hormones (estrogens)?
Yes	No	Do you use birth control pills?
Yes	No	Has a member of your mother's side of the family ever had cancer of the cervix, vagina, uterus, or ovary?
Yes	No	Did your mother take hormones when she was pregnant with you?
Yes	No	Have you ever had an ovarian cyst or tumor, a Dilatiation and Curettage operation (D&C or scraping), surgery of the female organs?
Yes	No	Have you had an early marriage — or intercourse beginning before age 18?
Yes	No	Have you completed the menopause?
Yes	No	Are you diabetic?
Yes	No	Are you obese?
Yes	No	Have you ever been pregnant?
Yes	No	Have you had several different sexual partners?
Yes	No	You don't have a Pap smear test as scheduled for your age.
Yes	No	Has a member of your mother's side of the family ever had breast cancer, cysts or tumors of the breast, or any breast surgery?
Yes	No	You forget to examine your breasts each month after your period.

Evaluation: Yes answers indicate susceptibility for cancer. It does not mean you will develop cancer, but that you should be alerted to the potential. Gain as much information about cancer and especially the often-cited "Seven Danger Signals."

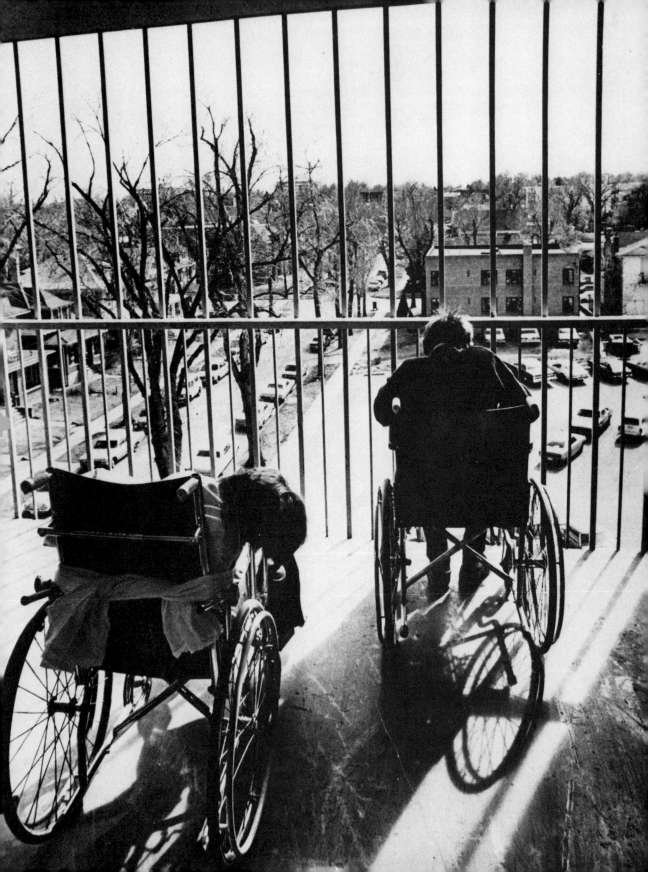

13

Chronic Diseases: Everybody Gets Something

ARTHRITIS

"Arthritis is man's oldest known chronic illness."[1]

Arthritis is an inflammation of the joints. It is not to be confused with rheumatism, which is an inflammation of connective tissue structures such as muscles, tendons, and ligaments, including joints. There is some overlapping in these definitions. If the muscles are predominantly involved, the condition is rheumatism. If the pain and swelling are in the joints and bones, it is arthritis.

The tragedy is that many people become crippled and stay crippled unnecessarily. Many do not understand that arthritis is seldom hopeless, and few seek and follow treatment that can either prevent disability in the first place or reduce it after it has happened. If you can learn the facts about arthritis, a great deal *can* be done about arthritis.

HOW ARTHRITIS CAN AFFECT A JOINT

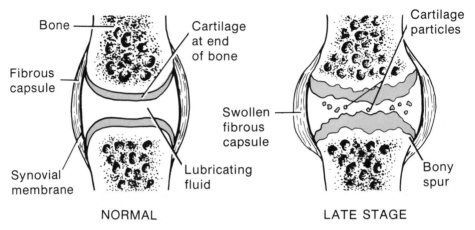

Figure 13-1.

The four major warning signs of arthritis are:[2] (1) persistent pain and stiffness on arising; (2) pain, swelling, or tenderness in one or more joints; (3) recurrence of pain, swelling, or tenderness, especially when they involve more than one joint; and (4) recurrent or persistent pain and stiffness in the lower back, neck, knees, and other joints. Unfortunately, aching and pains in the joints or around the joints can mean a host of things — not just arthritis. It is critical to be examined and diagnosed promptly if you experience any of the four warning signs of arthritis, because prompt treatment can help prevent a great deal of crippling.

To help cope with arthritis, try the following:

1. Take off extra pounds. Obesity adds stress and strain to joints and provokes and worsens arthritis.
2. Get a *sufficient* amount of rest — particularly important during periods when your joints are inflamed and painful. In the past, doctors recommended extensive bed rest, but experience has shown that long periods of inactivity can lead to deformity and can have an adverse effect on circulation and muscle tone.
3. Heat is usually beneficial in relieving pain, and a warm bath first thing in the morning can help victims of arthritis get going. Specific areas of pain can benefit from hot water bottles, heating pads, or heat lamps.

4. Depending on the type of exercise, movement can be either good or bad for arthritis victims. Any kind of exercise that puts undue strain on the arthritic joint or that may cause inflammation should be avoided. Most beneficial are exercises that allow the joints to move through their full range of motion without strain; swimming, especially in a heated pool, is considred to be excellent.
5. Medical attention, diagnosis, and treatment should *always* be obtained and followed. Arthritis, untreated and advanced, can and does lead to death.

DIABETES

In ordinary conditions, the body extracts a chemical called glucose out of foods. The glucose, or sugar, is used by the body for energy; a reserve supply is stored in various places in the body and is used as needed for reserve energy. The hormone insulin, secreted into the bloodstream by the pancreas, is essential in the process of breaking down and using glucose.

Figure 13-2.

BOTH PARENTS
DIABETIC

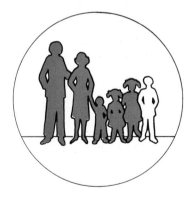

Odds: if I have four children,
three will have diabetes
or become diabetic.

ONE PARENT
DIABETIC

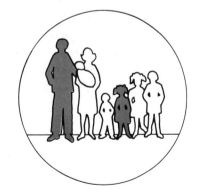

Odds: if I have five children,
one will have diabetes
or become diabetic.

INSULIN AND THE UTILIZATION OF FOOD

NORMAL PERSON

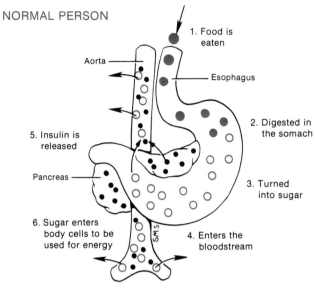

1. Food is eaten

Aorta

Esophagus

2. Digested in the somach

5. Insulin is released

3. Turned into sugar

Pancreas

6. Sugar enters body cells to be used for energy

4. Enters the bloodstream

DIABETIC

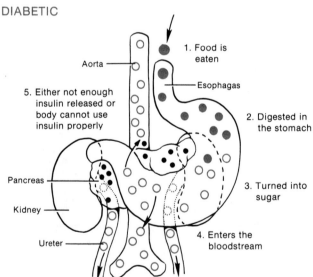

1. Food is eaten

Aorta

Esophagas

5. Either not enough insulin released or body cannot use insulin properly

2. Digested in the stomach

Pancreas

3. Turned into sugar

Kidney

4. Enters the bloodstream

Ureter

6. Sugar keeps building up in the blood. Finally it spills over into the urine and leaves the body.

Figure 13-3.

474

In diabetes, not enough insulin is available to complete this essential process. The insulin can be missing completely, can be present in insufficient supplies, or can be in a form that cannot be utilized by the diabetic. The result? The glucose accumulates in the blood and stays there until the surplus can be passed through the kidneys and out of the body with the urine. As a result, the body cannot use the glucose for energy and cannot store the surplus glucose as needed for reserve energy.

Anyone can develop diabetes, but certain risk factors lead to its development.[3]

1. **People whose relatives have diabetes.**
2. **People over the age of forty.**
3. **Women.** Two out of every three diabetics are women.
4. **People who are overweight.**

Since the earlier diabetes is diagnosed, the better, you should have frequent physical examinations if you fall into one or more of these risk groups; your physical examinations should always include a test for diabetes.

The typical list of symptoms of diabetes includes: excessive thirst, excessive urination, hunger, loss of weight, fatigue (tiring more rapidly and easier than usual), slow healing of cuts and bruises, changes in vision, intense itching, pain in the fingers and toes, or drowsiness. While these symptoms are the most usual, all of them will not appear in most cases. In many cases, the victim may experience only one or two. Also, you can have diabetes without having any symptoms at all. Diabetes is detected by blood and urine tests; one of the most positive signs is sugar in the blood and urine.

Most treatment regimes consist of dietary control, medication, injection of insulin, and exercise. In about one in three diabetics, diet alone is enough to keep the disease under control. Insulin, generally given by injection under the skin of the arm, abdomen, or thigh, helps lower the amount of sugar in the blood and helps the diabetic utilize some of the blood sugar more efficiently. It is critical that insulin be administered at the proper time of day and that it be administered in the proper dosage; mistakes in administration can lead to diabetic coma (too little insulin) or insulin shock (too much insulin). Either condition, unchecked, can lead to death. Diabetics are in good control if they feel well, are able to maintain normal weight on a well-balanced diet, have urine tests that are negative (do not indicate sugar content), and have normal blood tests.

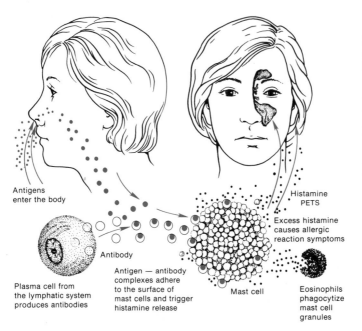

Figure 13-4. During specific antigen-antibody reactions, eosinophils migrate to the affected site, where they try to ingest and phagocytize the antigen-antibody complexes and neutralize the chemical mediators responsible for the reaction. Source: Patient Care, June 15, 1976.

Antigens enter the body

Plasma cell from the lymphatic system produces antibodies

Antibody

Antigen — antibody complexes adhere to the surface of mast cells and trigger histamine release

Mast cell

Eosinophils phagocytize mast cell granules

Excess histamine causes allergic reaction symptoms

Histamine PETS

ALLERGIES

Allergies are among the nation's most common and costly health problems.[4] Even though allergies cause few deaths, they have the capacity for making life miserable.

Individuals who have an allergy have developed an unusual sensitivity to some substance, known as an allergen, which does not bother most people.[5] The severity of symptoms resulting from this sensitivity ranges from mildly discomforting to, in rare cases, life-threatening. Common substances that may serve as allergens include foods, drugs, cosmetics, insects, molds, dusts, and pollens. Some of the most common include bees, ragweed, penicillin, chocolate, saccharin, pets, milk, fruits, and nuts.[6]

Scientists do not yet know what causes one person to develop an allergy to a substance that has no effect on other people. There is evidence, however, that an individual may inherit a tendency to become sensitized but not to any specific allergen.

Although allergy treatments tend to be individualized according to the substances to which the person is allergic, general procedures may be adapted for most allergies.

1. **Drugs.** Anti-inflammatory and antihistamine agents are the drugs most commonly used in the control of allergic reactions. Drug

Figure 13-5. Source: *U.S. News and World Report,* January 1973, pp. 40, 41.

EIGHT COMMON TROUBLEMAKERS PLAGUING ALLERGY VICTIMS

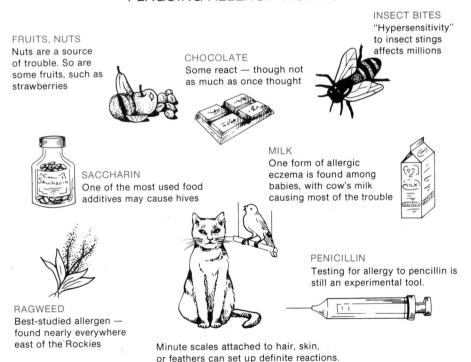

INSECT BITES
"Hypersensitivity" to insect stings affects millions

FRUITS, NUTS
Nuts are a source of trouble. So are some fruits, such as strawberries

CHOCOLATE
Some react — though not as much as once thought

MILK
One form of allergic eczema is found among babies, with cow's milk causing most of the trouble

SACCHARIN
One of the most used food additives may cause hives

PENICILLIN
Testing for allergy to pencillin is still an experimental tool.

RAGWEED
Best-studied allergen — found nearly everywhere east of the Rockies

Minute scales attached to hair, skin, or feathers can set up definite reactions.

Causes of allergy are myriad — depicted here are but a few. A physician frequently uses skin tests to help pinpoint the source.
Source: U.S. News and World Report, January 1973, pp. 40, 41.

SEASONAL DISTRIBUTION OF PLANT ALLERGENS

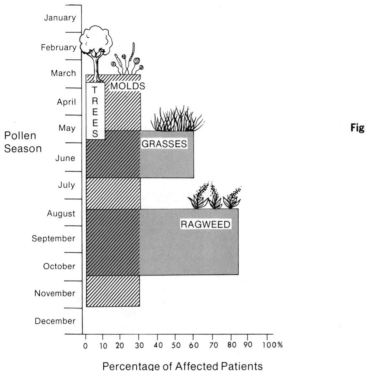

Figure 13-6.

therapy, however, has not been entirely successful in treating allergies, because individual response to the drugs may be erratic, and there may be undesirable side effects.

2. **Immunotherapy.** Immunotherapy or "desensitization" is accomplished by the injection of allergens known to trigger an allergic response under the skin.

3. With both seasonal and year-round allergies, partial control can be achieved through avoidance.

Hay Fever (Allergic Rhinitis)

The symptoms of hay fever include a stuffy nose with watery (not mucousy) discharge; red, itchy eyes; sneezing; a burning, itchy throat;

478

and occasional hearing impairment. There is never fever with hay fever. To tell the difference between a cold and hay fever, check for fever. If your hay fever is mild, it can generally be treated with over-the-counter remedies such as antihistamines or decongestants. You should always see a doctor if the hay fever is severe or if you experience pain or popping sounds in the ears; persistent coughing; difficulty in breathing; wheezing; or pain above the teeth, in the cheeks, above the eyes, or on the side of the nose. They generally signal complications or something more serious, such as asthma or sinus infection. Hay fever that is more severe may need to be treated by prescription antihistamines, anti-inflammatory drugs, and immunotherapy.

Bronchial Asthma

Asthma victims are generally extremely sensitive to allergens such

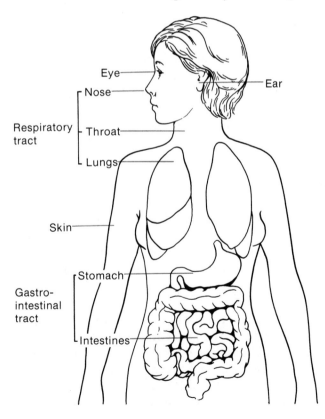

Figure 13-7. The sites of the body where allergic reactions most frequently occur are: the eyes; the ears; the respiratory tract — nose, throat, and lungs; the gastrointestinal tract — stomach and intestines; and the skin. Shock — collapse of the vascular system — can also occur.

as dust, pollens, fungi, animal dandruff, cold air, air pollutants, and even certain foods. The symptoms of asthma include coughing, wheezing, and extremely labored breathing. Because the victim cannot get enough air to properly oxygenate the blood, he develops a bluish tint of the skin, lips, and fingernails (called cyanosis). In severe cases, the chest appears to be overly expanded, and the victim gasps for air.

Most asthma begins in childhood; about 30 percent of all children who have asthma also have eczema (another allergic reaction). An infant who has both asthma and eczema has a greatly increased chance of having asthma as a permanent condition than an infant whose asthma is not accompanied by eczema. Approximately half of the children who have asthma when they enter kindergarten do not have it as adults; the attacks become less and less frequent and severe as time goes by. Only about 5 to 10 percent of childhood asthmatics still have severe asthma as adults. Even those who develop asthma as adults do not necessarily have it for the rest of their lives.

Most asthma can be controlled by one of the following means:

1. Controlling the environment (avoiding the irritants that affect the asthmatic and cause the asthmatic response).
2. Using antihistamines (which may provide relief for a small percentage of asthmatics).
3. Other drugs (i.e., bronchodilators and sympathomimetics).
4. Immunotherapy.

Anaphylactic Shock

Anaphylactic shock is a very serious manifestation of the allergic response. Anaphylactic shock occurs when the individual comes into contact with something to which he is extremely allergic. This exposure causes an immediate massive release of toxic, histaminelike substances by the mast cells. These chemicals overwhelm the body and may produce a potentially fatal reaction.

Anaphylactic shock may result in a variety of signs and symptoms that affect various parts of the body. In the heart and circulatory system, anaphylactic symptoms may take the following forms: weak, rapid pulse; low blood pressure; dizziness; restlessness; irregular heartbeats; and decreased cardiac output. When an anaphylactic reaction affects the skin, there may be itching and burning of the skin, especially around the face and chest; blueness around the lips; raised, hivelike patches with severe itching; swelling of the face and tongue; paleness; and swelling of the blood vessels just underneath the skin. In the gastrointestinal tract, anaphylaxis may produce nausea, vomiting, abdominal cramps, and diarrhea.

But by far the most serious symptoms occur in the respiratory system. Commonly there are spasms of the bronchioles; a painful, squeezing sensation in the chest; difficulty in breathing; bronchial obstruction; swelling of the larynx; and swelling of the epiglottis. In such cases, life-threatening breathing difficulties are due to the swelling of the larynx or severe bronchospasm.[7]

The following substances may produce an anaphylactic reaction in susceptible individuals:

1. **Insect stings.** Yellow jackets, honeybees, wasps, hornets, and other stinging insects such as the fire ant may cause anaphylaxis.
2. **Injected serums or drugs.** Sometimes the administration by injection of life-saving drugs or vaccines may cause anaphylaxis. Tetanus antitoxin and penicillin are two of the most common drugs associated with anaphylactic reactions.
3. **Foods.** Some food that commonly cause anaphylaxis are shellfish, fish, berries (especially strawberries), and milk. The anaphylactic reaction usually occurs more gradually, but it can become very severe.
4. **Drugs.** Even simple drugs like aspirin can cause an anaphylactic reaction. In fact, aspirin ranks with penicillin as one of the most frequent causes of drug reactions.

Treatment must be instituted immediately, because with the onset of circulatory and respiratory symptoms, death may occur within minutes or even seconds. To control the situation, drugs, such as epinephrine (and sometimes antihistamines and corticosteroids) can be used. There also may be a need for oxygen therapy and IV fluid administration.[8]

EPILEPSY

There are more than three million epileptics in the United States today; among neurologic disorders, only stroke is more common. Among adolescents and young adults, epilepsy is the most common chronic neurological disorder.

In epilepsy, the most common sign is a seizure — a temporary loss or impairment of consciousness. The seizure usually occurs without apparent cause, and it is usually accompanied by muscle movements that range from a slight twitching of the eyelids to violent shaking of the entire body.

The mechanism of epilepsy is an electrical malfunction of the brain. Epilepsy is like a sudden electrical storm in the brain that is comparable to a little bit of static electricity that builds up, involves a spreading number of brain cells, and finally erupts into lightning, sending currents throughout the body.

Causes of electrical malfunction include brain injury from trauma (such as an automobile accident), infection of the brain, or injury from a toxic substance; stroke or blood clot in the brain; metabolic disturbances; brain tumor; electrical shock (including lightning); and brain damage during birth due to difficult delivery that impairs oxygen to the baby. According to recent statistics, 20,000 new cases of epilepsy each year occur as a result of automobile accidents.

The intensity of the experience depends on the type of seizure. **Petit mal seizures** occur mostly in children and rarely occur in adult epileptics over the age of thirty. Petit mal seizures last only a few seconds at a time; there are only brief losses of consciousness, and the victims do not fall. Occasionally, slight jerking of the arms will accompany the seizure. As soon as the seizure passes, the child can continue with what he was doing before the attack occurred.

Grand mal seizures follow a classic pattern of an aura (called the prodromal phase) that warns of the attack, a cry (referred to as the epileptic cry), a fall to the floor, and a loss of consciousness. As the victim loses consciousness, the back stiffens, the muscles in the arms and legs stiffen, and the eyes roll upward. Rhythmic contractions of the large muscle groups of the body result in convulsions, and breathing often ceases, causing blue discoloration (cyanosis). There may be loss of bowel and bladder control, and some epileptics froth at the mouth. Because the muscles of the jaw tighten and clench, the epileptic may bite his tongue or cheek. The grand mal seizure usually lasts only a few minutes. When it is over, the victim is generally sleepy, exhausted, and confused. He usually has a headache and may have aching muscles, and many fall into deep sleep. Occasionally, the epileptic may suffer temporary paralysis of the arms and legs. The epileptic has no memory of the seizure, but may remember the aura.

482

Myths about Epilepsy

Myth	Facts
Epilepsy is passed on from father to son.	Most epilepsy is caused by brain injury.
All epileptics foam at the mouth and have convulsions.	Only those suffering from grand mal have this type of seizure.
An epileptic attack is easy to spot.	Not always. Victims of some psychomotor attacks have symptoms quite similar to drunkenness (slurred speech, unsteady gait, irrational behavior, etc.). Some victims of cerebrovascular disease exhibit symptoms similar to the epileptic's.
Epileptics can't drive cars.	Thirty-five states have no prohibitions against epileptics driving; others (with two exceptions) allow epileptics to drive if their seizures are fully controlled.
In most epileptics, seizures can be completely controlled.	If the ability to go two years without any seizure is taken as a criterion for "complete control," only thirty percent of epileptics fall in this group. However, eighty percent can have their seizures under control most of the time.
Most epileptics have only one form of epilepsy.	Two-thirds have two or more forms of seizure.
The type of seizure doesn't change.	It can change with age or with changes in body condition because the brain damage that causes it may improve or grow worse.
There is no surgical procedure for epilepsy.	Anterior temporal lobectomy can completely free certain types of epileptics from seizures. The operation takes from five to twelve hours and may cost $12,000.

Source: Helen K. Branion, "The Epileptic — How You Can Help," *RN*, Vol. 35, no. 6, p. 56.

The epileptic suffers no pain during the seizure; there is little danger unless the victim hits his head during the fall or unless the tongue blocks the airway, inhibiting breathing.

In **psychomotor seizures,** the electrical impulses of the brain act on the mental processes as well as upon the muscles. The individual has periods of activity that include picking at clothing; making chewing movements; lip smacking; removal of clothing; running or wandering around for several minutes; or, rarely, aggressive behavior. As the seizures begin, the epileptic often has the sensation of unpleasasnt odors or tastes. When the seizure is over, the epileptic has no memory of it.

In **focal seizures,** the epilepsy can be traced to one small focal area in the brain. Many focal seizures begin in one part of the body, and if they stay isolated to one small area, the victim often does not lose consciousness. Any focal seizure, however, may spread to involve the entire body, and the result is similar to a grand mal seizure. Focal motor seizures consist of jerking movements or stiffening of the muscles of a single part of the body, such as an arm, leg, or the face. The movements may persist for several minutes or more, or they may be momentary.

Treatment for epilepsy centers on controlling the condition with medication. If the cause is known and preventable (such as low blood sugar, an operable brain tumor, or excessive consumption of alcohol), treatment regimes center on eliminating the cause. In very rare cases, surgery is required to correct defects in the temporal lobe.

HEARTBURN

Heartburn — which has nothing to do with the heart — is one of the most common complaints of gastrointestinal origin. The lower esophageal sphincter (LES), a band of muscle at the end of the esophagus where it joins the stomach, functions to open and let food pass into the stomach. Normally, the LES closes when food is not passing through to prevent stomach contents from being regurgitated back into the esophagus. In some individuals, the LES is weak, and it opens and relaxes, allowing regurgitation of the stomach's hydrochloric acid into the esophagus, where it irritates the sensitive mucous lining of the esophagus. Current research is centering on the development of new drugs, chemical methods, and surgical methods of correcting weak or malfunctioning LES.

A peptic ulcer is a noncancerous, craterlike sore in the wall of the stomach or intestine; it erodes through the thin, inner mucous membrane lining of the stomach or intestine and into the deeper muscular wall.[9] Peptic ulcers occur only in those regions of the gastrointestinal tract that are bathed by the digestive juices secreted by the stomach and derive their name from the protein-digesting enzyme, pepsin.

Almost all peptic ulcers occur either in the stomach (gastric ulcers) or in the small intestine just below the stomach (duodenal ulcer). In the United States, duodenal ulcers are about eight times more common than gastric ulcers.

The hydrochloric acid and pepsin secreted by the stomach bring about the digestion of meat and other proteins as they reach the stomach. Under normal conditions, the mucous membrane lining of the stomach and duodenum is resistant to the digestive mixture, and no ulcer develops. In some people, however, this resistance breaks down, and an ulcer forms. The controlling factors, then, are the amount of acid and pepsin secreted by the stomach and the ability of the intestinal wall to resist erosion from the mixture.

Of these two factors, the secretion of too much acid and pepsin is by far the most important. The majority of people with duodenal ulcers and some of the people with gastric ulcers secrete much more acid than does the normal person. Excretion of excess acid is the most readily controllable by medical techniques.

The large middle portion of the stomach — called the body of the stomach — is lined with cells that produce acid and pepsin. Two important triggers stimulate these cells to secrete more acid: stimulation by the vagus nerve (as a response to hunger, the sight or smell of food, or tension and anxiety) and the presence of food in the lower part of the stomach. As a result, a person who is tense most of the time will secrete more acid — not only when there is food in his stomach, but when his stomach is empty as well, due to stimulation by the vagus nerve as it responds to anxiety.

Specific foods and many drugs can greatly increase the amount of acid and may also be directly irritating to the stomach and duodenal walls. Alcohol, coffee, and aspirin are notorious examples of this type of irritant.

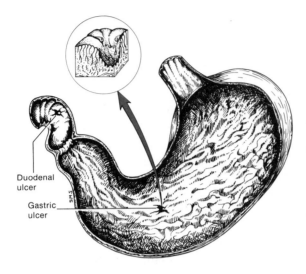

Figure 13-8. Excessive secretion of acid and pepsin is a leading cause of ulcers of the duodenum and stomach.

Duodenal
ulcer

Gastric
ulcer

Symptoms of ulcer can vary, but the most common, almost universal symptom of peptic ulcer is pain — usually steady, and often resembling a burning or gnawing in the stomach. The pain often feels like it is in a small area of the abdomen, usually somewhere between the navel and the lower end of the breastbone. The pain generally appears from thirty minutes to two hours after a meal, and it is usually relieved by eating or taking antacid. Some ulcer sufferers have pain of this kind that occurs off and on for years.

Almost anyone is at risk for developing a peptic ulcer. Ulcers can occur at any time from infancy to old age and are most frequent in people who are over twenty years of age. People in their thirties, forties, and fifties are slightly more prone to develop a gastric ulcer than are people who are sixty or older, but when it does develop in older people, it is generally more serious. Ulcers in this country occur more frequently in men than in women, although peptic ulcer is increasing in frequency among women. You are at particular risk of developing ulcer if you are under continuous strain of any kind, regardless of your age or sex.

Treatment for uncomplicated peptic ulcer is generally aimed at decreasing the amount of acid or irritants that inferfere with the normal healing process. There is usually some restriction in diet, and the amount and degree depend on the individual and the ulcer. One of the most important — and difficult — parts of therapy is to successfully reduce tension and worry. You should, among other things, avoid taking on more responsibilities and duties than time allows for, take time out for leisure, get a sufficient amount of rest, and avoid situations that you know are stressful. If you are unsuccessful in reducing the amount of stress that you suffer, your physician may prescribe a tranquilizer, a mild sedative, or even a term of hospital rest.

If you follow the recommendations of your physician, the ulcers should heal in four to eight weeks. This does not mean that you are cured. Ulcers are known to recur.[10] Being alert to this enables you to adjust quickly and bring the flare-up under control.

Notes

1. *How to Cope With Arthritis* (Washington, D.C.: U.S. Department of Health, Education and Welfare, 1976), DHEW Publication No. (NIH) 76-1092, p. 1.
2. *Arthritis: The Basic Facts* (New York: Arthritis Foundation, 1976), p. 6.
3. *The Facts About Diabetes* (New York: American Diabetes Association, 1966), pp. 4-5.
4. *Allergy Research: An Introduction* (Washington, D.C.: U.S. Department of Health, Education, and Welfare, Public Health Service, National Institutes of Health, 1972), DHEW Publication No. (NIH) 72-281.
5. Ibid.
6. *U.S. News and World Report*, January 1973, pp. 40-41.
7. Brent Q. Hafen and Keith J. Karren, *PreHospital Emergency Care and Crisis Intervention* (Denver: Morton Publishing Company, 1981).
8. Ibid.
9. U.S. Department of Health, Education and Welfare, *Peptic Ulcer* (Washington, D.C.: U.S. Government Printing Office, 1971), DHEW Publication No. (NIH) 72-38, pp. 4-7.
10. Charles S. Winans, "Living with a Duodenal Ulcer: A *Drug Therapy* Patient Guide," *Drug Therapy*, vol. 10, November 1980, pp. 57.

Self-Evaluation

Section A
Symptoms of Arthritis

Place a checkmark next to any of the following symptoms that you have now or that you have had in the recent past.

————— persistent pain and stiffness when you wake up in the morning

————— pain in one or more joints

————— swelling in one or more joints

————— tenderness in one or more joints

————— pain, swelling, or tenderness in one or more joints that comes and goes, recurring frequently and more often as time goes by

————— recurrent or persistent pain and/or stiffness in the lower back

————— recurrent or persistent pain and/or stiffness in the neck

————— recurrent or persistent pain and/or stiffness in the knees

————— fever

————— fatigue

————— loss of appetite

————— weight loss (unexplained)

————— swelling of lymph glands anywhere in body, especially in proximity to joints that are painful or swollen

————— pain in midabdomen

————— pain or stiffness in the joints that is relieved or lessened by soaking in a hot bath

————— limited range of movement in one or more joints

————— small nodes and lumps under the skin, especially in the hands and on the elbows

————— mild aching or soreness in one or more joints, unaccompanied by swelling

————— muscle weakness

————— joints that appear to be knobby

————— skin rash

————— inflammation of the eyes

————— joints that are hot and swollen

_____ sharp, needlelike pain in the big toe on either foot

_____ pain in the lower back accompanied by pain in the legs

_____ stiffness and rigidity in the spine

_____ reddening and swelling of the skin over a joint

Scoring: All of the above are signs and symptoms of arthritis in one of its forms. Each of the symptoms on the list, even in combination with other symptoms on the list, can be indicative of a number of other conditions, and medical diagnosis is essential. If you checked *any* of the above symptoms, and if they have lasted longer than two weeks, you should see your doctor.

Section B
Symptoms of Diabetes

Place a checkmark next to any of the following symptoms that you have now and that have persisted for longer than two weeks.

_____ fatigue

_____ excessive thirst

_____ excessive urination

_____ hunger, usually representing a marked change in normal appetite

_____ unexplained weight loss, especially accompanied by increase in appetite

_____ slow healing of cuts and bruises

_____ changes in vision

_____ intense itching anywhere on body that is unexplained by contact with irritating chemicals or poisonous plants

_____ pain in the fingers and toes

_____ drowsiness

Scoring: All of the above are symptoms of diabetes; if you checked more than one, you *may* be developing diabetes or you *may* have it now. Many victims of diabetes suffer only one or two symptoms, and many have no symptoms at all. The symptoms in the above list are also indicative of other disease conditions, so just because you checked one or more does *not* mean that you have diabetes; if you checked one or more, however, you should see your doctor.

Section C
Hay Fever or Cold?

If you are currently bothered by coldlike symptoms, circle those that apply to you in the columns below.

COLUMN A

red, itchy eyes
watery discharge from nose
burning itchy throat

sneezing without watery eyes

itchy nose

symptoms that drag on and on

COLUMN B

fever
mucousy discharge from nose
sore throat

sneezing that makes eyes water

symptoms that clear up in one to two weeks

Scoring: If you circled the responses in Column A, your problem is hay fever; those in Column B, and you have a cold. The most distinguishing features of hay fever are a thin, watery nasal discharge (as compared to the cold's thick, mucousy discharge) and the lack of fever.

Section D
Indications of Allergy

Place a checkmark next to any of the following symptoms that you presently have or that you suffer recurrently that persist longer than one week.

_____ coughing

_____ wheezing

_____ labored breathing

_____ skin eruptions characterized by itching

_____ skin eruptions characterized by swelling

_____ skin eruptions characterized by blistering

_____ oozing scales on the skin

_____ itchy, swollen areas of skin

_____ swelling of the tongue

_____ swelling of tissues inside the mouth other than the tongue

_____ swelling of the feet

_____ swollen welts anywhere on the skin

_____ inflamed and itchy skin

_____ a fine rash with or without itching

_____ inflammation of the eyelids

_____ purplish-red bruiselike marks anywhere on the body

_____ red, itchy eyes

_____ thin, watery discharge from nose

_____ burning, itchy throat

_____ itchy nose

_____ diarrhea

_____ constipation

_____ cramps following eating or drinking

_____ nausea and/or vomiting following eating or drinking

_____ swelling of unusual size or duration following an insect sting or bite

_____ hives following insect bite or sting

_____ overall itching following insect bite or sting

_____ tightness in the chest following insect bite or sting

_____ abdominal pain, nausea, and/or vomiting following insect bite or sting

_____ dizziness following insect bite or sting

_____ weakness following insect bite or sting

_____ speech difficulties following insect bite or sting

Scoring: Any of the above symptoms _may_ be an indication of an allergic reaction to food, drink, drugs, insect bite and sting, or may indicate a condition such as hay fever, contact dermatitis, eczema, or asthma. If you notice any of the above symptoms occurring in a pattern — especially at the same time of year every year or following exposure to the same elements (detergents, food, drinks, plants, cats or dogs, and so on), you should see your doctor.

Section E
Peptic Ulcer Symptoms

Place a checkmark next to any of the following symptoms you now have that have persisted longer than two weeks.

_____ a gnawing pain in the stomach

_____ a burning pain in the stomach

_____ pain in the stomach or abdomen that begins after eating

_____ pain in the stomach or abdomen that is eased by eating

_____ pain in the stomach or abdomen that is eased by taking antacids

_____ pain located between the navel and the end of the breastbone

Scoring: If you checked any of the above symptoms, and if they are made worse when you eat spicy foods, eat foods high in acid, take aspirin, or drink coffee or alcohol, you may be suffering from a peptic ulcer — especially if you are under a great deal of stress from school or work or home life. You should see a doctor if you checked any of the above symptoms and they are persistent.

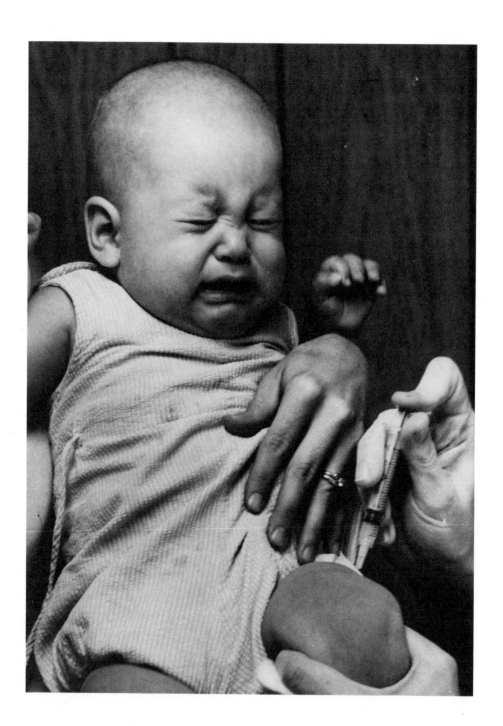

14

Infectious Disease:
Don't Get Bugged

Infectious diseases — or contagious or communicable diseases, as they are sometimes called — have been with us through history and will probably always be with us. Common usage has made all of the above terms interchangeable, but, strictly speaking, **infectious** diseases include any disease that is caused by a living organism, regardless of the way in which the disease is transmitted. A **contagious** disease, on the other hand, is one that is spread by direct contact.[1]

FACTORS DETERMINING DISEASE INTENSITY

Certain general factors affect the intensity of disease and its development, determining whether or not an individual who is exposed to the disease will become ill:

1. **Genetic makeup.**

2. **The environment.** The effects of the environment begin even before birth, when an unborn baby can be affected by infection that has invaded its mother's body. All of the elements of the natural environment — the type of soil, the amount of humidity in the air, the altitude, the bacteria found in the water supply, and various pollutants — can contribute to the spread of infectious diseases. Climate has a remarkable effect. When the climate is cold, large groups of people congregate indoors, in confined areas, increasing the incidence of airborne diseases. Central heating used in most homes and buildings during the winter dries out the nasal passages, making them most susceptible to infection. But during warm weather, people move outside and socialize more, increasing their chances of picking up disease in swimming water, spoiled food, or from insect bites.

3. **Stress.** All kinds of stress — physical, emotional, mental, and social — weaken the body and its natural defense systems, making it more prone to disease. Stress events that involve large numbers of people (such as floods, earthquakes, wars, or other calamities) can lead to epidemics as disease spreads through overcrowded areas where poor sanitation may exist.

4. **Economic status.** Characteristically, the poor suffer most from infectious disease due to a variety of reasons: they have less health education, they cannot afford good medical care (and, therefore, practice very little preventive medicine), they are exposed to rats and flies, and they often have inadequate clothing, food, and housing.

5. **Life-style.**

DISEASE-CAUSING AGENTS

In order for disease to exist, there has to be a **pathogen** — a microorganism that invades the body tissues, resulting in infection and disease. The pathogen lives and multiplies at the expense of the body and its tissues, often destroying tissue cells completely. Most pathogens are microscopic, but their size is not indicative of the damage that they cause: these tiny organisms cause the world's most dreaded and serious diseases

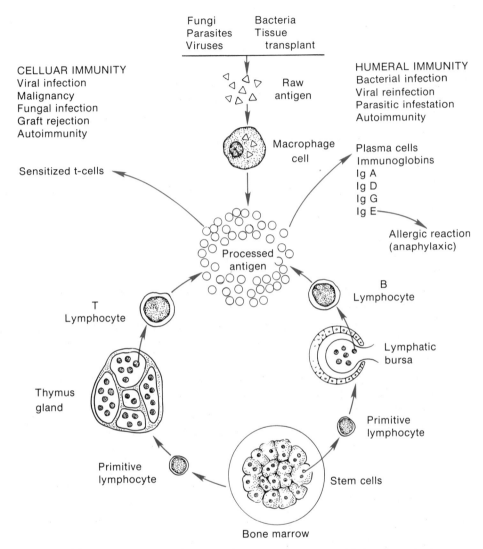

Figure 14-1. The differentiation of lymphocytes that serve each of the two major immune systems is shown here. The two types are the "B" cells (from "bursa," their supposed origin) of the humoral system, and the "T" cells (from "thymus" of the cell-mediated system). Source: *Patient Care*, January 15, 1975.

(such as polio and tetanus) as well as the world's most ordinary (such as the common cold). Pathogens include the following:

1. **Viruses.** The virus — the tiniest of all pathogens — is also the most

497

serious, partly because there is no effective treatment against it. Drugs that kill the virus also kill the healthy cells that have been invaded, and drugs that have been found effective against bacteria (such as antibiotics) have no effect against viruses.

2. **Rickettsia.** Rickettsia are so similar to bacteria in shape and appearance that they are distinguishable from bacteria only on the basis of their size: rickettsia are so tiny that they are barely visible under conventional mircoscopes. All rickettsia are transmitted by insects, ticks, and mites and are responsible for only a few serious diseases — typhus fever, spotted fever, and Q fever.

3. **Bacteria.** Hundreds of times larger than viruses, bacteria are still visible only under the microscope; the most plentiful of the pathogens, most, fortunately, are not harmful to man. Bacteria are found in abundance in the air, soil, and water; the human body itself harbors millions of bacteria, most of them harmless and some of them beneficial (such as those in the digestive tract critical to the digestive process). When the body is weakened, though, even the friendly bacteria can cause infection and disease.

4. **Fungi.** Primitive plants consisting of threadlike strands that produce a number of spores, fungi lack chlorophyll and must get their nourishment from organic matter — such as human cells. Fungi release an enzyme that digests and destroys cells, most often in the hairy, moist areas of the body. The most common diseases caused by fungi are athlete's foot and ringworm; fungi may also attack the external ear, scalp, beard, and groin.

5. **Protozoa.** Most diseases caused by protozoans are common only to areas of tropical climate and poor sanitation — among the diseases are malaria, amoebic dysentery, and African sleeping sickness. One protozoa — Trichomonas — causes a vaginal infection common to women throughout the United States.

6. **Parasitic Worms.** Largest of all the pathogens, the parasitic worms can be flat or round and range from a fraction of an inch to sixty feet in length. Complex multicellular animals, the parasitic worms attack tissues or organs and sap nutrients needed by the host.

STAGES OF DISEASE

There are four major stages of disease, marking the period from

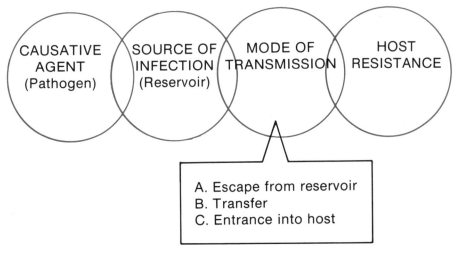

Figure 14-2. Breaking any one of these links in the infectious disease chain will halt the spread of disease.

entry of the invading organism into the new host to the period in which the disease subsides:

1. **Incubation Period.** Once the pathogen enters the new host, there is an incubation period — an interval between entry of the pathogen and the appearance of the first symptoms of disease. During this time period — which may be as short as a few hours or as long as several months or years — the pathogen multiplies in number until it is abundant enough to produce symptoms of the disease.

   While the length of the incubation period varies from disease to disease, the average incubation period is from a few days to a few weeks. The incubation period is a dangerous one: generally, the disease is not contagious during the early stage of the incubation period, but is highly contagious during the latter part of the incubation period — so a victim of disease is most likely to pass the disease on to others before he is even aware of its presence.

2. **Prodromal Period.** Another period of high contagion is the prodromal period — the period during which the first, vague, nonspecific symptoms appear. The victim usually suffers from fever, headache, and various aches and pains during the prodromal period, which lasts from a few hours to several days — the victim knows he is getting

INFECTIOUS DISEASES STAGES

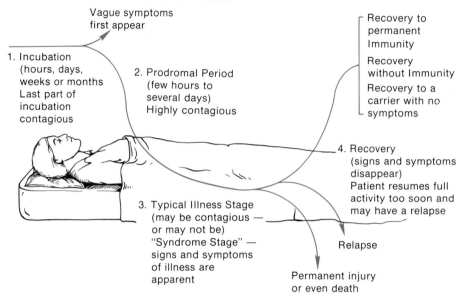

Vague symptoms
first appear

Recovery to
permanent
Immunity

Recovery
without Immunity

Recovery to a
carrier with no
symptoms

1. Incubation
(hours, days,
weeks or months
Last part of
incubation
contagious

2. Prodromal Period
(few hours to
several days)
Highly contagious

4. Recovery
(signs and symptoms
disappear)
Patient resumes full
activity too soon and
may have a relapse

3. Typical Illness Stage
(may be contagious —
or may not be)
"Syndrome Stage" —
signs and symptoms
of illness are
apparent

Relapse

Permanent injury
or even death

Figure 14-3.

sick, but the symptoms are not specific enough to allow identification of a specific disease.

3. **Typical Illness Stage.** A group of specific symptoms emerges at the end of the prodromal period, and the disease is at this point recognizable. The group of symptoms characteristic of the disease are often referred to under the phrase *syndrome*. While some diseases are still contagious at this stage, many are not — so the victim may not even be able to pass the disease to others once he is aware of its presence.

4. **Recovery Stage.** The recovery stage begins when the body defenses start to overpower the pathogens and the symptoms disappear. The recovery stage is another dangerous period in the disease: while the symptoms no longer exist, the pathogens are still present in the body. Many people, feeling much better and believing the disease to be conquered, resume full activity too quickly without allowing enough convalescing. Without adequate rest and recovery, the body defenses are weakened, and the pathogens again overpower the

500

body, creating a relapse of the original disease. Symptoms return, and the weakened body has even more difficulty eliminating the disease.

DEFENSES AGAINST DISEASE

The body has a number of methods of resisting disease — and they range all the way from natural defenses (such as the skin) to the immunity obtained from vaccinations.

Mechanical Defenses

The skin is one of the body's most effective barriers against infection and disease — when unbroken, the skin keeps out most pathogens. The respiratory passages also have their own system for removing pathogens: short, fine, hairlike bodies called cilia move a wall of thick mucous along the respiratory tract. The sticky mucous traps viruses, bacteria, foreign particles, dust, and other irritants that are inhaled; the cilia move the mucous to the back of the throat, where it is swallowed and then destroyed in the digestive process.

The digestive juices are only one of the body's secretions that fight disease and infection. Chemicals that can kill bacteria are found in the digestive juices and in perspiration, tears, saliva, skin oils, vaginal secretions, and the lacrimal secretions that bathe the eyes.[2]

White Blood Cells: The Body's Defenses

If a pathogen does successfully penetrate through the body's mechanical defense barriers and begin invading tissues, the white blood cells begin an attack on the pathogen. Also, the pathogen begins to produce **antigens** — certain chemical signals that alert the body's defense mechanisms to the presence of the invading element. By determining the exact chemical makeup of the antigens, the plasma cells produce a chemical **antibody** that neutralizes the antigen and robs the pathogen of its ability to produce disease. Some antibodies are small enough to cross

HOW IMMUNITY IS ACQUIRED

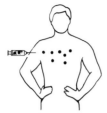

1 Live, attenuated virus
  (antigen) is introduced
  into the body and elicits
  a mild, subclinical infection.

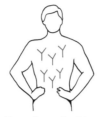

2 The antigen stimulates
  B lymphocytes to produce
  specific antibodies, which
  neutralize the virus.

Figure 14-4.

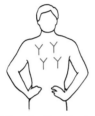

3 With time, the blood level
  of antibody declines, but
  since the body "remembers"
  the structure of the antigen,
  more antibody can be produced
  on a short notice.

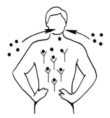

4 Subsequent invasion by the
  same virus following contact
  with an infected individual
  is therefore quickly repelled
  by existing as well as newly
  formed specific antibodies.

the placenta — so a developing fetus has the ability to fight off the pathogens that have invaded the mother's body.

Once the body produces antibodies to fight certain antigens, the body is protected for life against the same antigens. A person who gets infectious mononucleosis, for instance, will produce antibodies to fight that disease — and will then be immune from that disease. This kind of defense is called **active immunity** and results from the body's exposure to the disease and the body's defenses in fighting off the disease.

Effective against some infections is the process of **passive immunity:** the individual is injected with gamma globulin from the blood of an individual who has built up an immunity against the infection. Passive immunity is temporary, but it can help the body resist disease for a short period of time. Gamma globulin is most commonly used to protect family members when an individual develops infectious hepatitis.

Vaccinations and Immunizations

Of course, you do not want to be infected with every disease in order to be able to develop immunity. Some diseases, such as polio, tetanus, and typhoid, can kill before the host has a chance to develop antibodies that will ward off the next attack. The body can be protected against some diseases through a process of active immunity resulting from vaccinations and immunizations.

Vaccinations and immunizations work by introducing an antigen into the body that then stimulates production of the appropriate antibodies. There are three basic kinds of vaccine:

1. Weakened microorganisms — still alive but too weak to produce disease — are suspended in fluid and injected into the bloodstream. These microorganisms produce antigens, and the body reacts with antibodies. The Sabin polio vaccine is one of these.
2. Another vaccine is made up of dead microorganisms that are still capable of stimulating antibody production due to residual antigens. The Salk polio and most vaccines against influenza contain these dead microorganisms.
3. When bacteria release toxins into the body, they act as antigens to stimulate production of antibodies. A third type of vaccine uses the chemically inactivated toxins produced by bacteria; two examples are the tetanus and diphtheria vaccines.[3]

Vaccinations and immunizations should be given as early as two months of age (against diphtheria, tetanus, whooping cough, and polio) and should continue until the age of of sixteen (when a combined tetanus-diphtheria vaccine is given). Every adult should have a tetanus-diphtheria booster every ten years; the booster should be given if the individual gets a contaminated wound and has not had a booster for five years.

Vaccines have been developed against poliomyelitis, rubeola (measles), rubella (German measles), mumps, smallpox, yellow fever, some kinds of influenza, some kinds of encephalitis, cholera, typhoid fever, typhus, pertussis (whooping cough), Rocky Mountain spotted fever, diphtheria, and plague. A vaccine has also been developed that is effective against tuberculosis.

See Table 14-1, p. 517, for immunization guidelines.

TYPES OF INFECTIOUS DISEASE ■■■■■■■

Measles (Rubeola)

Called the "red measles," rubeola is one of the most serious diseases a child can have — complications include brain inflammation and death, and the measles can leave a child deaf and blind. Once, 90 percent of the red measles cases occurred in children under the age of ten; now, young adults account for more than 60 percent of the red measles cases in the United States. The problem? It is the older victim — those in high school and college — who are particularly vulnerable to encephalitis as a complication.[4]

German Measles (Rubella)

In children, the German measles is often so mild that in many cases it goes undetected. In other cases, it may be misdiagnosed as a simple cold or as some other mild disorder. But when German measles strikes a woman in the first trimester of pregnancy, the disease wrecks havoc on the fetus, resulting in cerebral palsy, blindness, congenital heart defects, cataracts, arthritis, encephalitis, deafness, and mental retardation. The woman may have a miscarriage, or the baby may die in the uterus.

Vaccination is recommended for previously unvaccinated adolescents and for women and girls who are not pregnant at this time. A woman should avoid pregnancy for three months after she has been vaccinated. It is a good idea to get a vaccination even if you think that you may have had the disease as a child.

Polio

Currently, millions of children under the age of fourteen are still unprotected from polio, and outbreaks still occur in the United States and other areas of the world. Adults who are exposed to unusual risk should be immunized, as should adults who were not immunized as children. The most widely used form of polio vaccination is the oral method. The vaccine is given in a series of four doses and should be started at the age of two months.

United States, Calendar Year 1980
Total Number of Reported Cases of Specified
Notifiable Diseases — 1,503,278

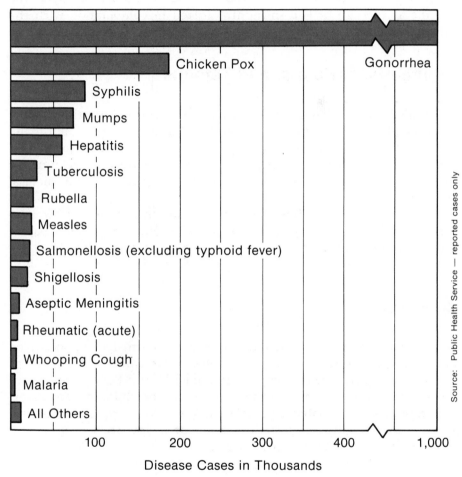

Chicken Pox

Gonorrhea

Syphilis

Mumps

Hepatitis

Tuberculosis

Rubella

Measles

Salmonellosis (excluding typhoid fever)

Shigellosis

Aseptic Meningitis

Rheumatic (acute)

Whooping Cough

Malaria

All Others

Source: Public Health Service — reported cases only

100   200   300   400   1,000

Disease Cases in Thousands

Figure 14-5.

Mumps

More than 16,000 children between the ages of five and ten get the mumps each year in the United States; complications among young children are usually mild or rare, but among young adults, the mumps can result in sterility (in males), deafness, and juvenile-onset diabetes.

Adult males who have never had the mumps should be immunized to prevent the complication of sterility. Children should be given the vaccine at the age of fifteen months (often in combination with the measles vaccine).

Diphtheria, Pertussis, and Tetanus

Called the DPT shot, one immunization affords protection against all three diseases. Diphtheria can result in paralysis, heart failure, and death if it goes untreated; pertussis, better known as whooping cough, can lead to brain damage, lung collapse, and convulsions; tetanus, or lockjaw, claims almost half of its victims despite excellent medical treatment.

Given in a series of five shots, the vaccine should be first administered to children at the age of two months. Adults can receive separate tetanus shots if they are wounded five years or more after the DPT series ended or more than five years after they received a tetanus shot.

Smallpox

Since it has been more than thirty years since smallpox has occurred in the United States, and since October 1977 saw the last case of smallpox anywhere in the world, the Public Health Service no longer recommends routine smallpox immunizations of children.[5] However, you should be vaccinated against smallpox if you are traveling to a country that requires such a vaccination or if you are traveling to a country that has a recent record of infection.

Typhoid Fever

Due to improving sanitation and other control measures, the number of typhoid cases has been steadily declining. Routine typhoid vaccination is not longer recommended in the United States. If you come into contact with a known typhoid carrier, if there is an outbreak of typhoid fever in the area where you live, or if you plan to travel to a country where typhoid fever is prevalent, you should be vaccinated. Vaccination is no longer recommended for areas that have been flooded or for children going to summer camps.

Yellow Fever

Yellow fever occurs today only in South America and Africa, and vaccination is recommended for persons over the age of six months who travel in areas where yellow fever still exists. (If you do require a vaccination for travel, you must receive it at a Yellow Fever Vaccination Center; such centers are listed with the World Health Organization.)

Bubonic Plague

Bubonic plague, a disease associated with wild rodents, occurs so rarely that vaccination is no longer recommended unless you travel to Laos, Cambodia, or Vietnam, where the disease has reached epidemic proportions. Those whose work brings them into contact with wild rodents in South America, Africa, Asia, or the western United States should receive vaccinations, as should laboratory personnel who work with plague-infected rodents or plague organisms. As long as you remain in a condition that may lead to infection, you should receive a booster shot every six to twelve months.

Viral Hepatitis

Persons living in households with hepatitis patients and persons who travel to tropical areas should be vaccinated with immune serum globulin (ISG) against hepatitis. The vaccination should only be taken if recommended by a physician.

Influenza

Although influenza shots were recommended for the general public for two or three years during the mid-1970s, they are no longer recommended for most people, partly because flu viruses change their makeup from year to year and partly because there are so many different strains of flu virus.

CYCLE RELATIONSHIP OF INFLUENZA
OUTBREAKS AND BUILDUP OF IMMUNITY

──────── Gradual buildup of antibody immunity to a particular strain.

─ ─ ─ ─ ─ Gradual buildup of immunity to mutant strain.

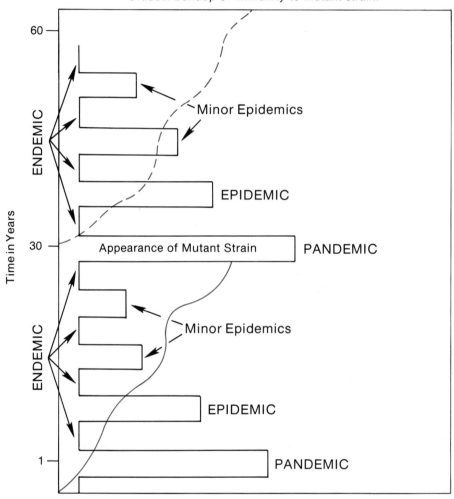

Incidence of Influenza

Source: American Druggist, October 1978, p. 72.

Figure 14-6.

508

Influenza vaccines are recommended for those who suffer serious consequences from the flu: children and adults of all ages who have chronic conditions such as diabetes, heart disease, kidney disease, chronic bronchitis, emphysema, asthma, or tuberculosis; adults over the age of sixty-five, since flu is often harmful to people in that age bracket and can lead to death; and those who are in extended-care facilities where outbreaks may infect large numbers of people.

About every ten years, there is a drastic change in the composition of the flu virus, and those who have built an immunity to previous strains of flu are infected. During those times, flu vaccinations are often administered to anyone who desires them.

Rabies

Only one to three cases of rabies are reported each year in the United States, but because the disease is almost always fatal, researchers continue in their efforts to further refine the rabies vaccine.

There is always a dilemma about how and if to treat a victim of a bite, because all forms of available treatment carry with them adverse side effects. In some cases, the vaccines themselves have resulted in death. Factors that determine whether an individual should be vaccinated including the following:

- The species of the animal that bit: carnivores and bats are much more likely than other kinds of animals to be infected.
- The presence of rabies in the area.
- The circumstances of the bite incident — if the attack was unprovoked, the chances are greater that the animal was rabid.
- The vaccination of the biting animal — it is not likely that a house pet that has been vaccinated for rabies will carry and transmit the disease.
- The type of exposure; scratches from a rabid animal or contamination of an open wound *can* result in rabies, but an animal bite is more likely to carry risk of infection.

Although the rabies vaccinations in the past involved a series of twenty-four shots in the abdominal area, recently, a new vaccine has been perfected and used to great success. This procedure involves only four to seven shots and may be administered in the arm.[6]

SEXUALLY TRANSMITTED DISEASES ━━━━━

In any single year, approximately eight to ten million Americans have some kind of venereal disease: gonorrhea, syphilis, genital herpes, or non-gonococcal urethritis.[7] All of these diseases have different symptoms and different courses of treatment, but they are all spread by sexual contact. Accordingly, those most affected by venereal disease are those in the most sexually active group — from fifteen to thirty years of age.

Figure 14-7.

GONORRHEA
Case Rates per 100,000 Population
Calendar Year 1980

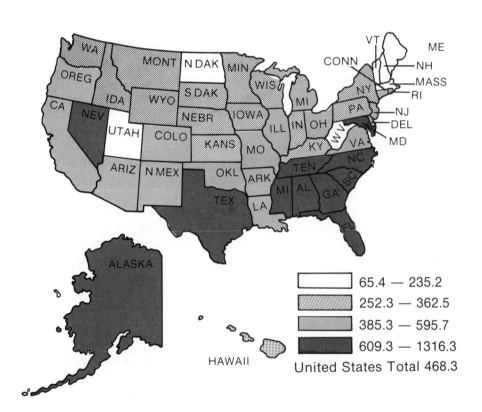

☐	65.4 — 235.2
▨	252.3 — 362.5
▧	385.3 — 595.7
▉	609.3 — 1316.3

United States Total 468.3

Gonorrhea

Gonorrhea accounts for approximately 2.7 to 3 million infections in this country alone; worldwide, there are approximately 100 million cases, and the number is rising. Gonorrhea has become the most common human bacterial infection — it now affects more Americans each year than measles, tuberculosis, hepatitis, whooping cough, and encephalitis combined. The Public Health Service estimates that one out of every fifty persons in the fifteen-to-nineteen-age group contracts gonorrhea each year. The absence of symptoms is one of the principal difficulties in its control: about 80 percent of the women and 20 percent of the men infected with gonorrhea have no symptoms, yet they remain contagious and can spread the infection to others.

Gonorrhea can almost always be traced to sexual contact with an infected person; rarely is gonorrhea contracted from an inanimate object, such as soiled clothing or toilet seats, because the gonococcus bacteria is extremely delicate and survives very poorly outside the human body. The bacteria is especially prone to die in open air or under significant changes of temperature.

Sites of Infection

While gonorrhea most commonly affects the genital area, it can settle in other sites of the body as the disease progresses.[8] Women commonly have rectal infections, which can occur without participation in rectal intercourse. Gonorrheal infections of the throat are common among men and women who engage in oral sexual activity. Gonorrhea that occurs at nongenital sites usually does not cause obvious symptoms and often does not respond to the same antibiotics that are effective in treatment of gonorrheal infections of the genitals. It is critical that the physician be informed of the full range of sexual activities so that treatment can be complete.

Symptoms

Typically, symptoms first occur in the lining of the genital and urinary tracts. In men, painful urination and discharge from the tip of the penis are common. Most of the time, symptoms appear about one week

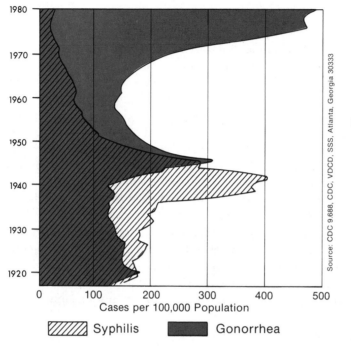

Figure 14-8.

Source: CDC 9.688, CDC, VDCD, SSS, Atlanta, Georgia 30333

Cases per 100,000 Population

⟍⟍⟍ Syphilis   ▓ Gonorrhea

after sexual relations with an infected person; sometimes the symptoms take longer to appear, however, and at other times no symptoms at all appear in men. In infrequent cases, the pus and discharge appear as soon as two days after exposure.

In women, infection of the urethra and the cervix is usual. Many women never develop symptoms of gonorrhea; those that do frequently suffer vaginal discharge and, rarely, painful urination. A newborn infant who passes through a mother's infected birth canal may acquire a potentially blinding infection of the eyes; as a preventive measure, physicians place silver nitrate drops in the eyes of all infants immediately following birth.

Treatment

Treatment for gonorrhea consists of two injections of penicillin given simultaneously with probenecid, an oral tablet designed to increase the effectiveness of penicillin. Ampicillin, an oral medication similar in chemistry and pharmacology to penicillin, may also be used in treatment. Those allergic to penicillin and ampicillin may be given tetracycline or spectinomycin hydrochloride.

Once treatment is begun, symptoms begin to clear up quickly, and the individual may no longer be contagious in as soon a period as twenty-four hours. Some stay contagious for longer periods, however, and follow-up examinations are important.

It is critical to take all of the medication that is prescribed. Symptoms may disappear within a day or two, and you may assume that you are better and quit taking medication. Even though symptoms may disappear, the infection will still remain. The entire course of antibiotics needs to be used. Since a certain dosage is required, a person should never attempt self-treatment.

In gonorrhea, as in all other venereal infections, early treatment is essential to success in cure. Many venereal diseases can have severe complications if treatment is not begun immediately. If you have any reason to believe that you may have contacted a venereal disease, or if you notice symptoms that appear to be venereal in origin, you should seek medical attention immediately. Prompt medical help can help ensure a quick cure, can prevent complications, and can keep you from infecting others without knowing it.

Syphilis

While syphilis is not as widespread as gonorrhea, it is one of the most devastating of the sexually transmitted diseases if it is left untreated. Partly because of diligent efforts to identify and treat possible carriers, syphilis is much less frequent than gonorrhea in North America.

Like gonorrhea, syphilis is spread by direct intimate contact with the lesions of someone in the infectious stages of the disease. Also like the gonococcus, the syphilis bacterium is fragile and is unlikely to survive outside the body long enough to permit contracting from inanimate objects.

Treatment

As with gonorrhea, treatment consists of penicillin injections given during a single visit to the doctor's office; the infected person is generally no longer contagious within twenty-four hours after treatment. Those

513

who are allergic to penicillin are given tetracycline, erythromycin, or cephaloridine. If early treatment is initiated, all signs of syphilis can be eradicated from the blood in six months or two years. In all stages of syphilis, the treatment will cure the disease, but the organ damage that accompanies the final stage cannot be reversed.

Genital Herpes

While gonorrhea and syphilis are both caused by a bacteria, other agents can also be transmitted sexually — including a virus that results in a condition called genital herpes, caused by the herpes simplex virus. One form of the virus — type 1 — is best known as the cause of cold sores and fever blisters that affect many individuals from time to time. The familiar lesions of type 1 herpes simplex virus can occur anywhere on the body and are most common around the mouth. Another kind of herpes virus — type 2 — causes lesions to develop most commonly on the genitals. While genital herpes is not as serious as gonorrhea or syphilis, herpes infections are quite painful and disabling; like fever blisters, they tend to recur.

The herpes virus is present in the fluid of the skin lesions, in some of the bodily secretions (including saliva and urine), and is spread by close contact — but not necessarily intercourse. Primary lesions tend to appear in those from the ages of fifteen to thirty, but recurring lesions (those that recur after the initial infection) may appear at any time later in life.

Symptoms

Genital herpes begins with a primary infection; the virus goes into hiding in certain parts of the nerve cells and reemerges spontaneously in response to sexual contact, menstruation, other infections, emotional stress, and nonspecific conditions. The primary genital herpes infection is usually more disabling than later recurrences.

Two to twelve days after exposure to the virus, a small sore or cluster of sores appear at the site of exposure — usually on the penis or in the urethra in men and on the cervix, in the vagina, or on the external genital area of women. The sore may be quite painful with local swelling, and there may be fever and other general body symptoms of infection. The symptoms of primary infection disappear in two to three weeks, and the virus may remain hidden for years before recurring.

The blisters that accompany primary infection may appear on the back, buttocks, hands, or other areas that have been infected. The blisters

Common Sexually Transmitted Diseases in the United States

Disease	Pathogen	Incubation Period	Symptoms	Possible Complications	Treatment	Immunity
Genital Herpes	Virus: Herpesviris (Herpes type II)	2 to 10 days after sexual contact	Blister-like sores usually on and inside the genital organs that reoccur often with genital pain and fever; can occur on body at virus contact points	Cannot be cured; can cause miscarriage, death to infected newborns, brain damage to newborns, and increased cervical cancer	No effective cure at present; symptomatic treatment only	None No vaccine
Gonorrhea	Bacterium: Neisseria gonorrhea (gonococcus)	2 to 9 days after sexual contact	Pus discharge from penis and vagina; painful urination in males (women often show no symptoms)	Pelvic inflammation in women; infection causes plugging of fallopian tubes in women and vas deferens in males resulting in sterility; Newborns develop eye infections	Penicillin, tetracycline, ampicillin (injections required)	None No vaccine
N.G.U. (non-gonococcal urethritis)	Bacterium: Chlamydia trachomatis	5 to 21 days after sexual contact	Men often have painful urination with pus discharge from penis. Women seldom exhibit outward symptoms	Males: Epididymitis and prostatitis resulting in infertility; Females: inflammation of the cervix and fallopian tubes resulting in infertility; Newborns: eye infections	Erythromycin, tetracycline (injections required)	None No vaccine
Syphilis	Bacterium: Treponema pallidum	10 to 90 days after sexual contact	Primary stage: chancre sores on or inside the genital organs or on body at infection contact. Secondary stage: body rash, fever, tiredness, loss of hair, mouth lesions	Organ disease and death; Unborns: congenital defects, brain damage, miscarriage	Penicillin, erythromycin, cephaloridine, tetracycline (injections required)	None No vaccine

usually break open shortly after they form, especially in women, and the resulting open sores are extremely painful. During recurrence, the only involvement is generally with the local lesion, which usually occurs in the same place as did the primary lesion. Some involve pain, but sores in the cervix, upper vagina, urethra, or prostrate produce no symptoms at all. Recurrences are usually healed within one to two weeks.

Treatment

Antibiotics, which are effective against bacterial infections, have no use in the treatment of viral infections; genital herpes treatment usually centers on the use of pain-relieving ointments, good genital hygiene, and the use of loose-fitting underwear.

To minimize the discomfort of genital herpes and to hasten healing of the sores, you should keep the infected area clean and dry; wash the infected area three or four times a day with a mild soap and water, and rinse thoroughly. Make sure that the area is completely dry. You can add

515

talcum powder or cornstarch to your underwear if you perspire heavily. Wear loose-fitting cotton underwear to prevent the spread of infection and to help keep the area dry; women should not wear pantyhose until the sores have healed, and neither men nor women should wear nylon underwear. Do not use ointments or creams unless they have been prescribed by your doctor.

Nongonococcal Urethritis

Also known as nonspecific urethritis, NGU is probably about twice as common as gonorrhea and is spread by sexual contact. Most of the NGU cases that are diagnosed are in men, but women are frequently infected, too. About half of the cases of NGU are caused by a rare bacterium called Chlamydia; the exact cause of the other half is unknown.

Symptoms

The symptoms of NGU in the male are the same as gonorrheal symptoms — discharge from the penis and painful urination — but they are usually milder. Some men who are infected have no symptoms at all. As with gonorrhea, women frequently have no symptoms; in some, irregular menstrual periods, genital irritation, vaginal discharge, or pain in the lower abdomen are present.

Treatment

Tetracycline is the best antibiotic to use in the treatment of NGU; erythromycin is a preferred alternative. Oral antibiotics must be taken four times a day for at least a week to clear up the infection. You must abstain from sexual intercourse until the infection has completely cleared up.

Table 14-1

Immunization Guidelines

AGE	DISEASE
2 months	DPT (diphtheria and tetanus toxoids combined with pertussis — whooping cough — vaccine); TOPV (trivalent oral polio virus vaccine)
4 months	DPT; TOPV
6 months	DPT; TOPV
12-15 months	Measles (may be combined with rubella — german measles — or may be a measles-mumps-rubella combination); mumps (may be given later, but before puberty); rubella (may be given later, but before puberty).
18 months	DPT; TOPV
4-5 years	DPT; TOPV
Every 10 years	DT (diphtheria-tetanus booster)

*Tetanus immune globulin or antitoxin is given following a wound if immunization history is incomplete or last booster was more than 5 years earlier.

Notes

1. Shirley Morrison and Carolyn Arnold, *Communicable Diseases*, 9th edition (Philadelphia, Pennsylvania: F. A. Davis Company, 1969), p. 4.
2. Franklin Top and Paul Wherle, *Communicable and Infectious Diseases*, 8th edition (St. Louis: C. V. Mosby Company, 1976), p. 4.
3. Margaret B. Tewinkle, "Immunization and Communicable Diseases," *Journal of Practical Nursing*, March 1974, pp. 22-25.
4. "Important! Get the Kids the Shots They Need," *Changing Times*, May 1979, p. 46.
5. Faye Peterson, "Vaccine Recommendations," *FDA Consumer*, July-August 1978, p. 14.
6. Stanley A. Plotkin, "Rabies Vaccination in the 1980s," *Hospital Practice*, November 1980, p. 69.
7. Basis for this section taken from U.S. Department of Health, Education, and Welfare, *Sexually Transmitted Diseases* (Bethesda, Maryland: National Institute of Allergy and Infectious Diseases, Public Health Service, National Institutes of Health, 1977), DHEW Publication N. (NIH) 76-909.
8. H. Hunter Handsfield, "What You Need to Know About VD," *Drug Therapy*, June 1979, p. 104.

Common Infectious Diseases

Disease	Pathogen	How Transmitted	Incubation Period	Characteristics of Occurrence	Signs and Symptoms	Prevention (See accompanying recommended immunization schedule
Chickenpox (varicella)	Virus	Spreads by air, through inhalation; droplets are directly or indirectly spread.	14-16 days	Occurs epidemically, mainly in winter and spring, before age 20; affects both sexes equally. Virus reaches skin from respiratory system via the blood. Virus can affect nerve pathways, causing the disease, "shingles," years after the infection.	Mild disease with fever and itching vesicular eruption. Papules make appearance about 24 hours after onset of fever. Lesions are most abundant over the trunk, but also on the face, and spread to mouth, throat, and extremities. Successive crops of lesions may be seen, with general involvement of lymph glands.	Immunizations (somewhat ineffective); Gamma globulin prevents some cases.
Diphtheria	Bacteria	Directly by droplet infection from respiratory discharges, and through contamination of hands, objects and occasionally, milk.	2-5 days	Endemic and epidemic, where child immunization measures have been neglected.	Abrupt fever, chilliness, malaise, sore throat. Whitish-grey membrane forms on tonsils and then thickens to form yellowish diphtheric membrane. Other areas may also be invaded. Cervical lymph nodes are swollen. Bacteria do not invade the tissues but produce toxins that cause heart and kidney damage.	Diphtheria-pertussis-tetanus toxoids (DPT) and diphtheria-tetanus toxoids (D-T) for pediatric use, and special tetanus and diphtheria toxoids (T-D) for adult use.
Hepatitis, infectious	Virus	Fecal or oral discharges contaminating food, water, or milk.	15-35 days	Occurs sporadically and in small local epidemics which have been traced to sewage-contaminated water or consumption of contaminated food, especially shellfish. It is believed that, like serum hepatitis, infectious hepatitis may also be transmitted by injection equipment.	Headache, fever, and anorexia (in most cases), shaking chills (in half). Nausea and vomiting. Malaise, myalgia (sore muscles), joint stiffness, sore throat, dull upper abdominal pain. Urine darkens. Jaundice. Most cases recover fully within four months. Disease tends to be mild in children and young adults; more serious in older adults.	Gamma globulin after known exposure is helpful but does not prevent the disease.

Disease	Agent	Transmission	Incubation	Occurrence	Symptoms	Prevention
Herpes Simplex	Virus	Presumably by direct or droplet contact, and maybe by indirect association.	Unknown	Primary herpes simplex is mainly a disease of childhood. In adults, herpes-like episodes may occur during attacks of pneumonia, meningitis, malaria, and other diseases. The virus lives in balance with most tissues and does not reveal its presence until some stress shifts the balance in favor of the virus.	The commonest form of the disease is characterized by painful blisters on lips and gums sometimes associated with fever, irritability, malaise, and swelling of glands. Symptoms may persist for 7 to 10 days. Other sites sometimes affected are the genitalia, and the conjunctivae and eye. It is likely that most herpes simplexlike attacks in adults are caused by other, as yet ill-defined, viruses.	
Infectious Mononucleosis	Virus	Direct contact, secretions.	4-14 days	Outbreaks in colleges, camps, and institutions, but generally appears sporadically. Typically affects young adults. Very little is known about the disease.	Malaise, fever, lymphatic enlargement (neck). Some have jaundice due to hepatitis (difficult to distinguish from infectious hepatitis).	
Influenza	Virus	Droplet infection, soiled articles, direct contact.	24-72 hours	Sporadic cases, local epidemics, pandemics. May affect up to 50% of population within period of 4-6 weeks. Each year the National Institutes of Health, after a careful survey of viruses recovered from recent influenza cases, decides what the exact composition and strength of influenza vaccine should be for the new season, and that becomes the new standard for all U.S. manufacturers.	Sudden onset, fever of 1-7 days, chills, listlessness, nausea, vomiting, prostration, aches and pains in back and limbs, coryza, sore throat, bronchitis.	Immunization for high risk individuals, i.e., those with diabetes, chronic respiratory diseases, heart ailments, advanced age.
Measles (Rubeola)	Virus	Respiratory discharges directly or indirectly	9-11 days	Most outbreaks in late winter and early spring. Epidemics run in 2 to 3 year cycles. Mainly a disease of children; mortality	Rhinitis, cough, mild fever, headache, malaise, fatigue, anorexia, conjunctivitis, eye sensitivity to light, and lacrimation. Rash usually	Immunization.

(continued on next page)

519

Common Infectious Diseases (continued)

Disease	Pathogen	How Transmitted	Incubation Period	Characteristics of Occurrence	Signs and Symptoms	Prevention (See accompanying recommended immunization schedule)
Measles (cont.)				is highest in those under 5 years old and in the aged.	appears the second to the fourth day.	
German Measles (Rubella)	Virus	Respiratory discharges directly or indirectly	9-11 days	Usually a childhood disease, it is fairly common in adults. One attack may confer life-long immunity. The age group usually affected is from 2 to 15 years. Permanent effects are rare except for damage to the unborn child when the mother is infected in the first 6 months of pregnancy.	Mild rash, slight fever, and swelling of lymph nodes. These symptoms usually appear from 14 to 21 days after exposure and last for 1 to 4 days.	Immunization; gamma globulin may curtail symptoms, the vaccine should not be given to pregnant women.
Mumps	Virus	Infected droplets or direct contact with salivary droplets from infected person.	17-21 days	Mumps occur most often in the 5-15 age group, but disease may attack adults. Because of the low degree of infectivity, many adults have not been exposed to the disease, and are susceptible. Many cases are asymptomatic.	Prodromal symptoms (fever, chilliness, malaise, loss of appetite, and headache) may or may not precede swelling of parotid gland. Swelling may affect one or two glands, with tenderness and difficulty in moving jaw. Testes, ovaries, pancreas or thyroid gland can also be involved.	Immunizations are available but do not offer full immunity.
Pertussis (whooping cough)	Bacteria	Inhalation of droplets or dusts from infected person.	7-14 days	Epidemic at 2 to 4 year intervals; endemic in winter and spring; mainly disease of infants and very young children; high mortality under six months of age. Highly contagious.	Mild cough becomes violent and spasmodic. Coughing is followed by loud whooping sounds as the individual attempts to breathe. Disease usually of 6 weeks duration in 3 stages approximately 2 weeks each. Catarrhal stage: upper respiratory infection with increasingly intense non-	Immunization.

Disease	Agent	Transmission	Incubation	Symptoms	Prevention
Pertussis (cont.)				productive cough and rhinorrhea; sometimes low-grade fever. *Spasmodic stage:* in 10 to 14 days cough becomes strangling and explosive, ending with characteristic whoop; thick, ropy mucus; vomiting; exhaustion; mental confusion. *Convalescent stage:* gradual decrease in severity of symptoms.	
Poliomyelitis	Virus	Nose and mouth droplets, as well as fecal contamination.	7-14 days	Children most susceptible; pregnant women vulnerable. Mild infections confer full immunity. There are three strains of virus.	Fever, headache, vomiting, malaise, sore throat, stiffness and pain in back, weakness, flaccid paralysis (in spinal type of disease). In bulbar type, respiratory paralysis, inability to swallow or talk clearly.
					Immunization with all three types of vaccine.
Tetanus	Bacteria	Usually, contamination of puncture or deep wounds.	4-12 days	This bacteria is found in the soil, but boiling is usually not sufficient to destroy. The disease is painful and fatality approaches 20%.	Tightness in neck, general irritability, stiffness of muscles, inability to open mouth. Convulsions and cyanosis. Extensor spasms in which the head and heels are bent backward, and the body forward.
					Immunization

Self-Evaluation
The Risk of Communicable Disease

Choose the response that most closely resembles your life-style.

Handwashing   **Score**

Never misses washing hands with soap and water — after getting
    up in the morning, after bowel movements, and before eating   0
Washes hands 3 times daily   1
Washes hands 2 times daily   2
Washes hands once a day   3
Seldom washes hands   4

Contact with Other People

Around few people each day   0
Shakes hands with several people daily, occasional hand
    to mouth, eye contact   1
Is in public contact work daily and close personal contact with
    infected persons, frequent hand to mouth, eye contact   2
Kisses others frequently   3
Around sick persons daily, handling infectious discharges   4

Sexual Contact

No sexual intercourse   0
Sexual intercourse with marriage partner only   1
Sexual intercourse with several others   2
Sexual intercourse with many others   3
Sexual contact with prostitutes, homosexuals   4

Water Source

Boils all water before drinking   0
Drinks mainly from State Health Dept.-approved water supply   1
Does #1 but shares drinking cups with others   2
Does #1, but drinks from unclean cups, glasses frequently   3
Does #1, but drinks from streams while camping
    or from unapproved water sources   4

Food

All food preserved under sanitary conditions   0
#0 plus meat is often not well cooked   1
#0 and #1 plus does not wash fruit before eating
    and/or flies allowed on food   2

Food (continued)

	Score
Frequently eats at unsanitary cafes, restaurants (daily)	3
#0 and #1 plus which it is not refrigerated	4

Immunization

	Score
Immunized against mumps, measles, rubella, polio, tetanus, influenza	0
#0 except for latest influenza	1
#0 except tetanus	2
Immunizations in #0 are not complete and/or current	3
Travels frequently or lives in a developing country with poor sanitation and personal hygiene	4

Nearness to Illness

	Score
Maintains strict distance from the ill	0
Near an ill person every week or two	1
#1 plus coughed or sneezed upon by sick	2
#1 plus buildings have poor ventilation	3
Daily near the ill (nurse, M.D., teacher, etc.)	4

Personal Hygiene

	Score
Uses own personal toilet articles	0
Does not bathe daily; shares towel	1
Inadequate sleep, rest, diet	2
Shares toilet articles (toothbrush, towels, etc.)	3
Puts fingers in mouth, eyes, nose. No hand washing after handling unsanitary articles	4

Contact with Animals

	Score
No pets or contact with farm animals or excrement	0
Keeps animals clean and house trained	1
No immunization of pets but clean and house trained	2
No immunization of pets, pets not house trained, seldom cleaned, seldom examined by vet	3
Pets allowed to roam, no immunization, close contact with pets, pets not clean nor house trained. Diseased pets	4

Contact with Insects/Rodents

	Score
House is insect and rodent proof	0
Lives in area where mosquito and rodent abatement programs function	1
No abatement program but some insects and rodents exist	2
Water impoundment, swampland, no abatement, trash accumulation prevalent	3

Contact with Insects/Rodents (continued)   **Score**

Hordes of mosquitoes, rodent harborage, evidence of disease
in animals and humans exposed to insects   4

Scoring

30+	=	living in squalor
20-29	=	expect to be ill frequently
10-19	=	can do better
0-9	=	living "clean"

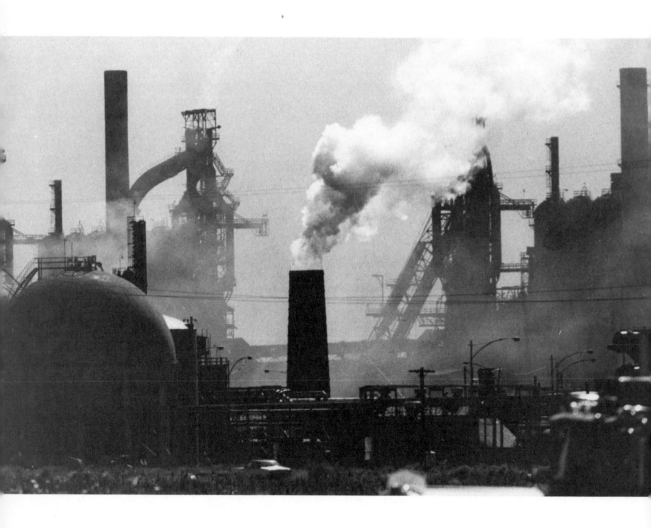

15
Environmental Hazards: Cleaning Up Your Act

Take a look around: if you are an average American, some serious threats to your health — even your life — are as close as the car you drive, the air you breathe, and the water you drink. Hazards present in the environment, including accidents, account for a weakening of defense systems that enable us to resist disease; in some severe cases, pollution and impurities actually cause disease. And traffic accidents kill about 50,000 Americans each year, leaving almost two million more injured and maimed.

ACCIDENTS

Accidents are the leading cause of death between the ages of one and thirty-eight; they account for roughly 50 percent of all fatalities among those one to twenty-four years of age. Many of these could be prevented through proper safety education and safe practices.

527

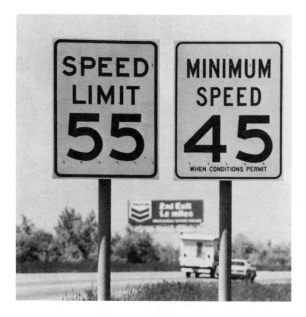

Most experts agree that the 55 mph speed limit has saved lives.

Motor Vehicle Accidents

Adolescents and young adults — those fifteen to twenty-four years of age — have the highest rate of death from motor vehicle accidents of any age group, accounting for one-third of all motor vehicle deaths. While prevention has primarily been aimed at driver education, experts estimate that deaths and injuries could be significantly reduced if any or all of the following factors could be employed:

1. **Reduce the number of vehicles on the road.**
2. **Lower speed limits.**
3. **Do not drink and drive.**
4. **Improve vehicle design.** Some design changes have been adopted: flexible bumpers, collapsible steering columns, padded hard surfaces, and recessing knobs and handles.
5. **Use of seat belts.** The most effective combination is the lap and the shoulder belt.
6. **Use of children's car seats.** Car seats that can be used as early as a newborn's trip home from the hospital are available in a number of styles and prices. A child should be restrained at all times; if there is no specially designed seat, an adult lap belt is better than nothing.

7. **Use of motorcycle helmets.** The motorcycle helmet has proved to be the most effective device for protecting riders from death or serious injury in a collision.

8. **Improve highway conditions.** The interstate highway system has halved the death rates compared to all other roads by eliminating crash-precipitating features such as sharp curves, steep grades, blind intersections, and uncontrolled access. All roads and highways could be improved by keeping these factors in mind and by physically separating opposing lanes of traffic, by removing fixed objects where possible, by shielding fixed structures (such as bridge abutments) with energy-absorbing barriers, by locating essential signs and poles at a sufficient distance from traffic, and by designing guardrails to guide vehicles away from hazards.

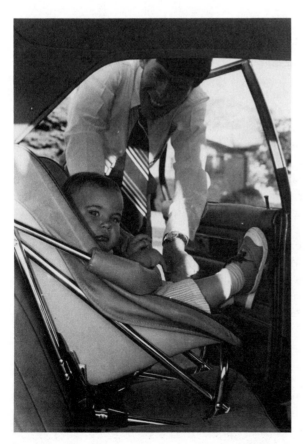

Child restraints are an act of love.

Falls

Preventing deaths and injuries from falls is contingent upon preventing the falls themselves. Some ideas for prevention include:

1. **Improve walking surfaces.** Keep snow and ice cleared from sidewalks and other areas where people walk; keep sidewalks and other walkways in good repair. Make sure that walkways are well illuminated, and provide handrails where possible and appropriate.
2. **Minimize the distance that people fall.** A simple, but effective, solution is to provide lower beds for the elderly.
3. **Modify surfaces against which people fall.**

Burns

Deaths and injuries from residential fires (and from scalds and electrical burns in the home) could be prevented or reduced through the following:

1. **Safe use of cigarettes.**
2. **Use of flame-proof clothing.**
3. **Use of fire-prevention devices.** Homes should be equipped with smoke detectors, and the furnishings and draperies should be of a flame-retardant material. You should make sure that you have an easy route of escape from any part of your home, and you should practice fire evacuation procedures to guarantee your ability to act quickly.
4. **Lowering of water heater temperatures.** Scalds — which usually happen in the shower or bathtub — account for about 40 percent of all hospital admissions for burns. Water heaters in homes, nursing homes, dormitories, and hotels should be equipped with automated cutoffs so that water temperatures remain below a scalding level.

Poisoning

You can prevent poisoning by keeping medications and cleaning solutions out of the reach of children and by keeping them in their original containers, clearly labeled. Toxic substances should be equipped with safety caps, and you should check to make sure that they are fastened tightly. Store toxic supplies away from food to avoid confusion. Never tell a child that you are giving him candy when you give him vitamins or medicine.

Poison control centers have been established across the nation to provide immediate information on poison antidotes and to instruct callers in poisoning emergencies. Find out the number of the center nearest you, and keep the number posted in a conspicuous place near the telephone.

Product-Related Accidents

Such seemingly innocent products as bicycles, glass, skateboards, roller skates, nails, knives, playground equipment, furniture, toys, electrical devices, and home swimming pools are the leading causes of death among consumer products. Survey the items that you are using at home. Discard products that are worn; examine toys carefully, and reject those with sharp edges, swallowable parts, or other safety hazards. Cover electrical outlets in your home, and fence your swimming pool; do not let children swim without supervision.

POLLUTION

Some pollutants poison the air; others get in the water and soil, where they eventually end up in the food that we eat. Some pollutants make us sick; a few can even kill us. It is important to eliminate pollution as an environmental hazard: besides the health advantages, we would realize financial savings, improved efficiency, and esthetic pleasure. Most important, we would protect our health and our very lives.

Air Pollution

Any time that the natural air gases (oxygen, carbon dioxide, etc.) are present in concentrations higher than normal — or any time that foreign gases are present — a state of pollution exists. Your reaction to particles of pollutants in the air depends a great deal on your general health and your individual circumstances.

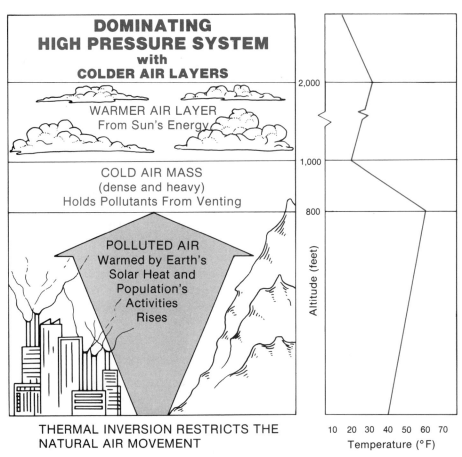

DOMINATING
HIGH PRESSURE SYSTEM
with
COLDER AIR LAYERS

WARMER AIR LAYER
From Sun's Energy

2,000

COLD AIR MASS
(dense and heavy)
Holds Pollutants From Venting

1,000

POLLUTED AIR
Warmed by Earth's
Solar Heat and
Population's
Activities
Rises

800

Altitude (feet)

THERMAL INVERSION RESTRICTS THE
NATURAL AIR MOVEMENT

10 20 30 40 50 60 70
Temperature (°F)

Figure 15-1. Normally, polluted air rises with the thermal lift and is dispersed at higher elevations. A thermal inversion interferes with the lift by establishing a lid of dense colder air at strategic elevations. Until this cold air is warmed by the sun and rising warmer air (called "burn off"), stagnant, polluted air remains trapped. Photochemical reactions take place within this trapped air, creating additional noxious gases that cause damage.

Air pollution's major effect on human health is the result of irritants acting on the respiratory tract. Research has proven the following results:[1]

1. Certain irritants, either gaseous or particulate, can slow down and even stop the action of the cilia — the hairlike cells that line the respiratory airways. The sweeping movement of the cilia propels the mucous — and the dirt and germs that are caught in it — out of the respiratory tract. When the action of the cilia is slowed or stopped,

the sensitive underlying cells of the respiratory tract are left without protection.

2. The irritants in pollution can cause the increased production of thickened mucous, which the cilia cannot move as easily out of the airways.

3. The airways become constricted, causing difficulty in breathing.

Figure 15-2.

AIR POLLUTANTS AND THEIR HEALTH EFFECTS

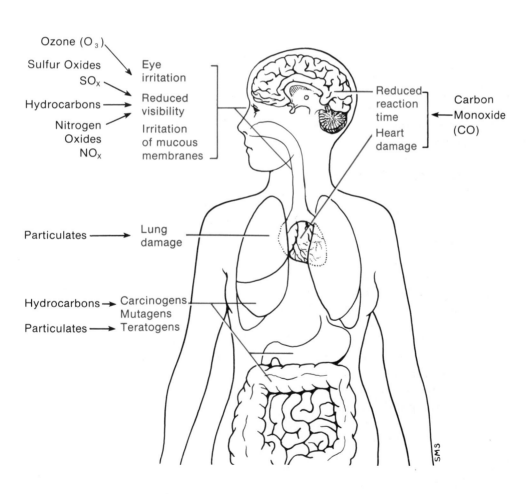

4. Pollutants can cause swelling or excessive growth of the cells that form the lining of the airways, resulting in airway restriction.
5. Pollutants can destroy the cilia and may even destroy several layers of underlying cells.

Because of one or more of these reactions, breathing may become more difficult, and foreign matter — including bacteria and other microorganisms — may not be effectively removed. The result? Frequent, severe respiratory infection.

Water Pollution

Clean water, one of a community's most valuable assets, is critical not only for drinking purposes, but for a vast number of industrial, agricultural, and recreational uses. Any pollution of water becomes a potential hazard to human health and safety, destructive to aquatic life, damaging to agricultural interests, esthetically deplorable, and a potential economic burden to society.

The major sources of water pollution and their health affects include the following:[2]

1. **Sewage and other oxygen-demanding wastes.** These include the obvious — human wastes — and the wastes from animals and from various manufacturing processes (such as food and meat processing, paper mill production, and tanning). Human wastes that eventually contaminate drinking water bring with them harmful bacteria, amoebae, and viruses that can cause typhoid fever, salmonellosis, cholera, bacillary dysentery, and amoebic dysentery.
2. **Disease-producing agents.** The bacteria, amoeba, and viruses that are carried into water by human wastes or by some industrial wastes (especially meat-packing operations and tanneries) include the polio virus (three distinct types), coxsackie viruses, infectious hepatitis viruses, and other viruses destructive to human health and life.
3. **Synthetic organic chemicals.** Toxic to fish and aquatic life and possibly harmful to humans, synthetic organic chemicals include detergents, household cleaning products, pesticides, synthetic industrial chemicals, and wastes from their manufacture. Some are highly poisonous at even low concentrations, and they resist conventional water treatment efforts.

534

4. **Inorganic chemicals and minerals.** There are many ways in which inorganic chemicals and minerals find their way into the water (i.e., irrigation water, highway salting, etc.). High concentrations of the pollutants have been linked with cancer, cardiovascular disease, and kidney problems.

5. **Radioactive substances.** Exposure to radiation in the water carries the same threats to health and life as exposure to ionizing radiation in any form.

Solid Wastes

Each American contributes approximately three to five pounds of disposable solid waste every day — mostly garbage from food preparation and refuse from cartons, containers, and newspapers. That in itself would not seem to pose such a problem — but when you then consider the bulk of items such as discarded automobiles, demolished buildings, and landscaping wastes, the problem becomes gigantic. And there are only three repositories for solid waste: the earth, its waters, and its atmosphere. Improperly managed, waste disposal into any of the three can lead to pollution of the earth's air and water.

The health hazard of solid wastes has long been recognized. Rats, flies, and other vermin breed freely in open dumps and then transport disease and economic burden to humans. Property loss and food damage due to rodent infestation is in itself extremely costly, but add to the problem a host of communicable diseases spread through improper solid waste disposal: typhoid fever, cholera, leptospirosis, dysentery, plague, trichinosis, and rat-bite fever.

Noise Pollution

Noise has always been around — but excessive noise deafens, and it is now recognized as a form of pollution and as a serious threat to health. The problem of exposure to noise has resulted in a premature loss of hearing among American youth. Today's generation of young adults will probably encounter hearing problems much more serious in their middle years than the present group of fifty- to sixty-year-olds.[3]

Excessive noise can alter endocrine, cardiovascular, and neurologic functions and can cause biochemical changes. Even a moderate, short

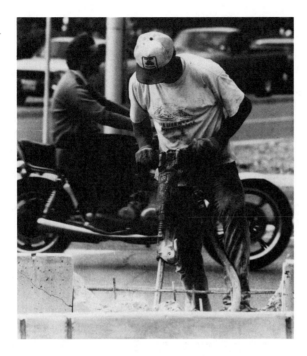

We are beginning to understand the adverse effects of excessive noise in the environment.

sound, such as a heavy truck passing on the other side of the street, can produce immediate effects in a susceptible individual. Blood vessels in the brain dilate, blood vessels elsewhere constrict, blood pressure rises, heart rate changes, pupils dilate, endocrine glands pour excessive hormones into the blood, and the stomach changes its rate of acid secretion. Most of these reactions are temporary — but if the noise persists, some could become chronic.

Continuous exposure to excessive noise can lead to irritability and increased susceptibility to infection, heartburn, indigestion, gastrointestinal malfunction, ulcers, high blood pressure, and heart disease. Workers exposed to unbroken high levels of noise exhibit a higher incidence of cardiovascular, ear, nose, throat, and equilibrium disorders than other workers.

In extreme cases, unwanted noise can lead to a complete breakdown of bodily function. Excessive noise has been linked to high mental hospital admissions, other psychological disturbances, losses in work performance, sleep disruption, annoyance, and irritability.[4]

536

Pesticides

Today, man is exposed to an ever-increasing number and variety of chemicals, among them pesticides. Although pesticide chemicals were known and used before World War II, their use has increased significantly. New, more toxic compounds, such as the synthetic organic pesticides, have largely replaced the older compounds. Little information is available to evaluate the hazards associated with use of the newer products. While society has reaped tremendous benefits from the use of pesticides, fungicides, herbicides, and plant growth regulators — such as prevention of vector-borne disease, control of insect pests, and increase in quantity and quality of foods and fibers — we need to be concerned with the unintentional effects of pesticides on human health and various life forms within the environment.

Certain pesticides can interfere with the functioning of the central nervous system; more than seventy-five different pesticide types have caused human poisoning, including damage to the human nervous system, respiratory system, digestive tract, skin, eyes, mucous membranes, metabolism, visceral organs, and the psyche.

Radiation

Increasing man-made radiation also poses a danger to health — most principally cancer and genetic disturbances. Apparently, some body tissues are particularly vulnerable to irradiation — the most susceptible are the young (particularly the unborn). The blood-forming organs, the thyroid, bone marrow, the breast, the lung, and the reproductive organs suffer the most damage from exposure to radiation.

Everyone receives radiation from natural sources over which he has no control. The remainder of our exposure comes from medical and dental x-ray machines, fallout from nuclear weapons testing, faulty color television sets, uranium mines and mills, uranium fabrication plants, nuclear power generating and fuel reprocessing installations, and various electronic devices. Many hospitals and laboratories commonly use radioactive isotopes in basic research and in patient diagnosis and treatment. Construction materials with radioactive properties have been used for homes, schools, factories, and other structures.

Despite this variety of sources, our exposure to radiation thus far has been quite low. Yet, we know little about the cumulative effects of even small amounts of radiation over long periods of time. Probably the greatest damage is suffered by the developing fetus. Any pregnant woman should have a lead-impregnated shield applied to her body before having routine dental x-rays or diagnostic x-ray examinations.

Radiation is not a clear-cut health issue — it poses serious risks to human life and health, yet it affords us certain benefits. For example, the same ultraviolet radiation that causes genetic mutations, fetal and infant deaths, and physical and mental deformities also destroys harmful bacteria in operating rooms, rendering the surgical environment sanitary. The radiation in color televison that can cause cataracts of the eye also brings us educational television, news and political information, and entertainment. The medical x-rays that can in large amounts result in leukemia, central nervous system cancer, bone tumors, thyroid cancer, and cancer of the lung allow us to diagnose and treat a host of medical conditions.

Notes

1. National Tuberculosis and Respiratory Diseases Association, *Air Pollution Primer* (New York: National Tuberculosis and Respiratory Disease Association, 1969), pp. 55-75.
2. Adapted from American Medical Association, *The Physician's Guide to Water Pollution,* 1973, pp. 9-10.
3. U.S. Environmental Protection Agency, *Effects of Noise on People,* (Washington, D.C.: Environmental Protection Agency, 1971), pp. 7-11.
4. Ibid.
5. Excerpted from Valorie Britain, "Radiation Benefit vs. Risk," *FDA Consumer,* September 1974, pp. 9-11.

Self-Evaluation

Section 1
Accident Susceptibility

Circle the number in the frequency column that best describes you. Respond to every statement.

	Usually or Always	Some-times/ Often	Seldom	Never
Motor Vehicle Accidents				
I drive above the posted speed limit.	3	2	1	0
I drive after drinking alcohol.	3	2	1	0
I drive without a seat belt buckled.	3	2	1	0
I drive more than 20,000 miles per year.	3	2	1	0
I drive or ride a motorcycle.	3	2	1	0
I drive or ride a motorcycle without wearing a helmet.	3	2	1	0
Falls				
My shower or bathtub is slippery.	3	2	1	0
I have stairs without an adequate rail.	3	2	1	0
I do not know how to fall.	3	2	1	0
There is inadequate lighting in my home or yard.	3	2	1	0
There is ice and snow on my porch or steps.	3	2	1	0
Drowning				
I swim alone.	3	2	1	0
I cannot swim ten yards.	3	2	1	0
I ride in boats without wearing a life vest.	3	2	1	0

Fires

I smoke cigarettes in bed.	3	2	1	0
I do not have a fire extinguisher.	3	2	1	0
I do not practice fire exit drills at home.	3	2	1	0
I do not have a definite plan for escape in case of fire at home.	3	2	1	0
I do not have a smoke detector.	3	2	1	0
I store matches and flammable materials improperly.	3	2	1	0
I overload my electrical circuits.	3	2	1	0

Poisoning

I have improper storage for medications, drugs, or toxic substances.	3	2	1	0
I leave any of the above uncapped.	3	2	1	0
I have household plants at home.	3	2	1	0

Firearm accidents

I am a hunter.	3	2	1	0
I store guns and ammunition together in an unlocked area.	3	2	1	0
I point a gun at another person.	3	2	1	0
I show off with guns.	3	2	1	0

Miscellaneous

I hang glide or skydive.	3	2	1	0
I snowmobile.	3	2	1	0
I play football.	3	2	1	0
I ski (either on snow or water).	3	2	1	0

I roller skate or ride a skateboard.	3	2	1	0
I live in an area where a natural disaster has happened or is likely to happen.	3	2	1	0
I fly in a private airplane.	3	2	1	0
I ride a bicycle.	3	2	1	0
I use a knife.	3	2	1	0
I am a mountain climber.	3	2	1	0
I use a trampoline without a spotter.	3	2	1	0
I climb ladders.	3	2	1	0
I light fireworks.	3	2	1	0
I swallow large slices of meat.	3	2	1	0

Scoring: Total the amounts of the numbers, that you circled to ascertain your likelihood of having an accident.

100-120 points	You are extremely susceptible to having an accident — and you will likely have one!
67-99 points	You are susceptible to having an accident.
46-68 points	You have an average susceptibility for accidents.
23-45 points	You are less likely than most people to have an accident.
0-22 points	You are an extremely safe person and are not likely to have an accident.

Use this test to your advantage — go back through it and pinpoint the items that are increasing your susceptibility to accidents, and then do something about it! You might even isolate certain sections where you seem especially headed for trouble.

Section 2
Your Car and Air Pollution

Answer the following questions based on the vehicle that you drive most of the time. Circle either "yes" or "no" for each one.

1. Does your engine stall frequently?	Yes	No
2. Is your engine hard to start?	Yes	No
3. Does your engine keep running when you turn off the ignition?	Yes	No
4. If your car has an automatic transmission, have you noticed it shifting erratically?	Yes	No
5. Can you detect the odor of oil or gasoline in the passenger compartment?	Yes	No
6. Are there dark deposits just inside the tailpipe?	Yes	No
7. Are there dark deposits around the tailpipe?	Yes	No
8. Does your car have sluggish acceleration?	Yes	No
9. Does your engine knock or ping?	Yes	No
10. Does your engine misfire?	Yes	No
11. Does your engine emit blue/black smoke upon acceleration?	Yes	No
12. Does your car use an excessive amount of either gasoline or oil?	Yes	No

Scoring: If you answered even one of the above questions "yes," your car could be a significant polluter of air! If you answered more than one question "yes," the probability is increased. To cut down on your personal pollution, make sure that the pollution control devices installed by the manufacturer are maintained at optimal performance, and keep your engine well tuned and timed. Make sure that you burn the proper fuel for your automobile, too.

Section 3
Personal Involvement in Ecology

Read each statement below carefully; on the line that precedes each statement, write "yes" or "no" as it applies to your situation most of the time. Answer each question.

_____ I participate in a carpool to work, school, or other regularly scheduled activities.

_____ I use the mass transit system to get to work, school, or to run errands.

_____ I avoid watering my lawn or garden at midday.

_____ I place litter and other waste in proper receptacles.

_____ I use pesticides only according to instructions.

_____ When I see an unacceptable environmental condition, I report it to the proper authorities.

_____ I control the amplification of my sound system so that music I listen to is below eighty decibels.

_____ I support bond issues for water and sewage treatment plants.

_____ I listen to the weather report daily to determine the quality of the air.

_____ I insist on appropriate shielding whenever I have any x-ray examinations (including dental x-rays).

_____ I immediately replace worn-out mufflers on my personal motor vehicles.

_____ I try to conserve water.

_____ I try to conserve electricity.

_____ I choose returnable bottles and reusable containers when shopping.

_____ I participate in local beautification projects.

_____ I keep my car well tuned and timed.

_____ I maintain the emission control devices on my personal motor vehicles.

_____ I recycle newspapers, cans, and glass.

_____ I walk or ride a bicycle on short errands.

_____ I keep the heat or air-conditioning in my home at the suggested limits.

_____ I observe posted speed limits.

Scoring: Count the number of statements that you answered "yes" to determine your participation in maintaining a balanced ecology:

5	You are interested in environmental protection.
10	You are concerned with improvement of the environment and with getting rid of pollution, both for yourself and others.
15	You are dedicated to environmental protection for your community.
21	You display an outstanding interest, concern, and dedication to fighting environmental pollution.

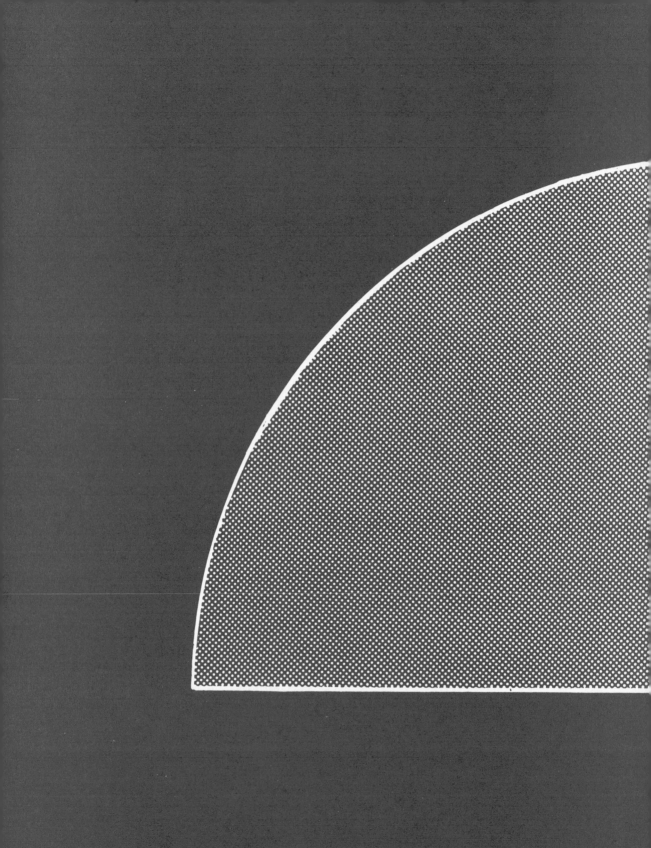

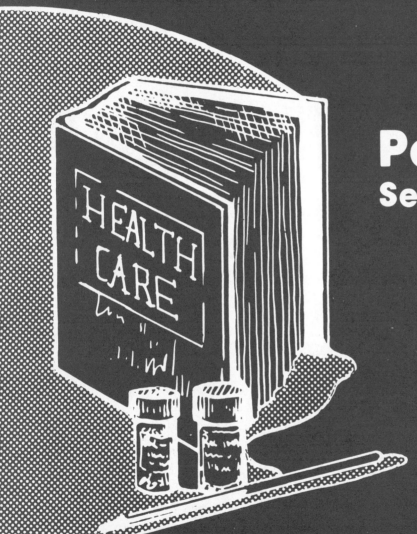

Part V
Self-Care

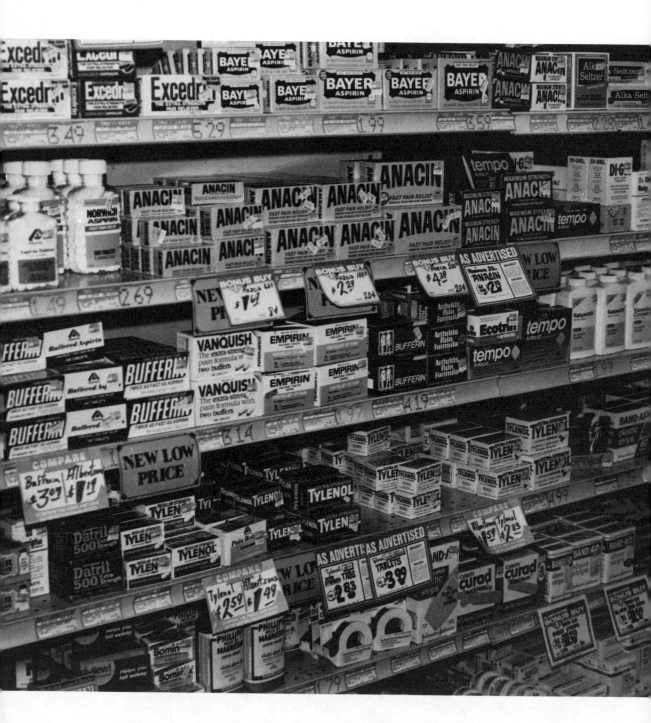

546

16
Consumer Health: Have It Your Way

With the recent interest in fitness, nutrition, and other positive approaches to well-being, the consumer has recognized his personal responsibility for his own health and is taking a more direct role in the decision-making process. Decisions relating to consumer health range in importance from selecting a toothbrush that may contribute to a sparkling smile to selecting a physician in whose hands you may place your life. With the abundance of sometimes conflicting information, these decisions are not always easy.

When a consumer purchases a health product or service, he is really attempting to buy a power that will have a positive influence on health. The question the consumer should ask is, "Will this product or service have that power; will it really work?" The consumer should also ask, "Is it economical; is it worth the price?"

SELECTING A PHYSICIAN

The physician is the gateway through which the patient must pass in order to gain access to the various services available to meet his health

547

needs. The ideal physician is one who is adequately trained to provide direct assistance to the patient. To locate a physician that will serve you best, begin by calling your county medical society and asking for the names of two or three family physicians, general practitioners, or family internists in your neighborhood. Ask the same question of the local medical exchange answering service and the administrator's office of your local hospital. When you call, describe the kind of medical service that you require (your age, how many children you have, or any special problems that you may have). Membership on the staff of an accredited hospital is essential. If hospital care is required, your physician is helpless if he has no hospital privileges. Seek the advice of people in the community who you respect and who have lived there for a number of years. Check with related professionals, such as dentists, nurses, and pharmacists. Select a physician who is available to your neighborhood or town, thus making medical care more readily accessible.

As a patient, you have certain rights:[2]

1. **The right to choose a physician.**
2. **The right to change physicians.**
3. **The right to privacy.** No one who is not involved directly in your health care should have access to any information about your medical condition or history unless you give specific permission.
4. **The right to full information.** You not only have the right to ask questions, but you have the right to complete, truthful answers.
5. **The right to know medical costs and fees, before you submit to treatment.**
6. **The right to a second opinion.** One prominent West Coast surgeon estimated that obtaining second and third opinions reduces the amount of unnecessary surgery as much as 60 percent.

Most physicians are of sufficient integrity to refer a patient to other personnel when the health problems are beyond the scope of their professional expertise. Although medicine today is highly specialized, the average patient is usually best served by the general practitioner or doctor of family medicine. Such physicians are generalists with a wide scope of training that enables them to deal effectively with 80 percent of the ailments commonly found in the population. When the general practitioner encounters a patient with problems demanding additional training, he refers him to the appropriate specialist.

548

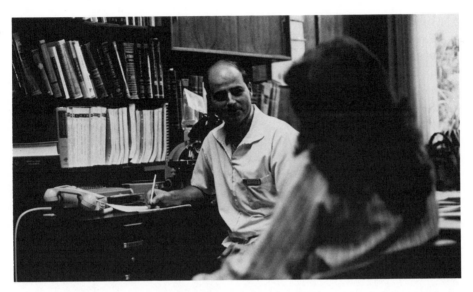

A very important step in preventive health care is the selection of a competent medical practitioner.

DO YOU NEED
AN ANNUAL CHECKUP?

Recent medical developments have caused doctors to question the need for an annual checkup of active, healthy people. You should certainly have an annual checkup (and sometimes one at more frequent intervals) if you or your doctor determine that you are a member of a high-risk group and that you have a good possibility of developing a medical problem.

If you do not run the risk of developing specific medical problems, you probably do not need a complete physical checkup every year. There are some exceptions to this rule:[3]

1. If you have been exposed to tuberculosis or if you live in an area where tuberculosis is common, you should be tested every year for the disease. While chest x-rays used to be the most common method of testing, you should ask for a tuberculin skin test instead to avoid unnecessary exposure to x-ray.

2. If you are a female over the age of of twenty-five, you should have a Pap smear every year. Women over twenty-five should also conduct breast self-examination each month and should have their breasts examined annually by a physician (this can be accomplished at the same time that the Pap smear is taken).
3. After the age of forty, you should be examined annually for glaucoma.
4. After the age of thirty, you should have an annual examination that includes urine cultures, urinalysis, and tests for blood in the stools (to detect cancer of the digestive tract, kidneys, or bladder).
5. Your blood pressure should be checked at least once a year regardless of your sex or age.

The following represents a schedule that may be used to determine when physical exams are necessary. Note that this schedule applies only if you are well, not on regular medication, have no complaints or symptoms, or have had tests to determine your state of health.[4]

- Infant: within twenty-four hours of birth, between the ages of two to four weeks, and at the age of one year.
- Toddler: every three to six months during the second year of life.
- Children from three to thirteen years: every two to three years.
- Teenagers: every four to five years.
- Young adults, ages twenty to thirty-four years: every five to seven years.
- Adults, ages thirty-four to forty years: every five years.
- Adults, ages forty to fifty years: every three years.
- Adults, ages fifty to sixty years: every two years.
- Adults, ages sixty to seventy years: every two years.
- Adults over age seventy-five: every year.

X-RAY EXAMINATION

Probably the most valuable and the most widely used tool for diagnosis is the x-ray — high energy electromagnetic impulses that cannot be seen or felt as they pass through the body.[5] In extremely high doses, x-rays are capable of severely damaging or destroying human tissue. The low doses required for most diagnostic tests will not damage normal tissue unless certain precautions are not taken or unless a patient receives too many x-rays.[6]

While the benefits of diagnostic x-rays outweigh the disadvantages, recent findings indicate that overexposure to x-ray radiation may trigger serious disease or tissue destruction, including cancer. As an x-ray passes through the body, some of the radiation is absorbed — more is absorbed by the dense body parts. The radiation, which is instantly dissipated into other forms of energy, can result in damage or destruction of cells from the transfer of energy. Most such damage is repaired by natural body processes, but some damaged cells can remain and cause serious problems as long as thirty years after exposure.

You can take measures to protect yourself against the potential harms of x-ray by doing the following:[7]

1. Keep accurate records of each x-ray that you have — the type of x-ray, the reason for the x-ray, the name of the dentist or physician that gave you the x-ray, and the date. Record the location of the facility where you received the x-ray so that you can obtain the x-rays if necessary.

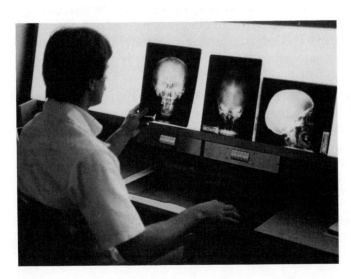

Wisely used X-rays are an invaluable tool in diagnosis.

2. Whenever your physician or dentist orders an x-ray, ask him to explain why the x-ray is necessary. If you are not satisfied with his reason, tell him that you feel that the x-ray is unnecessary. Find out if an alternate diagnostic method will work as well. Be sure to tell your doctor if you have had similar x-ray tests performed before.

3. If you are changing communities or physicians, ask for your x-rays. Some doctors or hospitals will release your x-ray file to you, and such files should be given to your new physician; they may prevent the need for further x-rays.

4. Chest x-ray screening programs for the diagnosis of tuberculosis are no longer recommended. If your employer requires that you be tested for tuberculosis prior to accepting employment, ask the doctor to give you a tuberculin skin test instead of a chest x-ray.

5. Dental x-rays are no longer recommended on a regular basis but should only be used in specific instances to diagnose a suspected problem that the dentist cannot diagnose in any other way. The American Dental Association has ruled that dental x-rays should *not* be a standard part of every dental examination.

6. If it does not interfere with the diagnostic procedure, insist that a lead shield be placed around your reproductive organs if you are having x-rays of the lower stomach, lower back, abdomen, or any area near the reproductive organs. In addition to causing sterility in some rare cases, exposure to x-ray may cause chromosomal damage that is then passed on to subsequent generations. Because the male's reproductive organs are located outside the body, it is particularly critical that a man request a gonadal shield if he is to receive x-rays of the abdomen or lower back.

7. If you are a woman and have any suspicion that you might be pregnant, tell your doctor before he orders diagnostic x-rays. Because x-rays are damaging to a fetus, you should not receive x-rays during pregnancy unless the x-rays are vital to saving your life. Even if you do not think you are pregnant, you should limit x-ray exposure to the first fourteen days of the menstrual cycle to prevent exposure to a fetus.

8. Never demand an x-ray if your physician seems reluctant. Some physicians have resorted to unnecessary x-ray to protect themselves against charges of malpractice.

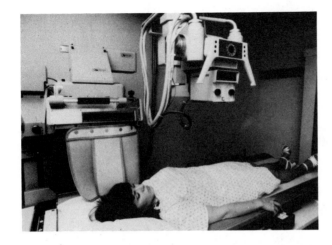

X-rays are particularly hazardous in early pregnancy when excessively used and when adequate shielding is not provided.

UNNECESSARY SURGERY

It is estimated that 2 million unnecessary operations are performed in the United States annually. Some physicians, through poor judgment or greed, perform needless operations on uninformed patients. However, many operations are done because *patients* insist upon them. Surgery has become so common and successful in the minds of the patients that they find it hard to believe that it would not remedy their medical problem.

Regardless of the reasons, it is apparent that patients need to become more informed concerning surgical matters. Every patient should ask the following when confronted with a surgical decision:

1. Is the surgery the only way to treat the medical problem?
2. Does the disease necessitate any treatment at all?
3. Is the surgeon qualified to perform this type of surgery?
4. Is the *individual* considered when the diagnosis is made?
5. Upon evaluation, do you feel that the surgery was recommended because *you* applied so much pressure to have it done?

If you still have questions or doubts, a second opinion from another physician often is in order. Many times, your own physician will encourage you to do this, or your insurance will require you to seek a second opinion. Studies have shown that second opinions have reduced the number of operations, but the long-term results are being questioned. Studies are now being done to determine whether patients who do not have surgery end up having it done later and if they require more extensive surgery.

MEDICAL INSURANCE

Health insurance is a means of providing some relief from the unexpected expenses associated with health care. It is not economically sound for insurance to pay for all health expenses, but it can help prevent a costly accident or illness from drastically changing the way of life of an individual or family.

To determine whether you are adequately covered by health insurance, check the coverage of your policy. It should include the following as a standard of minimum coverage.[8]

1. **Hospital insurance.** For a maximum deductible fee of $100, you should have hospital expense coverage that includes hospital room and board, the cost of general nursing care, and special diets for at least twenty-one days of continuous confinement. Your hospital policy should cover at least 80 percent of a semiprivate room charge (in some areas, insurance pays a flat rate per day, such as fifty dollars; this may not come close to covering the costs considering the rapidly increasing hospitalization expenses).

   Your policy should also cover at least 80 percent of the costs for surgery, recovery room fees, equipment (such as wheelchairs), intensive care, drugs, vaccines, intravenous preparations, dressings, plaster casts, oxygen, anesthesia, physiotherapy, chemotherapy, x-rays, electrocardiograms, radiation, or other customary hospital services rendered in connection with your hospitalization. Your hospital policy should also cover outpatient services on the day surgery is performed or for a period of up to twenty-four hours following an accident, and should cover at least 80 percent of the emergency room charges.

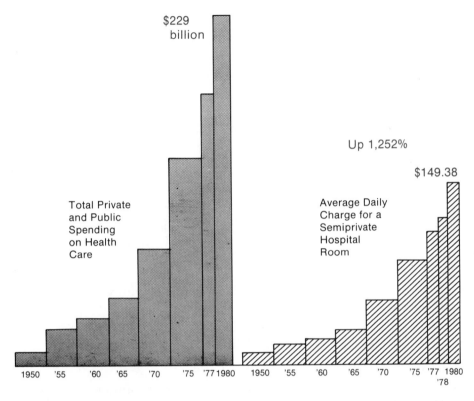

$229 billion

Total Private and Public Spending on Health Care

Up 1,252%

$149.38

Average Daily Charge for a Semiprivate Hospital Room

1950　'55　'60　'65　'70　'75　'77 1980

1950　'55　'60　'65　'70　'75　'77 1980
'78

Figure 16-1. The costs of health care have risen dramatically since 1950, as illustrated here.

2.　**Medical insurance.** Your policy should cover at least 80 percent of all surgical charges (including pre- and postoperative care by a physician), at least 80 percent of anesthetic charges, and at least 80 percent of all in-hospital medical services (including the physician's fee for a bed patient).

3.　**Major-medical insurance.** Your policy should include maximum benefits of at least $10,000. You should have coverage for laboratory tests, x-rays, drugs, radiation therapy, artificial limbs, treatment, and therapy performed outside a hospital. If you are at risk of developing a critical disease and your risk is extremely high, you may want to consider taking out a catastrophic illness policy in addition to your regular health insurance (such a policy, for example, would cover expenses incurred from cancer).

SELECTING A DENTIST

The training of a dentist is as scientifically based as that of a medical doctor, since considerable skill and dedication are required to provide quality dental care. Evaluating good dental practice is usually more difficult than determining good medical care. Most patients are satisfied with a physician if he makes them feel better. However, good dentistry extends considerably beyond the point of comfort and, in fact, is more closely equated with keeping teeth.

In general, a patient must look for a dentist who will provide the following services:

1. He provides a thorough examination.

2. He is concerned about and relieves pain.

3. He is concerned about the proper care and maintenance of baby teeth. The child's first visit to the dentist should occur around two years of age. Subsequent regular dental care should be directed at saving teeth, be they baby or permanent.

4. He puts in fillings that will last. Temporary fillings are occasionally appropriate but may be a gimmick for setting up another visit and collecting another fee. If permanent fillings crack or are lost, the dentistry was inadequate.

5. He helps prevent periodontal disease. The dentist's major contributions to preventing this problem are meticulous scaling and cleaning of the teeth and advice or counsel on plaque control and on what the patient can do to prevent and alleviate the condition.

6. He applies advanced techniques in his practice. Appropriate use of high-speed drills (risky for deep decay close to the pulp cavity), use of new resin adhesives for inlays, repair of broken teeth, replacement of teeth that have come out, and application of sealants for cracks and

fissures, which are the sisters of decay, are all new approaches to effective dentistry.

7. He educates the patient concerning proper nutrition and its effects on good dental health. He explains the role of excessive sugar in promoting dental caries and gum disease and elaborates upon the importance of proper cleaning of the teeth by flossing and brushing.

THE CHIROPRACTIC PHYSICIAN

One controversial area in health services today concerns chiropractic. According to the Chiropractic Fact Sheet prepared by the National College of Chiropractic, chiropractic may be defined as the diagnosis and treatment of human ailments without the use of drugs, medicine, or incisive surgery. It is a nonmedical, nonsurgical form of therapy utilizing manipulation of the spine and other articulations, clinical nutrition, physical therapy, psychological counseling, hygiene, and sanitation in the prevention and treatment of disease.

Chiropractic is *not* a branch of medicine. Chiropractics are not licensed medical doctors; by law they cannot prescribe drugs or perform surgery. They are not allowed to practice in any hospital accredited by the Joint Commission of Accreditation of Hospitals. Their treatment is usually confined to spinal and soft tissue manipulation. The limitations of chiropractic training would seem to cast doubt on its potential for delivering adequate health care.

Physicians maintain that the idea of illness being derived from a malposition of spinal bones is ridiculous; that chiropractics have not done scientific research for eighty-five years to support its claims; and that chiropractic is potentially dangerous because it may well aggravate some serious conditions and delay urgent medical attention to others. Chiropractics accuse the medical profession of economic and professional jealousy, of operating out of conservatism. They claim that chiropractic is clinically, if not scientifically, proven and point to many years and hundreds of thousands of satisfied patients.

For those who choose to use the services of a chiropractor, read the following advice:

1. Avoid any practitioner who makes claims about cures, either orally

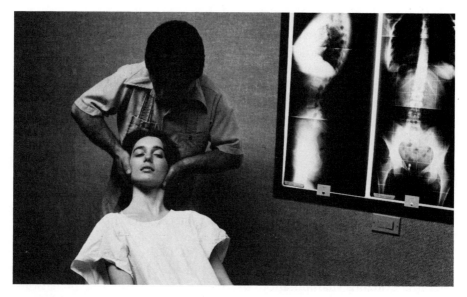

Chiropractic procedures are controversial because of inadequate supportive research evidence.

or in advertising. Anyone who implies or promises guaranteed results from treatment should be held suspect.

2. Beware of chiropractors who ask you to sign a contract for services. A written agreement is not customary practice.

3. Reject anyone advertising free x-rays. Radiation should not be used as a lure.

4. Do not make advance payments.

5. Do not be pressured by scare tactics, such as threats of "irreversible damage" if treatment is not begun promptly.

6. See a physician as well and find out what he or she has to say about the problem.

7. Only go to a chiropractor for back ailments or muscle pain, not for organic or visceral disorders.

8. Be wary if the chiropractor involves himself in anything other than muscles or bones.

9. Do not give up any medication that you are already taking just on a chiropractor's say-so.

10. Determine whether the chiropractor who you are considering has ACA (American Chiropractic Association) membership.

QUACKERY

The dispensing of false or misleading information is a form of quackery. The word "quack" is a short form of the dutch word "kwakzolver" (quacksalver), which means one who quacks boastfully, like a duck, about his medical remedies. Other definitions include "a medical imposter" and "one who promises health benefits which he cannot deliver."

Quackery in its various disguises has encroached into many areas of health and medical care. Nutritional quackery is one of the most prevalent forms with its false claims about dietary supplements, natural foods, and food processers. Cosmetic quackery is also big business, and it includes everything from sexual rejuvenation to curing baldness. The claims made for many over-the-counter medications are often flirting with quackery. There are also many fraudulent health schemes that are promoted so that they can be sold and distributed through the mail.

Recognizing Quackery

Most quacks are friendly, well-dressed, attractive people who approach you in a most sympathetic and kind way. Some have offices in reputable buildings. Many hire nurses and receptionists. So how can you recognize a quack? Some of the following characteristics are common:

1. **Secret remedies.** They claim to know of the latest discoveries and have access to their use. Secret remedies are usually worthless.

2. **Quick cure.**

3. **Guarantee of cure.** Science has not progressed to the point where it can guarantee results — there are simply too many unpredictables and individual variables. Even with the guarantee, the quack seldom refunds any money.

4. **Testimonials.** Testimonials may be fakes, may be bought, or may be given by people who only thought that they had a disease and were cured.

5. **Claims persecution.** He claims that the medical association, government agencies, and research institutions are persecuting him. He clamors for medical recognition, but he avoids scientific evaluation of

the products and methods that he claims are superior.

6. **Discredits accepted procedures.** Since a quack may not be able to legally use drugs, surgery, laboratory, or other proven procedures, he tries to discredit them.

7. **Low-cost diagnosis.** He may invite patients to mail in a description of their symptoms, and he will make the diagnosis and prescribe the proper medication for food supplement. Not even the most skilled physician can make an accurate diagnosis by mail or phone.

8. **Questionable degrees.** He may display his diplomas in a conspicuous manner in order to create an illusion of credibility. Certificates can be obtained for a price, and degrees are granted from schools that are nothing more than a "diploma mill." The so-called "school" may be a short course workshop, a correspondence course, or merely a post office box.

OVER-THE-COUNTER DRUGS

Over-the-counter drugs — those that can be purchased without a prescription — are the most widely used drugs in the country today. But just because you can get them without a prescription is no reason to believe that they are harmless or that they should be used any time. Some are safe and beneficial in relieving minor symptoms, but none should be taken continuously for long periods of time. They can never "cure" disease — they only relieve the *symptoms* of disease. If those symptoms continue, it is a sign that you should seek medical attention.

To protect yourself when considering over-the-counter drugs in general, remember the following:

1. Get into the habit of reading labels carefully, and make sure that the drug is the right one for your symptoms. Be especially careful if you have any allergies.

2. Keep advertising in the proper perspective. Do not expect more from the drug than it can be reasonably expected to deliver. Remember: no drug can make you look younger, can make you lose weight, or can relieve a headache in two minutes.

3. Follow directions. The label contains important information regarding who can take the drug, the conditions under which the drug can be taken, whether it is safe to drive your car when you are

taking the drug, and whether the drug is safe for children.

4. Ask questions. If you are confused or unsure about which product to buy, ask a pharmacist — he cannot legally diagnose disease or prescribe medication, but he can (and will) advise you about over-the-counter drugs. If you are unable to consult a pharmacist, call your doctor.

5. Before you take more than one drug at a time, ask your doctor about consequences of mixing medications. Some drugs just do not mix; others can create serious — even fatal — reactions.

6. Do not drink alcohol and use drugs simultaneously. Sleeping pills and antihistamines are only two of the drugs that result in extreme drowsiness when combined with alcohol; in some cases, coma results.

7. If you have children, check for safety packaging. Keep medications out of the reach of children, and ask your pharmacist to package drugs in child-proof packaging. When buying over-the-counter drugs, choose those that have child-proof caps.

8. Do not change packaging without consulting your pharmacist. Some drugs are packaged in a certain way to preserve their potency and freshness. Your pharmacist can tell you whether you can safely switch containers.

9. Stop taking the drug immediately if you notice that you are suffering from adverse reactions.

10. Be careful that you do not overdose. Over-the-counter drugs that are completely safe in normal doses may cause kidney disease, enzyme imbalance, or even accidental poisoning and death if taken in large doses.

PRESCRIPTION DRUGS

It is obvious that you can take an active role in choosing which nonprescription drugs you will buy. But there is no reason to think that you are totally helpless when it comes to prescription drugs. You can provide your doctor with information — and you can ask him questions — that will help him to prescribe the best medication for your needs.

You should give your doctor the following information before he fills out your prescriptions:

1. If you have *ever* had an adverse reaction to any drug, no matter what

you were sick with at the time. Your doctor would be interested in finding out that you had an allergic reaction to penicillin, for instance — there are other drugs that he might have considered giving you that are closely related to penicillin.

2. If you are allergic to any foods.

3. If you are taking any other drugs (this includes over-the-counter drugs or prescription drugs prescribed for you by another doctor). Certain drugs clash — it is important that your doctor know what else you are taking.

4. Whether you drink alcohol, coffee, or tea. Alcohol and caffeine can greatly affect the actions of a prescription drug and can even cause loss of consciousness or coma when mixed with certain drugs.

5. About any other medical conditions that you have. Certain prescription drugs that work well for one medical condition might be dangerous to another. Your one set of symptoms might disappear, but you might become even sicker in the bargain.

Paying Less for Drugs

What specifically can you do to help save costs when you need prescription drugs? Follow these suggestions:

1. Talk to your physician about prescription drug prices. If he knows that you are aware of price differences and that you care about them, he may make an effort to help you save money.

2. Ask your physician to prescribe drugs under their generic names. If he is unwilling to do so, ask him to explain why he thinks the brand-name medicine is best.

3. There is something even better than having your physician write out a prescription for a drug under its generic name: if he is aware of manufacturers' costs, have him write out your prescription for the brand that is the least expensive.

4. If your physician puts you on a long-term program of drug therapy, ask him to prescribe large doses at once. This not only saves you the inconvenience of extra trips to the pharmacy but will save you money. You do need to take one caution — check with the pharmacist and determine the drug's expiration date (many medications lose potency and effectiveness after a certain shelf life). If the drug expires before you will have the chance to use it up, buy a smaller quantity even if you have to pay more.

5. Comparison shop! There are wide differences in prices among pharmacies even in the same city.

Use Your Drugs Safely

There are many things that you can do to make better use of prescription drugs by using them safely. Consider the following suggestions:

1. Do not pressure your physician into prescribing a drug if you do not really need it.
2. Never take prescription drugs on your own.
3. Do not take a friend's prescription drug just because your symptoms are just like his.
4. Do not give anyone else — even a family member — your prescription drug unless your physician tells you to. It is against the law.
5. Do not change the dose or timing of your drug unless your physician tells you to.
6. If you start to suffer serious side effects that your physician warned you about, get in touch with the physician as quickly as you can. Or, if a drug is not doing what it is expected to, notify your physician.
7. Do not stop taking a prescription drug without letting your doctor know.
8. Do not take *any* drug while you are pregnant or nursing a child unless your doctor specifically tells you to. Make sure that your doctor knows that you are pregnant or nursing before he prescribes a drug for you.
9. Do not take more medications than you have to.
10. Never take any drug in the dark. If you get up in the middle of the night to take your medicine, turn on the light and make sure that you have the right bottle.
11. Do not mix medications in the same container. Potency may be destroyed — and if the medications look alike, you may take the same drug twice.
12. Learn the name and correct spelling of each drug that you are using.
13. Ask your doctor what dietary adjustments you can make to help your drug work better. Some drugs, for instance, are neutralized by milk — if you know that, stay away from dairy products.
14. If you are scheduled for surgery, tell your dentist, surgeon, or

anesthesiologist about *all* of the drugs that you have taken in the last several weeks.

15. If you get pregnant while you are taking any kind of a drug, inform your doctor immediately.

16. Keep a written record of all drugs that you take and all vaccines you receive during the entire nine months you are pregnant. Include the name of the drug, how much you took, the dates you took it, and what you took it for.

17. Keep the same kind of written record for all drugs to which you are allergic. Do the same for members of your family.

18. Tell your doctor about *any* allergy you have — not just allergies to drugs.

19. Call your doctor immediately if you think that you have taken an overdose.

20. Clarify with your doctor whether it is safe to drive a car or operate machinery while you are taking your prescription drug.

21. Ask the doctor if you can safely drink alcoholic beverages while you are taking the drug.

Notes

1. Lewis Miller, *The Life You Save* (New York: William Morrow and Company, 1979), p. 28.
2. Jean E. Laird, "Know Your Rights as a Patient," *Family Weekly*, November 13, 1977, p. 32.
3. Donald M. Vickery and James F. Fries, *Take Care Of Yourself: a Consumer's Guide to Medical Care.* (Reading, Massachusetts: Addison-Wesley Publishing Company, 1976), p. 12.
4. Miller, *The Life You Save*, pp. 56-57.
5. "X-Ray Hazards — Real and Imagined," *Sci/Di*, March 1979, p. 82.
6. "The New Worry Over X-Rays and What You Can Do About It," *Good Housekeeping*, July 1979, p. 221.
7. "Growing Debate Over Dangers of Radiation," *U.S. News and World Report*, May 14, 1979, p. 26; Public Health Service, *We Want You to Know About Diagnostic X-Rays* (Rockville, Maryland: U.S. Department of Health, Education, and Welfare, DHEW Publication No. (FDA) 73-8048, 1973).
8. "Health Insurance Policies: Why It's Hard to Pick a Good One," *Changing Times*, December 1978, p. 8.

Self-Evaluation

Section 1
What Do You Know About Your Health Insurance?

Instructions: If you have a health insurance policy, answer the following questions the best you can from memory. If you do not have health insurance coverage, answer the questions based on the policy that you would be most likely to have.

1. Check all of the following that apply.

    _____ I have no health insurance.

    _____ I am covered by the student health center plan on campus.

    _____ I have purchased additional student health insurance.

    _____ I am covered by my parent's health insurance.

    _____ I am covered by a government health service program.

    _____ I have another provision for paying for emergency health care.

2. Is your insurance a group plan or an individual policy?

    Group _____ Individual _____ I don't know _____

3. Is the policy guaranteed renewable?

    Yes _____ No _____ I don't know _____

4. Will the policy generally cover preexisting conditions?

    Yes _____ No _____ I don't know _____

5. Does the policy have a waiting period?

    Yes _____ No _____ I don't know _____

6. Does the policy have many exclusions?

    Yes _____ No _____ I don't know _____

7. Does the policy have a grace period?

    Yes _____ No _____ I don't know _____

8. Are the claims easy to process?

    Yes _____ No _____ I don't know _____

9. When benefits are paid, who gets the money?
The doctor or hospital directly _____   The insured _____
I don't know _____

10. What are the limitations on what the policy will pay?
There is a deductible _____   There is coinsurance _____
There is a flat fee _____   Dollar limit _____
Time limit _____

11. Does the policy cover both accidents and illness?
Yes _____   I don't know _____   Accidents only _____

12. What does the policy cover?

	Yes	No	I Don't Know
Hospital Admissions	____	____	____
Surgical Expenses	____	____	____
Anesthesia	____	____	____
Physicians Hospital Fees	____	____	____
Physicians Office Fees	____	____	____
Major Medical Expenses	____	____	____
Ambulance Transportation	____	____	____
X-ray and Laboratory Work	____	____	____
Prescription Medications	____	____	____
Physical Therapy	____	____	____
Dental Injuries	____	____	____
Maternity Benefits	____	____	____
Emotional Illness and Alcoholism	____	____	____
Disability Income	____	____	____
Private Room If Required by the Physician	____	____	____
Private Duty Nurse If Required by the Physician	____	____	____
Care in an Extended Care Facility If Required	____	____	____
Physical Examinations and Other Preventatives	____	____	____

Section 2
Are You An Intelligent Health Consumer?

Instructions: Rate yourself on a scale of 1-5 on each of the following statements. If the statement is nearly always true, mark a 5 in the blank; if the statement is nearly always false, mark a 1 in the blank; or if your position rests somewhere in between, indicate it by marking a 4, 3, or 2 in the blank.

1. You are well informed and know where to obtain the information needed to make sound decisions. _____

2. You are wary of providers of health services and can distinguish the competent practitioners from the inept and pseudopractitioners. _____

3. You are skeptical of health-related advertisements and can distinguish between what is definitely known about a product and the exaggerated claims made for the product. _____

4. You do not accept statements appearing in books and articles at face value and do not take for granted the information from a single source. _____

5. You select doctors with care and question fees, diagnoses, and treatments to clarify your understanding and to validate the information. _____

6. You have some means of financing unexpected health costs, yet you act in an economically responsible manner so as not to contribute to increased health care costs. _____

7. You will report apparent wrongdoing to the appropriate agency and be willing to testify if necessary to bring frauds to justice. _____

8. You will support social reforms that will promote the efficient delivery of safe and effective health products and services. _____

Scoring: Add the numbers for the eight statements. The higher the score the more intelligent you are as a healthy consumer. **TOTAL** _____

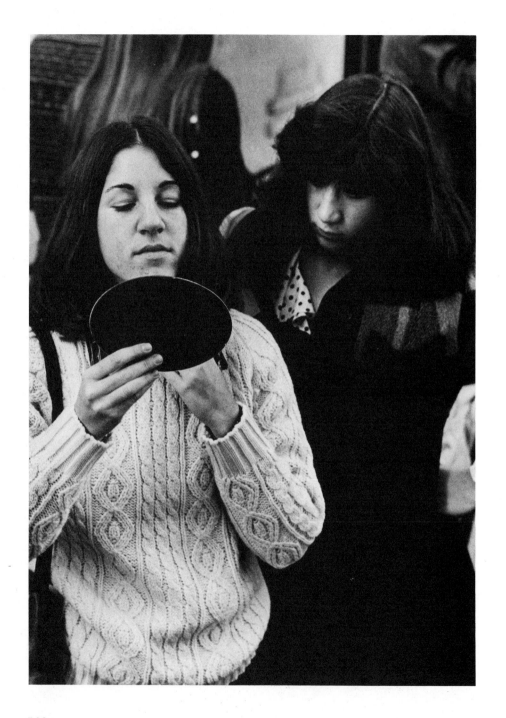

568

17
Self-Care:
To Each His Own

Self-care involves the idea that individuals can and should assume more responsibility for their own health. The push is to avoid unnecessary operations, overmedication, and needless visits to the doctor. The essence of self-care, then, is control, responsibility, freedom, expanded options, and improved quality of life. Other reasons why people are beginning to turn to self-care are as follows:

1. Widespread dissatisfaction with present medical care.
2. The fact that personal behavior and environment will help to improve health and to promote disease reduction.
3. The movement from acute to chronic disease orientation.
4. The desire to save money on health expenses.
5. The desire to be able to make better decisions concerning one's own health and the health of one's family, which leads to a certain joy of independence.

If you have ever gone to the doctor with symptoms that have turned out to signal the flu or mononucleosis, you know that most of the treatment depended on you — on what you did after you got home to take care of yourself. While a doctor's diagnosis is important to rule out the possibility of serious disease, there are many things that you can do to treat yourself in cases of mild illness and many ways in which you can take care of common problems.

If you know how, you can also measure your own vital signs, assess your own symptoms, and report your own history of illness to a doctor, enabling him to make a more accurate diagnosis. All of these add up to skills that will enable you to take a more aggressive role in your own health and well-being.

SIGNS OF CRITICAL ILLNESS

In certain cases, you should not attempt self-treatment; certain symptoms indicate illness too critical to be treated without skilled medical help.

Certain conditions are marked by signs and symptoms that should be referred to medical help. Such conditions are as follows:

1. Acuteness — the signs and symptoms are so severe that they cannot be endured (for example, chest pains or abdominal pain).
2. Persistence — the signs and symptoms persist for a few days or a week (for example, headaches).
3. Recurrence — the signs and symptoms return without a clear-cut cause (for example, diarrhea or other intestinal upsets).
4. Unusualness — the signs and symptoms raise doubts.

MEASURING VITAL SIGNS

Measuring vital signs is an important part in determining a health problem — whether you are examining yourself or someone else. You should be careful to use proper equipment and follow correct methods in order to get an accurate reading of temperature, blood pressure, pulse, or respiration.

Taking Temperature

Generally, a change in temperature is an indication that something is amiss, although "normal" temperatures in different individuals may vary slightly.

Before taking a temperature:

1. Wash your hands.
2. Check the thermometer for breakage; make sure that there are no cracks in the thermometer, especially in the mercury bulb (ingestion of mercury can lead to mercury poisoning).
3. Cleanse the thermometer with a disinfectant (alcohol is a good one), and rinse it with soap under cool running water.
4. If the thermometer reads above 95° F, shake it down: grasp the top end tightly, and shake the thermometer with a snapping motion. Keep your wrist loose, and make sure that you don't hit the thermometer against anything. Shaking it over a bed may help to prevent breakage in the event the thermometer is dropped.
5. Make sure that the patient has not had hot or cold liquids or been smoking — all of which can alter the temperature. If he has, wait for thirty minutes to an hour for the temperature to normalize.

You need to decide whether to take an oral or rectal temperature. The most convenient place for taking a temperature is the mouth — but it should not be used if the patient is unconscious, irrational, restless, delirious, or combative; if the mouth is parched or dry; if the mouth is inflamed; or if the patient is a child or infant who may bite the thermometer accidentally.

Use these steps in taking a temperature:

Oral

1. Place the mercury end of the thermometer under the tongue; ask the patient to keep his mouth tightly closed, but not to bite the thermometer with his teeth. His lips should stay tightly closed. The bulb of mercury should touch the base of the tongue.
2. Leave the thermometer in the patient's mouth for three minutes.
3. Remove the thermometer and read it. Normal oral temperature is 98.6°F (37°C).

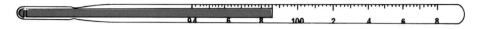

Figure 17-1.

Rectal

The thermometer used to take a rectal temperature has a short, blunt bulb as opposed to the long, slender bulb of the oral thermometer. To take a rectal temperature:

1. Lubricate the mercury tip of the thermometer with a water-soluble lubricating jelly.
2. Insert the thermometer about one and one-half inches into the rectum.
3. Hold the thermometer in place for about three minutes. If the patient is a baby, place him face down on your lap. Insert the thermometer, and hold in place with the thermometer between your fingers, your hand across his buttocks, while your other hand gently steadies the child across his back. This minimizes the danger of an active infant suddenly rolling over and breaking the thermometer.
4. Before attempting to read the thermometer, wipe it clean, removing any lubricating jelly and fecal matter (start at the top of the thermometer and wipe toward the bulb). Normal rectal temperature is 99.6° F (37.5° C).

To read a thermometer:

1. Hold the thermometer horizontally so that the numbers are on the bottom and the lines (calibration) are on the top.
2. Hold the thermometer at eye level, and slowly rotate the thermometer between the thumb and index finger.
3. Watch the area between the lines and the numbers until you see the mercury; notice where the mercury ends.
4. Rotate the thermometer to see which number is closest to the point at which the mercury ends. Count how many lines past the number the mercury extends.
5. The temperature reading is the whole number (100) marked by the long line, plus one-tenth for every short line (if the mercury ends three short lines beyond 100, the temperature is 100.3).

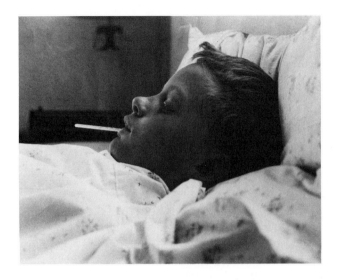

After you have read the thermometer, shake it down again. Rinse it under cold running water and soap, wipe it with rubbing alcohol, and allow it to dry thoroughly before you put it away.

Taking the Pulse

The pulse is the alternate contraction and expansion of an artery that corresponds to the contraction and expansion caused by the heartbeat. It is taken most easily at the wrist, using the following procedure:

1. Place your middle fingertip over the artery on the thumb side of the patient's wrist.
2. Move your finger around gently until you locate the pulsebeat.
3. Exert enough pressure so that you can feel the pulsebeat, but not so much pressure that you obliterate it.
4. *Never* use your thumb to take a pulse: the thumb has a pulsepoint and may conflict with the patient's pulsebeat, causing you to get confused and count the wrong beats.
5. When you are able to feel the pulse plainly, count the beats for one minute.

6. Record the number of beats per minute, as well as other characteristics of the pulse: whether it is strong or feeble, rapid or slow, and regular or irregular.

Normal resting pulse rates are:

Men	60-70	
Women	70-80	
Children over seven years of age		80-90
Children from one to seven years		80-120
Infants	110-130	

The classification of pulse in adults is as follows:

60 and below	Slow or subnormal
60-80	Normal (men and women)
80-100	Moderate increase
100-120	Quick
120-140	Rapid
140 and up	Running (hard to count)

Measuring Respiration

Respiration is the breathing in of air and the exhaling of gases from the lungs. A respiration, then, is one breath taken in and one let out.

A number of factors can cause the respiration rate to vary: exercise, fever, and activity all cause an increase in the respiration rate. Resting or sleeping reduce the rate. Normal rate is between fourteen and twenty respirations per minute. In taking respiration, it is more important to record the *kind* of respirations than the number: note, for instance, that the breathing is shallow, labored, or snorelike.

You should observe or count respirations when the patient is unaware that you are doing so; if he knows that his respirations are being counted, he may breathe abnormally.

Taking Blood Pressure

To read blood pressure, you need a device called a *sphygmomanometer* (blood pressure cuff) and a stethoscope, both to measure the force exerted on the arteries during heartbeat. Many factors can influence blood pressure: injury, internal bleeding, age, emotional excitement, weight, physical rest, shock, or disease.

The systolic pressure — the pressure exerted as the heart beats or contracts — is the number expressed above the line; normal is about 120. The diastolic pressure — the number recorded below the line — is the measure of the pressure on the arteries as the heart rests; 80 is about normal. A slight variation from these "normal" figures is insignificant; wide variations can be cause for alarm.

To take blood pressure:

1. Have the patient lie down or sit comfortably. You can use either arm; the arm should be bare.

2. Explain the procedure to the patient before you start to avoid nervousness and anxiety (causing blood pressure to climb).

3. Place the cuff around the patient's arm, above the elbow. The cuff should fit well in proportion to the patient's arm.

4. Make sure that the valve on the bulb is fully closed (turned clockwise).

5. Find the arterial pulse on the bend of the elbow; if necessary, use the stethoscope to find the pulse.

6. Keep your fingers on the pulse while you inflate the cuff by pumping on the rubber bulb until the pulse disappears. Note what number appears on the scale of the mercury apparatus.

7. Position the disc of the stethoscope over the area where you felt the pulse before it disappeared; position the earpieces of the stethoscope in your ears (with the earpieces directed upward).

8. Hold the stethoscope disc snugly in position with one hand while you continue pumping the cuff with the other.

9. Pump the cuff until the mercury on the scale is about 30 points above the point where you felt the pulse disappear.

10. Loosen the valve slightly, and permit the pressure to drop slowly. Listen *carefully* for the first sound of a beat: the number on the scale when you hear the first beat is the systolic pressure. (If you think that you missed the first beat or are unsure, tighten the valve again and pump the cuff up; repeat the method, listening carefully.)

11. Continue to deflate the cuff slowly until the last heartbeat is heard. When you hear no more blood flowing, the number on the scale is the diastolic pressure.

12. Open the valve completely, and allow the cuff to fully deflate.

THE COMMON COLD ▬▬▬▬▬

Few illnesses cause so much loss of productivity and so much personal discomfort as the common head cold. Everyone is familiar with the symptoms: headache, runny nose (with thick, mucousy discharge), red and watery eyes, sore throat, sneezing, and a general feeling of fatigue. Sometimes there is fever (rarely more than one degree over normal), aching muscles, or a cough. A cold may last only two or three days and should not last longer than a week.

Antibiotics are not effective against colds, because colds are caused by viruses. Some over-the-counter remedies are available and can be used if they make you feel more comfortable. One of the most important aspects of cold treatment is rest. Stay in bed for at least a day; stay there longer if you can. Your body will recover its healing abilities more quickly if you give it the rest that it needs. If you have a hard time developing an appetite while you are ill, just drink water. Blow your nose very gently to keep from forcing infectious matter into your ear canals and sinuses. When you blow your nose, allow both nasal openings to remain unblocked, and blow with only mild pressure.

If your throat is sore or scratchy, gargle with warm water — either plain or slightly salted (use about one-half teaspoon of salt to eight ounces of warm water). The cause of many sore throats that accompany colds is the draining of mucous along the sensitive tissue of the throat, and regular gargling can clear the throat of such secretions. You may also try sipping warm broths, such as bouillon.

If you develop fever, take two aspirin every four hours. Aspirin can also relieve muscle and body aches. If you cannot take aspirin, check with your doctor for a suitable substitute.

Dispose of your tissues in a covered container to prevent the spread of contamination to others in your household. Use separate dishes, utensils, and drinking glasses, and wash them as soon as possible after use with hot, soapy water. Keep your hands clean, and wash them before handling other household items.

Warmth is one of the best treatments for the aches and pains of colds. Soaking in a tub full of hot water is helpful in relieving aching muscles and joints.

There are a number of things that you can do to prevent a cold.

1. Avoid people who have colds. Try to stay away from crowds of

Facts and Fancies about Catching Colds

Careful scientific investigation has debunked many firmly held beliefs about the causes of colds — fatigue, wet and chill, for example, seem to have no effect. But some of grandmother's cautions have been upheld, such as the advisability of covering sneezes and coughs. Below is a selection of presumed facts, some true, some false and some still in doubt.

Children catch more colds than anyone else.
True. Not only do young children suffer more colds, but parents with young children get more colds than other people their age.

Kissing is a sure way to spread a cold.
False. Colds are rather difficult to catch by way of the mouth. University of Wisconsin researchers tested couples, asking that in each couple, the cold-stricken partner kiss the unafflicted one for 90 seconds. Only one caught cold.

Adults tend to get fewer colds as they grow older.
True. The older a person is, the more likely it is that he already has had a particular cold virus and has some immunity to it.

Smokers catch more colds than nonsmokers.
False. Several studies have shown that both groups are equally susceptible. However, their symptoms differ. Smokers develop coughs more often than nonsmokers, and the cough persists longer, nonsmokers more often have a sore, scratchy throat.

Adults whose tonsils were removed in childhood get worse colds than those who still have their tonsils.
False. Laboratory experiments with volunteers given virus-laden nose drops showed that a tonsillectomy affected neither susceptibility to colds nor the severity of colds that were contracted.

Hay-fever sufferers get particularly bad colds.
True. Experiments on those afflicted with this allergy indicated that their colds were more severe than those of other people.

Introverts suffer worse colds than outgoing, extroverted personality types.
Probably true. When volunteers at Britain's Common Cold Unit were rated with standard psychological tests, scientists found introverts did indeed get worse cold symptoms than extroverts. Introverts also spread more virus particles, another indication that their infections were more severe.

Ongoing stress, such as a high-pressure job, increases vulnerability to colds.
Probably false. Studies at the Common Cold Unit found that sudden psychological jolts, rather than continuing stress, heightened susceptibility to colds. The true culprit seems to be the stress associated with change itself, whether the change is positive or negative; thus any major disruption of routine — even a pleasant diversion such as a vacation — increases the risk of a cold.

Library of Health — Coping with the Common Cold, by Wendy Murphy. Editors of Time-Life books. © 1981, Time-Life Books, Inc.

people during the winter. The most sure way of catching a cold is direct contact with others who have colds.

2. Get enough sleep. Your body's resistance level is lowered when you go without the sleep and rest that you need. If the air where you live is dry (especially during the winter), sleep with a humidifier or vaporizer — the dryness will dehydrate the bronchial passages, crippling their ability to trap dust and bacteria in the nose and throat.

3. Get enough exercise. Your body stays in its optimum condition when you are exercising. Be sure to dress warmly if you exercise outdoors, but do not get so exhausted that you perspire and get damp.

4. Eat a well-balanced diet, and get the proper amounts of nutrients from the four basic food groups. Like sleep, proper nutrition helps build body defenses.

5. Keep your hands clean, and wash them often; keep them away from your mouth, eyes, and nose. Many colds are literally picked up from virus-infested objects and transmitted to the victim via the hands.

COUGHING

A cough is a reflex mechanism that acts as a defense to clear the breathing passages of mucous; even when voluntary, a cough is caused by a reflex action and is desirable if it acts to clear matter from the breathing tubes.

A productive cough is one that is accompanied by copious amounts of sputum — it can be yellow, green, or brown material and may be streaked with blood, depending on the cause of the cough. A dry (or nonproductive) cough usually is a hacking cough that brings up no sputum; it is characteristic of bronchitis, pneumonia, and the early stages of tuberculosis and follows inhalation of a foreign body.

In general, administer aspirin to reduce fever (do not administer aspirin if there is no fever, since aspirin does not act in any way on the cough), and increase the humidity in your home with a vaporizer, humidifier, or steamy shower.

If you have postnasal drip that is irritating your throat, take a decongestant every four hours; an over-the-counter cough syrup may help contain the cough and should be taken every four hours. Do not take antihistamines, because they dry out the lining of the throat and bronchial passages. If your throat is irritated, gargle with warm salt water (one teaspoon of salt to eight ounces of warm water) or suck on throat lozenges or hard candy if your throat is dry and tickly. Increase your fluid intake — especially important if you have a fever.

Do not rest too much — lying in bed can actually cause you to cough more. Smokers should discontinue their habit.

You should contact a doctor immediately if blood is coughed up; if the cough produces large amounts of thick, foul-smelling, yellowish or greenish sputum; if you have a fever of more than 102° F; if you have a fever of over 100° F that lasts longer than three days; if your cough lasts longer than ten days; if your cough worsens instead of improves after twenty-four hours of treatment; if you have pain other than a mild headache; if you have a sore throat; if you suffer from excessive weakness; or if you have to maintain treatment longer than a week.

SORE THROAT (PHARYNGITIS)

A sore throat — usually an extension of the common cold, tonsilitis, adenoiditis, or sinusitis — is the most common complication of the common cold. Eighty percent of all colds are caused by irritants or viruses; strep throat is caused by bacteria.

Sore throat can result from prolonged irritation to the throat, overindulgence in alcohol, overuse of the voice, exposure to irritating smoke, bacterial infection, fungus infection, viral infection, postnasal discharge, shouting, swallowing irritating foods, or diseases like measles or acute tonsilitis. An acute sore throat should run its course within a few days to a few weeks.

Strep throat is characterized by yellow or white mucous spots on the throat, swollen glands in the neck, and a fever over 101° F. While you are running a fever, you should stay in bed; take two aspirin every four hours for reduction of fever. Even after you have recovered from fever, rest frequently in a cool room. Keep the home — and especially your sleeping room — humid with the use of a vaporizer. Rest your voice as much as you can.

To relieve throat pain, gargle with a solution of one teaspoon of salt in eight ounces of hot water (not to exceed 120° F) every two hours. Frequent sips of hot liquids (at least six eight-ounce glasses a day) can help to break up mucous in the throat and relieve throat pain. Sucking on a throat lozenge, a cough drop, or a hard candy can keep the throat moist and the mucous moving.

If it is painful to swallow, drink as many fluids as you can, and eat a soft diet. Avoid smoke-filled rooms, and if you are a smoker, stop. You should call a doctor if your throat is red and raw, if your tonsils are red or enlarged or covered with a whitish material, if you run a fever over 101°F, if you experience a severe headache, if you develop chest pains, if your sore throat lasts longer than fourteen days, if you develop earache, if you experience abdominal pain, if you have a history of kidney infections, if you experience shortness of breath, if you develop a cough, if a skin rash develops, if you see white or yellow patches on the throat, or if someone in your family has been exposed to a strep infection.

INFLUENZA

Also caused by a virus and resistant to antibiotic treatment, influenza affects the linings of the respiratory tract and the tissues of the nose and throat. Some of the same viruses that cause common colds can cause the flu.

Some people can have a flu infection and never suffer symptoms; however, most victims come down with symptoms within twenty-four to forty-eight hours following exposure. The flu lasts anywhere from three to ten days; there is usually fever (101° to 106° F), cough, fatigue, muscle aches, chills, headache, and gastrointestinal distress.

The fever rarely lasts more than a few days, but other symptoms continue through the course of the illness. Cough and general feelings of fatigue may continue for several weeks after the illness is over. A prominent feature of the flu is severe pain under the breastbone, caused by destruction of cells lining the trachea.

Treatment for the flu is basically the same as for the common cold: get plenty of rest, drink lots of fluids (fruit juices if you can), stay warm, and take measures to avoid spreading the infection.

The flu may develop into pneumonia, although it is not common. At risk are individuals with heart disease or chronic respiratory disease, such as asthma or emphysema; if you are at risk, you should remain under a physician's care during the course of the flu.

The basic steps that you take to prevent catching a common cold will also help you resist the flu. In addition, avoid exposure to tobacco smoke (due to its drying effects on the respiratory linings).

Flu shots generally immunize against the most serious strains of the flu, and they are not recommended for the entire population. You *should* get flu shots if you are prone to have serious complications from the flu; if you are essential to community life (generally policemen, firemen, health care personnel, military personnel, and teachers); or if you live in an environment where an epidemic would be likely (a dormitory, nursing home, or military camp).

INFECTIOUS MONONUCLEOSIS

Called the "kissing disease," infectious mononucleosis strikes most often at college students and is caused by the Epstein-Barr (EB) virus, rendering it unresponsive to antibiotic treatment. Mononucleosis results in symptoms appearing anywhere from two weeks to three months following exposure; the disease is transmitted by direct salivary contact (hence, the name "kissing disease").

Mononucleosis develops slowly, and early symptoms are usually vague. Most include a general complaint of "not feeling good," headache, chilliness, puffy eyelids, and loss of appetite. As the disease progresses, the familiar symptoms appear: fever (generally from 101° to 105° F, lasting for five days to two weeks), sore throat, swollen lymph glands in the upper part of the body, and cough.

Mono affects primarily the blood, with a profusion of white blood cells and a number of atypical cells (called Downey cells) present in the blood. Blood tests are able to help in diagnosis and can help physicians tell the difference between mono and the diseases that it resembles: strep throat, meningitis, diphtheria, acute appendicitis, rubella or measles, cancer, and leukemia. Mono perhaps most resembles infectious hepatitis and diphtheria if only symptoms are taken into account.

Treatment for mono centers on treatment of symptoms. Bed rest is probably one of the most important, since it gives the body's healing mechanisms a chance to work. You should take measures to relieve individual symptoms: aspirin for fever and aches, hot baths for muscle and body aches, lozenges or gargles for sore throat, and well-balanced foods with plenty of liquids. Your doctor can prescribe medication for nausea if it is severe and can recommend cough remedies.

Mononucleosis can last anywhere from two weeks to one year; many victims do not feel their normal energy and health return for two to three months after the disease has actually run its course. Once you have had mono, you develop an antibody to the EB virus, and reinfection is extremely rare. Those who resume activity before the disease has run its course may become overly tired and may suffer a relapse of symptoms, but such a relapse is from the original infection and does not represent a new infection.

Studies indicate that the severity and duration of the infection depend on the individual's general state of health at the time of exposure. The best preventive measures include getting adequate rest and sufficient exercise, eating a well-balanced diet, and paying prompt attention to general infections or minor diseases that could lower your resistance.

DIARRHEA ━━━━━━━━━━━━

Diarrhea is a symptom — not a disease. The agent that results in diarrhea may vary, but the mechanical process is the same, no matter what the cause: the food is not completely digested in the intestinal tract. The function of the small intestine is to digest food, and the function of the large intestine is to absorb fluid and moisture from the waste products to maintain the body's ideal fluid balance. If, for any reason, the food is only partially digested or the fluid is not absorbed from the waste matter, the stools are runny and/or soft and are moved through the intestinal tract rapidly.

Painful gas and abdominal distention may accompany diarrhea.

Diarrhea can be caused by any of a number of factors:

1. Ingestion of contaminated food, resulting in food poisoning (Salmonella), causes diarrhea that is sudden and violent. Symptoms usually begin twelve to twenty-four hours after ingestion of the food, and the diarrhea lasts for one to five days.

2. Certain viral and bacterial infections also cause diarrhea. Symptoms include abdominal cramps, fever, frequent vomiting, and upper respiratory problems that resemble a cold. With most cases of bacterial or viral diarrhea, there is an overpowering urge to empty the bowels or bladder, but attempts to do so are generally ineffectual. The diarrhea is watery and sometimes contains specks of blood and shreds of mucous.

582

3. Drinking water that contains microorganisms to which you are not adjusted can cause diarrhea that comes on suddenly, accompanied by nausea and abdominal cramps.

4. A broad spectrum of drugs can cause diarrhea; among them are antibiotics, laxatives, antacids, and sulfates. Onset of the diarrhea is sudden; there is great rectal urgency, and severe abdominal cramps.

General treatment includes bed rest, drinking plenty of fluids, and eating foods that contain salt and minerals to replace those lost in diarrhea. Fluid replacement is particularly important to prevent dehydration. There are three main elements in over-the-counter diarrhea medication:

1. **Kaolin and pectin.** Kaolin, a gelling agent, is usually combined with pectin in diarrhea medication; the gelatin in kaolin helps you produce more solidly formed stools (the effect of the pectin is unknown).

2. **Paregoric.** Paregoric is a mild narcotic preparation; it is available in most states without a prescription. Paregoric stops the propulsive, wavelike motion of the intestines.

3. **Bulk-forming compounds.** Diarrhea medicine that contains bulk-formers serves to increase the mass of the stools and reduce their water quality.

In some cases, prescription drugs may be needed. With a bacterial infection, for instance, antibiotic treatment is needed. In cases where the diarrhea is caused by drugs, often discontinuance of the drug will clear up the diarrhea.

You should report any cases of diarrhea that last longer than four days to your physician; viral and bacterial diarrhea may last as long as twenty-one days and can be serious unless treated with medication.

CONSTIPATION

Constipation is one of the most common medical problems. A daily bowel movement is not essential to good health; metabolism and digestive rates differ among individuals, and what is normal for one person would be abnormal for another. Generally, doctors consider fewer than three bowel movements a week to be constipation — especially if those bowel movements are hard and difficult to pass.

Most constipation is temporary and resolves itself within a few days; it can be caused by a number of factors and is not considered serious. Constipation that persists for more than a few days should be checked by a doctor — it may be due to a serious medical problem, such as an abdominal obstruction or tumor.

The causes of constipation are varied, but the mechanism is the same regardless of the cause. It generally takes one to five days for food to move through the entire digestive process; when that process is slowed up, either because of poor muscle tone in the colon or because of inadequate bulk in the waste matter, too much moisture is absorbed from the fecal matter, and the stool becomes hard and difficult to pass. Among others, factors that cause constipation include change in diet, certain medications, travel, and unusual stress.

If you suffer only from occasional bouts with constipation, and if they are usually single incidents, your constipation is probably not serious. If there are any other factors, you should check with your doctor to rule out the possibility of serious disease before you attempt self-treatment.

One form of treatment — dietary in nature — is also a form of prevention. Adding fiber (roughage) to your diet can both ease and prevent constipation. Try adding bran to cereals and other foods; substituting whole-grain breads and cereals for what you usually eat; eating more fruits and vegetables, especially the skins and pulpy parts; and eating nuts and seeds, such as almonds, walnuts, cashews, pumpkin seeds, sunflower seeds, or pecans.

Resist the temptation to use laxatives. Laxatives can reduce the action of the intestinal walls, especially those in the colon, until they completely lose their motility; at that point, the individual must have a laxative in order to have a bowel movement. Drink plenty of fluids. Water is good in stimulating the bowels; you might also try fruit juices as a result of the added nutrition. You should drink a beverage with every meal, and you should drink fluids at regular intervals during the day.

Increase the amount of exercise that you get. A sedentary life-style can be an important contributing factor to constipation. Walking, biking, swimming, or any other form of regular exercise will help improve any problems with constipation.

584

A common infection of the eye area involves a sty — a pus-filled sac that generally develops around an eyelash. To relieve the sty, first remove the eyelash with a pair of tweezers; if the sty does not begin to drain, soak it with hot, moist compresses until it comes to a head and begins to drain. If mild inflammation accompanies the sty, bathe the area with a weak, warm solution of sodium bicarbonate.

A second common eye infection is conjuctivitis, sometimes called pink eye. The lining of the eyelid (the conjunctiva) gets red and inflamed; the eye often waters, and the white of the eye turns pink. The disease is highly contagious, so take care not to spread it; use your own towel and washcloth, and keep others from using the same ones. Bathe your eye with warm, sterile (previously boiled) water; if the condition does not clear up immediately, see your doctor.

When you watch television, do not do it in a dark room. Do not turn up the brights, either — experts advise watching television in a room with soft overall lighting for the best possible results and the least amount of eyestrain.

When your eyes do get tired, splash cool water on them, and take some time out. If possible, lie down for a few minutes and place a cotton ball saturated with cool water over each eye; the cotton balls act both to screen out light (thus providing the eye with a rest) and to refresh your eyes.

If you are going to be outside in the bright sun — especially if you are near water or snow — wear sunglasses to cut down on glare. Neutral gray or sage-green lenses provide for the greatest glare control coupled with the best perception and keenest vision. Make sure that the tint is dark enough to do some good: if you look in the mirror and can see your eyes through the sunglasses, the glasses are not dark enough. Wire frames are the best, because you can bend them gently to obtain the best fit.

Some kinds of lenses do not offer the greatest amount of protection. While photochromic lenses are designed to darken as the light intensity increases, the darkening process is triggered by ultraviolet rays — not by glare. These kinds of glasses will darken very little in an automobile, because most windshields are designed to filter out ultraviolet rays. On the other hand, plastic lenses will not filter out the infrared rays of the sun.

It is possible to become addicted to sunglasses: if you wear them when you should not, the mechanisms in your eye that help the pupil dilate and constrict get lazy, and they rely on the sunglasses instead to do their work for them. Respect your eyes — wear the sunglasses only to cut excess glare and reduce the strain of extremely bright light.

A discussion of eye care would not be complete without an explanation of eyewear used for the correction of visual defects. Of the 110 million Americans who need corrective lenses, about 12 million wear contact lenses. Convenience; improved visual correction; improvements in fit, design, and materials; and lengthened wearing time have all contributed to the growing popularity of contacts.

The chart that follows compares hard and soft lenses with eyeglasses. It will show you some of the advantages and disadvantages of each type of visual correction that can be used.

Examining the Pros and Cons of Contacts and Eyeglasses

SOFT LENSES		HARD LENSES		EYEGLASSES	
Advantages	Disadvantages	Advantages	Disadvantages	Advantages	Disadvantages
Excellent for sports or outdoor activities - rarely "pop out" of eye.	Less durable than hard lenses - wear out in a year or two and must be replaced.	Can be worn for years.	Lenses likely to pop out on contact and thus easily lost.		Weight of lenses - particularly of high-powered lenses.
Foreign particles do not get lodged under lenses.			Foreign bodies can get under lenses.		
	More expensive than hard lenses and eyeglasses.		More expensive than than eyeglasses. Chemicals more expensive than for soft lenses.	Less expensive than hard or soft lenses. No daily upkeep or maintenance.	
Invisible on the eye.					

Examining the Pros and Cons of Contacts and Eyeglasses

SOFT LENSES		HARD LENSES		EYEGLASSES	
Advantages	Disadvantages	Advantages	Disadvantages	Advantages	Disadvantages
Do not cause spectacle blur.	Rarely cause corneal edema.	Lens stable and bio-compatible.	May cause corneal abrasion and corneal edema.		
	Must be asepticized daily.				
Equal or better vision than glasses.	Ophthalmic examination every six months.	Equal or better vision than glasses.	Ophthalmic examination every six months.		Distorted image size.
Greater peripheral vision.		Greater peripheral vision.			Limited peripheral vision.
No blind spot.		No blind spot.			Blind spot from frames.
Natural image size.		Natural image size.			
Can be worn occasionally for a few hours at a time.	Usually not suitable for patients with astigmatism.	Correct for astigmatism.	Not good for part-time wear.		
Initially comfortable.			Break-in period of 2-3 weeks.		
	Must be removed when patient uses eyedrops or topical medication.				
Protective guard for the cornea.		Protective guard for the cornea.			

Types of Eye Medications

Three main kinds of eye medications are available for over-the-counter purchase:

1. **Vasoconstrictors (decongestants).** These medicines, most in drop form, contain many of the same decongestant properties used to fight the common cold. The vasoconstrictor action works to shrink the blood vessels in the eye, resulting in relief from congestion and swelling.
2. **Artificial tears.** Drops that act as "artificial tears" help people who suffer from irritation or dryness of the eyes by lubricating and soothing the eye. Medicines acting as artificial tears also contain preservatives, antiseptics, and viscosity agents (that help thicken the liquid).
3. **Eye washes.** These are used to lubricate and soothe the eye, but they contain no thickening agents. The fact that they are not as thick makes them better for irrigating the eyes and for washing out foreign matter.

EARS

"Never stick anything smaller than your elbow into your ear."

Well, it is good advice, and it merits repetition here: a large percentage of the injuries leading to hearing loss in the United States result from people who — for reasons of cleanliness or relief from pain or itching — stick cotton swabs, bobby pins, pencils, fingernail files, or toothpicks into their ears. It is no wonder that the ear, with its delicate construction, is injured — sometimes permanently — by something as apparently innocent as a cotton swab: the ability to hear depends on a precise balance of pressure between the air outside and inside the eardrum.

Blocked Ear (Excessive Wax)

The most common cause of conductive hearing loss, excessive ear wax is not a disease but may be a contributing factor in deafness and infection. Wax is normally produced in the auditory canal and is eventually excreted from the ear; excessive amounts may act as a medium for bacteria growth or may partially or completely block the ear canal — resulting in a decrease in hearing or a sensation of fullness or pressure in the ear. Accumulated water in the ear after swimming or bathing can make the wax swell and can cause the sudden onset of symptoms.

Never try to remove ear wax from your ear by poking at the wax with a device. Such efforts will only serve to compact the ear wax against the eardrum. You should not use ear drops without your doctor's prescription and instruction, since they could be dangerous in case of a perforated eardrum.

A doctor should be consulted for every case of excess ear wax; the doctor is equipped to remove the ear wax safely and effectively and to cleanse the ear canal.

Earache

Earache results from ear infection, usually infection of the middle ear, and is usually secondary to a common cold or sore throat. An earache may result when violent nose blowing forces infected mucous into the ear canals leading to the inner ear, or may result when there is a blockage of the canals that does not permit proper drainage from the ears. Earaches are common in children, because their eustachian tubes (the canals connecting the throat to the middle and inner ear) are narrow and do not permit proper drainage.

Pain, of course, is the primary symptom of earache; it is a throbbing, sharp, penetrating, constant pain. (Pain may be absent in some serious cases, with only other symptoms present.) There is usually impaired hearing, a feeling of fullness in the ears, ringing in the ears, and dizziness. Infants who have an earache usually tug at their ears, rub their ears, or roll their head with a drilling motion; they usually cry, with agonizing shrieks.

Apply heat for pain relief; you can use a hot water bottle, electric heating pad, or heated glass (heat a juice glass under running hot water, place several paper towels saturated with hot water in the glass, and hold the bottom of the glass against the ear; make sure not to invert the glass over the ear, because hot water from the paper towels will run into the ear). If you have your doctor's permission, use warm ear drops in an ear that has no discharge.

If you have a fever, rest. Take oral decongestants, and use a nose spray four times daily for two days. Use a vaporizer to keep the air moist. Unless your doctor specifically tells you to, you should not take aspirin; it may mask important pain that serves as an indicator of the progression of infection in the ear.

Call your doctor if you experience an increase in pain or headache despite your treatment; if you experience drainage from the ear canal or the symptoms of perforated eardrum; if you have a fever higher than 102°F; if you develop convulsive twitching of the facial muscles; or if you are dizzy. You should always consult a doctor if the patient is under the age of three.

CARE OF THE TEETH AND MOUTH

Cleaning teeth and gums is the key to preventing all major gum diseases and the *only* way to prevent dental decay. Proper and effective cleaning includes the use of flossing techniques, and the correct brushing procedure.

Flossing

There are many places in your mouth that your toothbrush can't reach: spaces in between your teeth, areas along your gum line, and the rear surfaces of your back molars. These places still need to be cleaned — they're major sites of plaque buildup and frequent sites of oral and dental disease. Flossing will enable you to clean the areas your toothbrush can't reach or can't properly clean.

Follow these easy steps:

1. Hold the floss between your thumbs and forefingers. There should be about an inch of floss between your two hands; use your thumbs and forefingers to guide the floss as you proceed.
2. Insert the floss between two teeth with a gentle sawing motion. Never snap the floss down into the gums — you'll cut or bruise them. As the floss approaches the gum line, curve it tightly in a C-shape against the tooth and gently slide it into the space between your gum

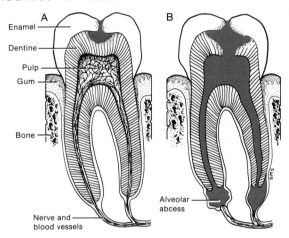

Enamel

Dentine

Pulp

Gum

Bone

Nerve and
blood vessels

Alveolar
abcess

Figure 17-3. Caries, or dental decay, is the most common disease of Western man. Bacteria collect in the fissures of the teeth and produce acid from refined sugar. The acid eats into the enamel. Decay then spreads more rapidly through the softer dentine. When the pulp becomes infected, irritation of the nerve leads to toothache.

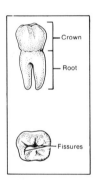

Crown

Root

Fissures

Figure 17-2.

and your tooth; continue sliding it gently until you feel a slight resistance.

3. Keep the floss held tightly against the tooth; scrape the side of the tooth as you move the floss away from the gum and back toward the chewing surface of the tooth.

Don't get discouraged at first; as you break up the plaque deposits and as you remove the bacteria, your gums will get sore and might bleed. This tenderness will probably continue for the first five or six days, or until you have succeeded in removing the stubborn deposits. As the plaque is removed, your gums will heal and will stop bleeding. If you

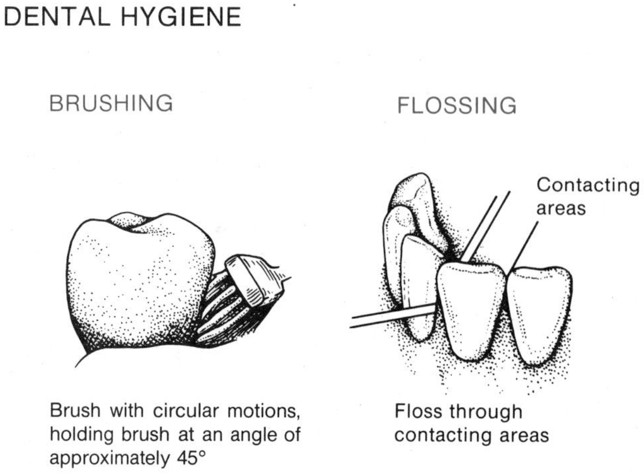

BRUSHING   FLOSSING

Contacting
areas

Brush with circular motions,   Floss through
holding brush at an angle of   contacting areas
approximately 45°

Figure 17-4. Without adequate dental hygiene, bacteria collect in the crevices and fissures of teeth, setting up caries or tooth decay. Regular brushing helps prevent tooth and gum disease, while use of dental floss helps clear bacteria and debris from between the teeth.

discontinue flossing, your gums may swell up and start to bleed again due to fresh plaque and bacteria deposits.

If the bleeding from flossing doesn't stop after a week, consult your dentist. It's important to floss every day to keep the plaque from building back up.

Basic Brushing

The key to good toothbrushing, of course, begins with a good toothbrush. Yours won't do the job properly if it's worn down or missing bristles — you need to replace your toothbrush often.

It's best if you brush your teeth after each meal, but you should make sure that you brush them at least once a day. Your toothbrush can be either manual or electric: both kinds are effective. You may find that an electric toothbrush makes brushing easier if you are handicapped or have arthritis; in addition, children may be delighted by the novelty of an electric toothbrush and may brush more often.

While oral irrigators — devices that shoot a high-powered stream of water that can be directed along the gum line and between teeth — are *not* substitutes for regular brushing or flossing (oral irrigators can't remove plaque by themselves); they are useful in helping remove food particles, in stimulating the gums, and in aiding cleaning for those who wear orthodontic braces. Make sure you adjust the water pressure to a safe level — water that's too strong can damage the delicate tissues of the gums.

Your choice of toothpaste depends on personal taste, but you should choose a toothpaste that contains flouride to give you the maximum protection against dental decay. Read the labels on different brands of toothpaste; some flouride toothpastes are effective in preventing up to 30 percent of the cavities in children.

Correct brushing procedure includes the following steps:

1. Angle your toothbrush so that it rests with the bristles along the gum line — an area where many cavities are prone to start and where plaque buildups can be particulary stubborn.
2. Move the brush back and forth with short strokes; you should use a gentle scrubbing motion. Concentrate on only a few teeth at a time — don't try to clean the whole side of your mouth at once. The toothbrush is designed to clean only a few teeth at a time, so change position frequently and concentrate on only one or two teeth.
3. When you have finished cleaning the inner and outer surfaces, thoroughly scrub the chewing surface.
4. To slightly freshen your breath, brush the surface of your tongue gently. Don't exert too much pressure: brushing vigorously can cause the papilla-like taste buds to lengthen, creating tiny traps for bateria and food particles.

ACNE

Acne is a plugging or congestion in the sebaceous glands. While there is no one single cause of acne, a specific case of acne may be aggravated by one or more factors that either lead to the development of the acne initially or that make it worse once it has developed.

A prominent cause of acne is hormonal change which occurs chiefly during adolescence and which causes the sebaceous glands — responsible for the outbreaks of acne on the face, chest, and shoulders — to be more active, secreting increased levels of sebum. Testosterone — found in both men and women — seems to be the most influential hormone. Another important cause is the suspicion that the cells lining the follicles of acne-prone individuals are abnormal. Because of the nature of these follicles, the dead cells are not sloughed off but instead accumulate along the

ACNE: A LOOK BELOW THE SURFACE

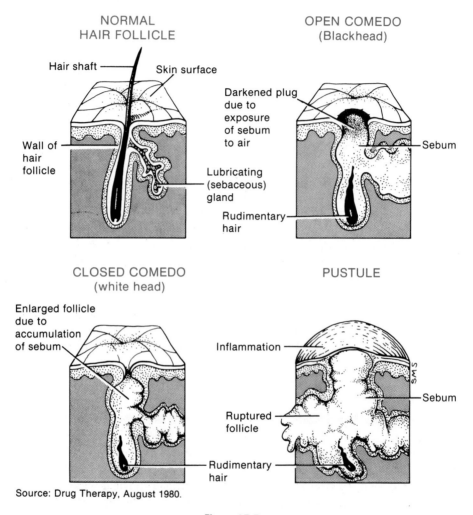

Source: Drug Therapy, August 1980.

Figure 17-5.

follicle walls, where they form layers that block up the pores. When these layers of dead cells combine with bacteria, the pore (follicle) becomes inflamed, resulting in a pimple (the medical term for this condition is *papule*). If the condition progresses, pus fills the papule (now called a *pustule);* if the pustule is left untreated, the result is a large and deeply

594

embedded cyst. The hormonal activity directly preceding a girl's menstrual period can cause acne to temporarily flare up.

A third cause in the aggravation of acne seems to be irritation. If you have a spot on your chin where you consistently have a pimple, it may be because you frequently rub that spot while you watch television or do homework. Such friction or irritation from the hair could be the cause for serious outbreaks along the hairline or forehead.

Still another cause of acne is stress. Stress generally is not the primary cause but is a secondary cause that plays a major part in aggravating already-present cases of acne.

Cleanliness can be a factor in controlling acne. Because excess sebum can be the cause of most acne, oil that is not removed from the face, chest, and shoulders by bathing can aggravate the acne by further clogging the pores. Oily creams and makeup foundations can also aggravate an acne problem.

You have probably heard all the stories about chocolate, nuts, cheese — and all the other foods that are supposed to cause acne. Researchers now believe that a well-balanced, nutritional diet can help the general condition of the skin, which will, of course, make it less prone to acne. Beyond that, food plays no part in the development or aggravation of acne.

A last significant cause of acne is hereditary. You can inherit the tendency to go through more violent hormonal changes during adolescence, the tendency to accumulate dead cells along your follicle walls, or the tendency to develop acne during childhood (sometimes as young as the age of three years). Treatment for prepubescent hereditary acne is long-range and difficult, and early diagnosis and treatment are essential.

Acne is a difficult disease to treat, both because the causative factors are difficult to isolate and because each individual reacts differently to treatment regimens. The most usual treatment consists of one or a combination of the following:

1. Cleanliness. In mild cases of acne, you should wash your face with mild soap and lukewarm water once in the morning and once in the evening; in more severe cases, you should add an afternoon wash. Do not use hot water — it tends to irritate your skin and make the acne worse. The same thing applies to many brands of deodorant or performed soap — use a mild soap that will not harm or irritate your skin (an antiallergy soap is a good one to use). When you are finished, pat dry — do not rub — with a clean towel.

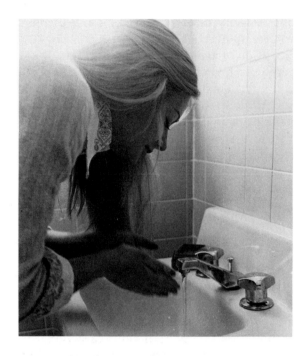

Cleanliness is especially important in controlling acne.

2. If your acne is severe, try soaking your face for a few minutes before you wash it; use a washcloth saturated with warm (not hot) water. Such soaking will help open your pores and soften any plugs that may have moved to the surface.

3. Whatever you do, *do not* pick at or squeeze your pimples! If you leave pimples alone, most will heal or disappear with time. If you attempt "treatment" yourself via squeezing or picking, you may cause a breakdown of the follicle walls, leading to spillover of pus into surrounding tissues and resulting eventually in deep scarring and tissue destruction. Squeezing can also cause infection.

4. It is best to avoid using cosmetics. They can act as an irritant. If you must wear some type of cosmetic, use one that has a water base instead of an oil base. Make sure that you remove the cosmetic before you go to sleep, and never wear it longer than necessary. You should also avoid using lotions or skin creams that have an oily base, and you should not use hair setting lotions, sprays, or creams that are oily.

5. The sun and its ultraviolet rays are an excellent natural treatment for acne — so getting out in the fresh air and sunshine may help

improve some cases. You should take every precaution, however, against getting a sunburn — overexposure to the sun can lead to permanent damage to the skin.

6. If your acne is particularly severe, if it resists your efforts at treatment, or if it becomes extremely disfiguring, you should seek medical attention from either a general practitioner or from a dermatologist.

IMPROVING THE QUALITY OF SLEEP

Both sleeping and dreaming are critical to maintaining a proper balance of health. There are a number of things that you can do to improve the quality of sleep and to help you over temporary periods of insomnia or other sleep disturbances.

Evaluate your situation carefully before you decide on a method of self-treatment for sleep problems. Any of a number of factors can influence the way (and amount) you sleep. For instance, it is normal for elderly people to sleep less hours and to sleep more lightly than other people. Those with certain physical illnesses — especially allergies, asthma, ulcers, epilepsy, or disease involving the spine (particularly lumbosacral disease) — are apt to have difficulty in sleeping soundly through the night.

Once you have ruled out a physiological disorder as the cause of sleeplessness, try any of the following to improve the quality of your sleep (these are effective, too, in helping normal sleepers to sleep even better):

1. Try to get on a schedule. Decide an appropriate "bedtime," and aim toward retiring each night at that time. Do not try to go to bed if you are wide awake, though — it is important to associate bedtime with a feeling of drowsiness.

2. Do things that are relaxing right before you go to bed. Read, watch television, or listen to music — but make sure that the book is soothing, that the television program is relaxing (no murder mysteries!), and that the music is calming. If you get stimulated easily, you should do these activities while you are lying in bed. Watching a

soothing television program, for instance, while you are lying in bed helps you associate relaxation with your bed and with sleep.

3. Keep physically active. You should exercise regularly to keep your body systems functioning well — a condition that is especially conducive to sleep. You should not exercise, however, within two hours of your bedtime: the exercise is too physically stimulating, and exercise that close to bedtime tends to interfere with the deeper stages of sleep. Exercise programs carried out on a daily basis in the morning or afternoon, however, improve sleep.

4. Cut down on external stimuli that interfere with your sleep. If you are in a communal living situation (such as a dormitory), you may decide to use sleeping masks or earplugs to help screen out light and sound. You should not, of course, attempt to sleep in a room where there is a lot of activity.

5. Take a warm bath right before you go to bed. The water should be lukewarm (comfortable enough not to be cold), not hot: hot water is stimulating and serves to awaken your senses and make it difficult for you to fall asleep.

6. Open some of the windows in your bedroom. A cold room is more conducive to sleep than a warm one. You should make sure that, in winter, you have enough bedclothes to keep cold drafts of air from making you ill, but even in the coldest weather, the fresh air will aid sleep.

7. Avoid stimulants during the several hours preceding your bedtime. Tobacco, alcohol, coffee, tea, and cola drinks all act as stimulants that, taken within a few hours of bedtime, can make it difficult for you to fall asleep.

8. Observe how you react to eating prior to bedtime. For some people, eating a light snack or small meal serves to relax and make it easier to fall asleep; for others, eating may lead to drowsiness that leads to sleep but may lead to the inability to stay asleep or the tendency to awaken early.

9. Do not take naps in the evening. Even if you seem to require a nap during the morning or afternoon, stay awake during the evening. Napping too close to bedtime will make you less tired, making it more difficult for you to fall asleep.

10. Eliminate sources of anxiety. If you have recently had a quarrel with a friend, and the quarrel is making you uneasy, set things straight before you try to go to sleep. If you are worrying about a letter that

you need to write, get up and write it — do not lie in bed worrying about it.

11. Think of peaceful relaxing things. Do not occupy yourself with your problems at bedtime — think instead of your joys, your triumphs, things that you are looking forward to.

12. Try practicing some relaxation techniques. Deep breathing is a good one. Draw in a deep breath through your nose, hold it for several seconds, and exhale it through your nose, as slowly as you can. Wait a few seconds before you take another breath. Then start to imagine your body unwinding, bit by bit. First your scalp relaxes. Then your face. Then your neck, and so on, until your entire body is physically relaxed.

MENSTRUAL CRAMPS

Dysmenorrhea — menstrual cramps — affect half of the female population under the age of twenty-five and occur just before and during the menstrual period. Dysmenorrhea is caused by congestion or inflammation of the pelvic tissues or by obstruction of the menstrual flow. This can be due to infection, long-standing anxiety, sex pressures, a sedentary life-style, constipation, or general lack of exercise, but in many cases the cause is unknown. Menstrual cramps are no longer a problem after a woman gives birth once, possibly due to dilation of the cervix and stretching of the uterine muscles.

Cramps that are continuous but that worsen during the menstrual period may be due to infection of the cervix, gonorrhea, or other diseases that should be treated by a physician.

Signs and symptoms include mild to severe pain in the lower abdomen with headache, irritability, mental depression, malaise, fatigue, mild nausea, or occasional vomiting. Bowel function is normal, and there is usually no fever. Pain sometimes runs down the legs and thighs and can result in a low backache. The victim may be pale and sweating; the menstrual flow may be either copious or scant. Cramps last about twelve hours from onset to resolution.

Get adequate rest, and avoid constipation. Exercise daily, and pay special attention to stretching the abdominal muscles. Avoid situations that bring on nervous tension. Take aspirin for pain, and apply hot compresses to the abdomen; remove restrictive clothing. A hot water bottle usually works well. Avoid getting fatigued.

HEADACHE

Headache is the most common symptom of mankind. Ranging from mild to severe, headache can cause pain that is general or regional, concentrated or intermittent, penetrating or throbbing, radiating or pressured, or bursting. Headache can stem from any of a number of causes — most of them organic (brain tumor, high blood pressure, neck injury, head injury, low blood sugar, allergy, infection, or dental problems) or environmental (sun glare, loud music, freezing temperatures) in nature. There are three general types of headaches: migraine, sinus, and tension.

Migraine Headache

Two-thirds of those who suffer migraines inherit the trait, and 80 percent of all migraine sufferers are women. The migraine headache is caused by the vessels in the brain first constricting, then dilating. The pressure of swelling blood vessels causes intense, throbbing pain to suddenly appear and worsen, usually on only one side of the head and usually in the same location each time. Other symptoms include nausea and vomiting, irritability, blurred vision, sensitivity to light and sound, constipation or diarrhea, redness and swelling of the eyes and nasal lining, elevated blood pressure, temporary blindness, blind spots, chills, tremor, dizziness, and excessive urination. The headache generally lasts from two to forty-eight hours.

Try to sleep or rest in a dark room. Do not bend your head forward or move or stop suddenly. An ice pack on your head can sometimes afford some relief, take aspirin to help relieve pain. There has been recent emphasis on the benefits of relaxation — such as yoga, transcendental meditation, and biofeedback — in migraine therapy. Massage of the head and neck may also be helpful in reducing pain.

600

Sinus Headache

Congestion, nasal blockage, inflammation, allergy, nasal polyps, the common cold, upper respiratory infections, tooth abscesses or infection, fatigue, poor diet, alcohol, and smoking all cause the sinuses to inflame, resulting in sinus headache. Sinus headache tends to be worse in damp weather and during times of heavy pollution.

Pain, usually moderate, dull, and aching, occurs over the sinuses, usually between the eyes. The pain is most severe in the morning and lessens throughout the day. Accompanying symptoms include difficulty in breathing, low-grade fever, irritability, sore muscles, or a stiff neck.

Stand erect with your head steady, or sit in an upright position in bed. Apply hot or cold compresses to the area that is causing pain. Get as much rest as you can, and do not drink alcohol. Do not smoke. Reduce the dust in the atmosphere as much as you can; a humidifier will reduce dust and will increase the moisture content of the air.

Avoid using over-the-counter nasal sprays or decongestants without your doctor's approval.

Tension Headache

One-third to one-half of all headaches are brought on by worry, anxiety, strain, muscle tension, or depression. Prior warning in the form of nausea, weakness, fatigue, or visual disturbance may precede a tension headache. The pain — which may last for weeks, months, or even years — is dull, steady, and throbbing; the steady, pressing ache is almost like having on a hat that is too tight. Accompanying symptoms may include nausea, diarrhea, fatigue, loss of appetite, sleeplessness, inability to concentrate, ringing in the ears, dizziness, or runny eyes. In addition, the muscles of the jaws, neck, back of the head, and temples may become tense and tender.

To gain relief from a tension headache, massage the scalp and the back of the neck; apply hot packs (moist heat) to the head, and take hot baths. Get extra rest. Lie down with your eyes closed and your head supported; take aspirin with milk or food (to prevent stomach upset). Eliminate anything that may be causing stress or strain; change your activities often, and get as much fresh air as you can.

Self-Evaluation

How Well Prepared Are You
to Provide Self- and Family-Care?

Section 1
Equipment

Circle the number 5 after each of the following that you currently have in your home. If you do not have the item, circle the 0.

1.	fever thermometer	5	0
2.	stethoscope	5	0
3.	sphygmomanometer	5	0
4.	textbook on self-care	5	0
5.	first aid kit	5	0
6.	vaporizer	5	0

Scoring: Total the amounts of the numbers that you circled and remember this score.

SECTION 2
KNOWLEDGE

Circle T if the statement is true and F if the statement is false for each of the following statements:

T	F	1.	Self-care involves the idea that individuals can and should assume more responsibility for their own health.
T	F	2.	A doctor should be consulted if signs and symptoms returns without a clear-cut cause.
T	F	3.	Normal rectal temperature is 98.6°F (37°C).
T	F	4.	The thermometer used to take an oral temperature has a short, blunt bulb.

T	F	5.	You may use any of your five fingers to take a pulse.
T	F	6.	You should observe or count respirations when the patient is unaware that you are doing so.
T	F	7.	A person's expected normal systolic blood pressure can be determined by adding 100 to his age.
T	F	8.	The common cold is best treated by aspirin, lots of fluids and plenty of rest.
T	F	9.	Antihistamines are one of the best treatments for a cough.
T	F	10.	Strep throat is characterized by yellow or white mucous spots on the throat, swollen glands in the neck, and a fever over 101°F.
T	F	11.	An illness lasting anywhere from three to ten days accompanied by *high* fever, cough, fatigue, muscle aches, chills, headache, and gastrointestinal distress is probably the common cold.
T	F	12.	Bed rest is probably one of the most important forms of treatment for mononucleosis.
T	F	13.	Diarrhea is a common human disease.
T	F	14.	Fluid replacement is especially important when treating diarrhea.
T	F	15.	You should report a case of diarrhea to your physician only after it has persisted for at least 2 weeks.
T	F	16.	A daily bowel movement is essential to good health.
T	F	17.	Adding fiber to your diet can both ease and prevent constipation.
T	F	18.	To relieve a sty, first remove the eyelash with a pair of tweezers.
T	F	19.	Conjunctivitis is characterized by a red and inflamed lining of the eyelid and a watering and "pink" eye.
T	F	20.	The most common cause of conductive hearing loss is sticking a small object in the ear.
T	F	21.	A doctor should be consulted for *every* case of excess ear wax.

T	F	22.	Taking aspirin is the best treatment for earache.
T	F	23.	Chocolate, nuts, and cheese cause acne and therefore should be avoided by teenagers.
T	F	24.	Stress tends to aggravate already-present cases of acne.
T	F	25.	Taking a hot bath prior to going to sleep improves the quality of one's sleep.
T	F	26.	Cramps that are continuous but that worsen during the menstrual period should be brought to the attention of a physician.
T	F	27.	The migraine headache is caused by the vessels in the brain first constricting, then dilating.
T	F	28.	Pain, usually moderate, dull and aching, occurring over the sinuses and usually between the eyes is indicative of a sinus headache.
T	F	29.	Kaopectate is used in the treatment of constipation, whereas diarrhea is treated with milk of magnesia.
T	F	30.	Antibiotics are helpful in the treatment of viral infections.
T	F	31.	Viral infections usually cause symptoms in many parts of the body while bacterial infections rarely do.
T	F	32.	Pain that extends beyond the low-back area suggests a need for consulting a physician.
T	F	33.	Abdominal pain accompanied by black or bloody stools should be diagnosed by a physician.
T	F	34.	Lying in bed is the ideal cure for a cough.
T	F	35.	The normal resting pulse rate in infants is 60-80 beats per minute.

Scoring: Give yourself 2 points for each correct response. True statements include 1, 2, 6, 8, 10, 12, 14, 17, 18, 19, 21, 24, 26, 27, 28, 31, 32, and 33. Statements that are false include 3, 4, 5, 7, 9, 11, 13, 15, 16, 20, 22, 23, 25, 29, 30, 34, and 35.

Now add the scores together from Sections 1 and 2 to obtain your total score.

80 - 100 points	You should be well prepared to provide self-and family-care.
56 - 79 points	Minor equipment purchasing and a review of the preceding chapter and other self-care literature should bring you up to date.
0 - 55 points	Major equipment purchasing and intensive study of the preceding chapter and other self-care literature are definitely needed here.

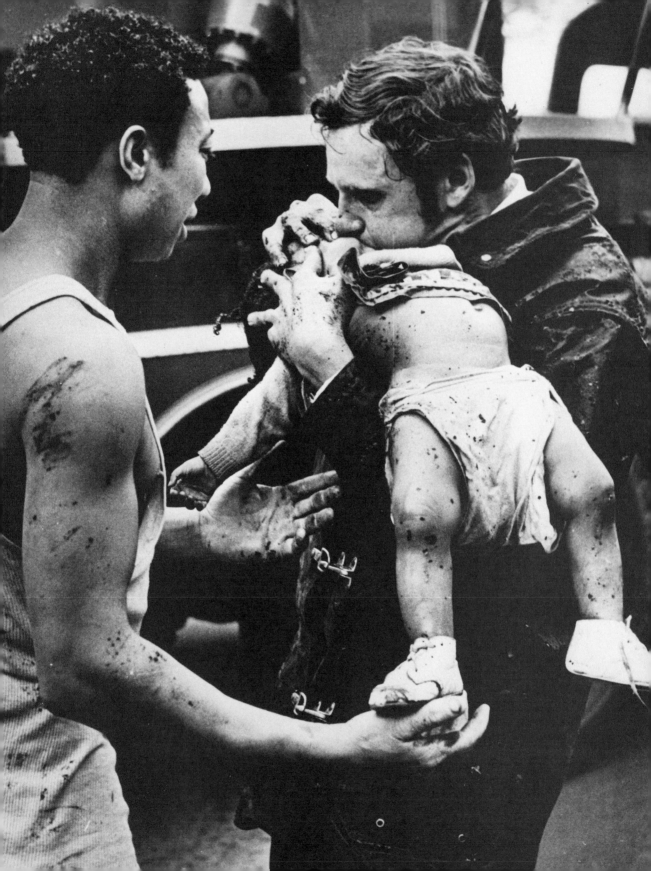

18
Emergency Care: Ready or Not

Illnesses, accidents, and injuries often happen with little or no warning. In many such cases, prompt and efficient action on the part of the first person to see the victim may mean the difference between a speedy recovery and chronic disability (or death).

First aid is the *emergency* treatment that is offered before professional medical help arrives at the scene. Bear in mind, though, that all first aid cases do not require professional medical help. In cases of severe injury, first aid is performed to prevent death by: preventing further injury, counteracting shock, restoring breathing, controlling bleeding, and removing poisons (with some exceptions).

While each emergency case will be different, the following general rules apply to situations where first aid is required:

1. Recognize your limitations. Do not attempt a procedure that is complicated if you are unfamiliar with it or if, for some reason, you cannot properly perform it.

2. Evaluate the victim rapidly before you begin any kind of first aid work. Check him over thoroughly; if you pay attention only to the broken arm that is obvious, you might miss a third-degree burn on the back of the leg.

3. Keep the victim lying down (an essential in shock control) *unless* he is vomiting, bleeding from the mouth, experiencing breathing difficulties, or in severe shock. A victim of severe shock should be kept on his back with his head lower than his body (unless there are head and/or chest injuries), while a victim of an injury should be left with his head level with his body until the extent of injuries is determined.

4. Do not move a victim unless you must.

5. Remove only clothing that is necessary — do not offend the victim or bystanders with unnecessary immodesty.

6. If the victim is conscious, reassure him. If you can, keep him from seeing his own injury.

7. Do whatever you can to prevent infection. Never touch an open wound or a burn with your fingers or with other objects that have not been sterilized. It is preferable to use sterile bandages or compresses. There is one important exception to this rule: if a person is severely bleeding and no sterile bandage is available, use whatever you can to stop the bleeding (including your hand, a piece of your clothing, or a piece of the victim's clothing).

8. Never try to feed an unconscious person any solid or liquid food — he may choke to death.

9. If you must move a victim due to environmental dangers, carefully assess the possibility of a broken bone (including back injury). Make sure that the affected part is completely immobilized before you move the victim.

10. If you move a victim on a litter or stretcher, always move him feet first — no matter what kind of an injury he has. Moving a victim feet first allows the carrier by the head to keep a constant watch for breathing problems.

11. Do not try to do too much. Keep the victim safe and comfortable (as much as possible), and take measures to reverse life-threatening situations (such as bleeding), but do not try to be heroic when unnecessary.

12. Keep bystanders away from the victim. You may need to enlist the help of others to accomplish this, but it is a critical part of first aid.

Shock is a state of circulatory deficiency associated with depression of vital bodily processes. It is a condition in which the cardiovascular system fails to provide sufficient blood circulation to all parts of the body. Lives have been lost due to this reaction of the body to physical and emotional trauma. Although only one area of the body may be injured, the body as a whole reacts to the injury and attempts to recover as a whole.

Some of the most common causes of physical shock may include: severe loss of blood, intense pain, severe or extensive injury, burns, anxiety, poisonous gases, surgical operations, excessive heat or cold, poison, certain illnesses, and intense emotion.

Since shock follows all injuries in some degree, treatment for shock should be given after every major injury. Shock may appear immediately following an injury, or symptoms may not show until hours later, so do not wait to treat for shock until symptoms appear. In fact, treatment for shock should be instituted before other injury treatment except asphyxia and severe hemorrhage. Even though a victim's injuries may not be fatal in themselves, they can be fatal when combined with shock.

Physical Signs and Symptoms of Shock

A victim who is in shock will manifest the following symptoms:

1. A dull, chalklike appearance to the victim's skin, regardless of color.
2. An anxious or dull expression.
3. Closed or partially closed eyelids; dull, lackluster eyes, dilated pupils.
4. Shallow, irregular breathing.
5. Weak, rapid pulse.
6. Cold, moist skin.
7. Shaking of the arms and legs as if chilled.
8. Vomiting.
9. Complaint of thirst.

In addition, the victim may be partially or totally unconscious. And if he is conscious, his responses to questions may be slow or irrelevant to the question.

Figure 18-1.

The Physiology of Shock

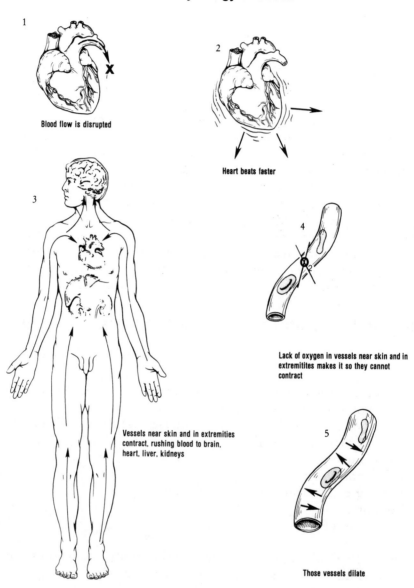

1 Blood flow is disrupted

2 Heart beats faster

3 Vessels near skin and in extremities contract, rushing blood to brain, heart, liver, kidneys

4 Lack of oxygen in vessels near skin and in extremitites makes it so they cannot contract

5 Those vessels dilate

610

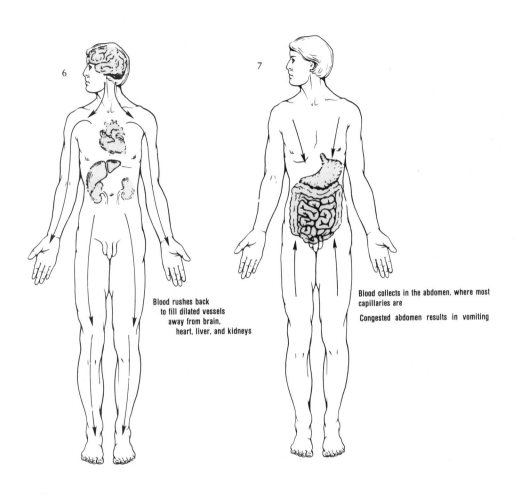

6

Blood rushes back
to fill dilated vessels
away from brain,
heart, liver, and kidneys

7

Blood collects in the abdomen, where most
capillaries are

Congested abdomen results in vomiting

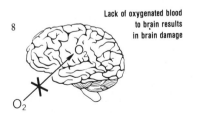

Lack of oxygenated blood
to brain results
in brain damage

8

O_2

611

First Aid for Shock

First aid should be given immediately to eliminate stoppage of breathing, hemorrhage, or severe pain as causes of shock. Then, the victim should be positioned properly. Lie the victim flat with his heart lower than the rest of his body, if possible. The only exception to this position is if the victim has a skull fracture, if there is severe bleeding from the head, or if there is a heatstroke or suspected stroke. When in doubt about correct positioning, keep the victim lying flat.

If the victim is nauseated and vomits, turn his body to one side. Keep his mouth and face wiped clean. If neck or spine injuries are suspected, do not move the victim unless it is necessary to protect him from injury or to give urgent first aid. In addition, loosen any tight clothing that the victim may be wearing at the neck, chest, and waist. Keep the victim warm and dry. Sometimes it is just as helpful to place blankets or materials under the victim to prevent loss of heat to surfaces below him as it is to cover him. Do not add extra heat to raise the surface temperature of the body. Heat draws the diverted blood supply back to the skin from more vital organs, thus robbing them of critically needed blood.

No particular harm will be done if you allow the victim to moisten his lips and mouth with cool water, if it will make him more comfortable, but in general, there is no need to give him anything to drink unless you are in a position where medical personnel will not be available for an excessively long period of time. Do not give fluids to victims who are unconscious, are having convulsions, are vomiting or are likely to vomit (they may aspirate fluid into the lungs), are likely to require surgery or anesthetic, appear to have abdominal injury, or have brain injury (additional fluids in the body may cause the brain to swell).

Take measures to relieve pain. A long-accepted, but false, generalization is that all extensive injuries are associated with severe pain and that the more extensive the injury, the worse the pain. In reality, severe and even fatal injuries may be considerably less painful than a mashed fingertip, which can cause agony. Another generalization is that with similar injuries, everyone experiences the same amount of pain. This, too, is incorrect. Also, those who would not be in much pain from a wound when rested, relaxed, and confident might experience severe pain from the same wound if exhausted, tense, and fearful. People in shock tend to feel less pain. But pain, unless relieved, may cause or increase shock. To help relieve pain, support the injury, and adjust tight or uncomfortable clothing or bandages.

Continue treatment as long as there is evidence of shock. Keep the victim down and quiet. Never allow a person in shock to sit up; additional strain will be placed on his heart and circulation. People in shock tend to relapse. Watch for it, and renew shock treatment immediately.

Always reassure the victim that his injuries are understood and that he will get the best possible care. Also tell him of plans to get medical help or plans to move him to a place where medical assistance is available.

PULMONARY RESUSCITATION

The respiratory (pulmonary) system and the circulatory system are vital body systems. If either fails for more than a short time, death will follow quickly. In terms of first aid, respiratory and circulatory emergencies must be treated at once in order to preserve life and prevent irreparable body damage.

Opening the Airway

The most important factor in successful resuscitation is the immediate opening of the airway. The two main procedures for clearing the airway are the head tilt and the jaw thrust.

To clear the airway with the head tilt method, lie the victim on his back. Remove all pillows or padding from under his head. Gently lift the neck from beneath with one hand, and with your other hand, tilt the head backward with pressure on the forehead. This will extend the neck and lift the tongue away from the back of the throat. Maintain the head in this position at all times. Most often, breathing will resume spontaneously if the victim's head is tilted backward.

If the head tilt method does not open the airway, additional displacement of the jaw is necessary. From a position at the top of the victim's head, place your fingers behind the angles of the jaw. In one movement, force the jaw forward, tilt the head backward, and retract the lower lip with your thumbs to allow breathing through the mouth and nose. If breathing does not resume, immediately give artificial respiration.

Figure 18-2. When breathing stops.

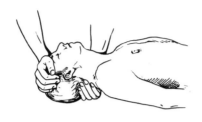

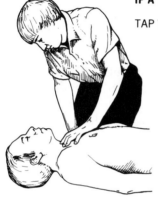

IF A VICTIM APPEARS TO BE UNCONSCIOUS

TAP VICTIM ON THE SHOULDER AND SHOUT, "ARE YOU OKAY?"

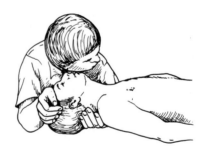

IF THERE IS NO RESPONSE

TILT THE VICTIM'S HEAD, CHIN POINTING UP.
Place one hand under the victim's neck and gently lift. At the same time, push with the other hand on the victim's forehead. This will move the tongue away from the back of the throat to open the airway.

IMMEDIATELY LOOK, LISTEN, AND FEEL FOR AIR.
While maintaining the backward head tilt position, place your cheek and ear close to the victim's mouth and nose. Look for the chest to rise and fall while you listen and feel for the return of air. Check for about 5 seconds.

614

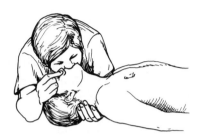 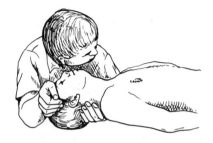

IF THE VICTIM IS NOT BREATHING

GIVE FOUR QUICK BREATHS.
Maintain the backward head tilt, pinch the victim's nose with the hand that is on the victim's forehead to prevent leakage of air, open your mouth wide, take a deep breath, seal your mouth around the victim's mouth, and blow into the victim's mouth with four quick but full breaths just as fast as you can. When blowing, use only enough time between breaths to lift your head slightly for better inhalation. **For an infant,** give gentle puffs and blow through the mouth *and* nose and do not tilt the head back as far as for an adult.

If you do not get an air exchange when you blow, it may help to reposition the head and try again.

AGAIN, LOOK, LISTEN, AND FEEL FOR AIR EXCHANGE.

The mouth-to-nose method can be used with the sequence described above instead of the mouth-to-mouth method. Maintain the backward head-tilt position with the hand on the victim's forehead. Remove the hand from under the neck and close the victim's mouth. Blow into the victim's nose. Open the victim's mouth for the look, listen, and feel step.
Source: American National Red Cross

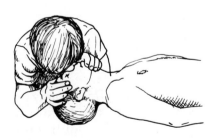 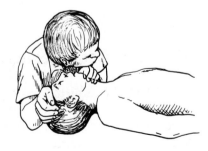

Mouth-to-Mouth Resuscitation

In case of respiratory emergencies, do not waste time! Begin artificial respiration at once. Place the victim on a flat, firm surface, and kneel at the victim's side (either one) or close to his head. Place one hand under the victim's neck to maintain the head position in the maximum backward tilt. Pinch the victim's nostrils together with the fingers of your other hand, and continue to exert pressure on the forehead to keep the head tilted backward. Open your mouth widely, and take a deep breath.

Make a tight seal around the victim's mouth, and blow in until his chest rises. Make sure that you see the chest rise.

Initially breathe into the victim four quick, full breaths without allowing the lungs to completely deflate between breaths. Remove your mouth and watch the victim's chest fall as he exhales passively. Repeat this cycle once every five seconds until adequate breathing is restored (twelve to fifteen times per minute for adults; about twenty times per minute for children).

To determine whether you are adequately ventilating the victim's lungs, watch the chest rise and fall. Feel in your own airway the resistance and then compliance of the victim's lungs as they expand. Feel and hear the air escape during expiration.

If the victim begins to breathe of his own accord, adjust your timing to his breathing rhythm. Do not fight his attempts to breathe. When the victim has regained consciousness and breathing is restored, treat the person for shock immediately. After breathing has begun, watch the victim closely; the breathing may stop again. In such a case, you will need to begin artificial respiration immediately. If it is necessary to move the victim before he is breathing normally because of extreme weather conditions or other dangers, continue artificial respiration while he is being moved.

Mouth-to-Nose Resuscitation

When the mouth is clenched shut or other circumstances make it impossible to force air into the mouth, mouth-to-nose respiration may be used. To perform mouth-to-nose respiration, maintain the backward head-tilt position with your hand on the forehead. Seal the mouth shut with your other hand. Open your mouth widely, take a deep breath, seal your mouth tightly around the victim's nose, and blow into the nose. If possible, open the victim's mouth to allow air to escape during exhalation.

For children and infants, do not make the backward head-tilt as extensive as for adults and large children. Seal both the mouth and nose of an infant or small child with your mouth when forcing air into the lungs. Blow into the mouth and nose every three seconds (about twenty breaths per minute). Blow with less pressure and volume than for an adult or large child. Small puffs of air will suffice for infants.

CARDIAC ARREST AND CARDIOPULMONARY RESUSCITATION

Cardiopulmonary resuscitation is an emergency first aid procedure that combines artificial respiration with artificial circulation. It is used in first aid emergencies where both circulation and breathing have stopped. When cardiac arrest occurs, certain body reactions warn the first-aider that the victim may need artificial circulation: absence of a carotid (neck) or femoral pulse, dilated pupils of the eyes, unconsciousness, limp body and flaccid skin, cyanosis, and no perceptible heartbeat.

The administration of external cardiac compression requires special training. The method can be hazardous, and there have been reported injuries to patients such as damage to the heart and liver, internal bleeding, multiple rib fractures, and puncture of the lungs. In untrained hands, the risk of injury is increased. For cardiopulmonary resuscitation training, contact your local chapter of the Heart Association, Red Cross, or enroll in a first aid course at your college.

HEART ATTACK

Heart attack is a term for a medical condition called coronary thrombosis. It is the sudden blocking of a heart artery by a stationary blood clot, or thrombosis. The leading cause of heart attacks is arteriosclerosis (hardening and thickening of the arteries), which cuts off the blood supply to a particular area of the heart muscle. Most heart attacks occur when people are resting or working quietly.

617

Heart attacks are difficult to identify and can only be diagnosed by a physician, but a physician should be called immediately when the following symptoms appear:

1. Severe, painful sensation of pressure in the front of the chest, sometimes spreading to the left arm and often lasting for hours. Some attacks are accompanied by nausea and vomiting and may be mistaken for acute indigestion.
2. Unexplained sweating.
3. Sudden, intense shortness of breath.
4. Loss of consciousness (occasionally).

When you suspect that a victim has had a heart attack, get him in the most comfortable position (usually semireclining or sitting up). Many heart attack victims have difficulty breathing when lying flat. Reassure the victim — he will be extremely frightened. Call a physician immediately. Do not allow the victim to walk — there should be a minimum of exertion.

If the victim is under medical care, he may have drugs on hand that should be administered. Keep the victim warm and loosen his clothing. Do not give him anything to drink.

If he stops breathing, administer mouth-to-mouth resuscitation. And if the heart stops functioning, begin cardiopulmonary resuscitation *if you are trained.*

CHOKING

Choking almost always involves food — usually meat. When food is inadequately chewed, when food is eaten too quickly, or when the eater begins to concentrate on other activities (such as the dinner table conversation), a piece of food may lodge in the throat in a location that prevents breathing.

If the object or food that caused the choking can be seen in the throat, pass the forefinger into the throat alongside the tongue, and try to withdraw the object. Be careful not to push the object farther back into the throat. If the object is a mass of food, try removing it by grasping with the fingers. If it cannot be so removed, perform the Heimlich Maneuver.

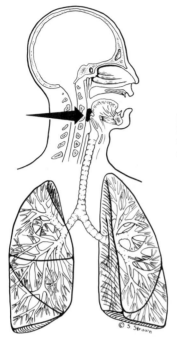

Figure 18-3. Asphyxiation due to aspiration of a large piece of food, usually meat, with total blockage of the airway (cafe coronary).

Heimlich Maneuver

A maneuver developed and recommended by most physicians suggests that the rescuer stand behind the victim, holding him with both arms around the waist, at or just above the beltline. The rescuer grasps one of his own closed fists firmly, then squeezes hard while allowing the victim to slump forward, head and arms dangling. There is always some residual air trapped in the lung, and the pressure below the diapragm compresses this air.

If the victim has already collapsed, the rescuer need not pick him up. The rescuer straddles the legs and places both hands, one on top of the other, just below the diaphragm, and pushes sharply upward. The procedure is repeated if necessary, and, if possible, a bystander should be ready to retrieve the ejected food so that it is not inhaled again.

619

Back Blows

Slapping the choking victim sharply on the back between the shoulder blades can be attempted if the Heimlich maneuver is not effective. You can perform this technique whether the victim is standing up, sitting down, or lying on the floor. Blows to the back should be forceful, quick, and applied in rapid succession.

If the victim is sitting or standing, stand at the side of and slightly behind the victim. Slap the victim's back — over the spine between the shoulder blades — with the heel of the hand. Support the victim by placing your other hand on his chest. Position the victim's head lower than his chest if you can to utilize gravity.

Do not pat the victim gingerly — you need to hit him forcefully with a series of pounding blows delivered in quick succession.

If the victim is lying down, kneel beside him. Roll him onto his side so that he is facing you and so that his chest is snug against your knee. Deliver sharp blows with the heel of your hand, stroking the victim on the back (over the spine and between the shoulder blades, as you would if the victim was standing or sitting).

If the victim is an infant or small child, place him face down across your forearm. Make sure that the child's head is lower than his chest. If the obstruction is only partial, or if the child can breathe adequately when he is sitting up, do not place his head lower than his chest. Deliver sharp blows to the child's back, much as you would for an adult. Keep in mind that a baby is not as large as an adult. If you are unable to dislodge the food without striking the child too hard, you will probably need to try one of the other two techniques.

HEMORRHAGE — CONTROL OF BLEEDING ━━━

External Bleeding

In first aid, the control of bleeding is secondary in importance only to maintenance of air passages and restoration of breathing. To control bleeding, cover the wound with heavy compresses, and apply direct pressure with the hand or a triangular bandage. Ten to thirty minutes of direct pressure should stop the bleeding. If the victim is moved, make sure that a bandage is applied to maintain pressure. Pressure dressings should not be replaced even when they are saturated. Replacing dressings releases pressure on cut vessels, interferes with coagulation, and increases chances of contamination. When bleeding is severe and a dressing is not immediately available, place your hand directly over the wound and exert direct pressure. Do not waste time trying to find a dressing.

If possible, lie the victim flat. Raise the wounded part of the body above the rest of the body unless bones are broken or unless the victim has a head injury, suspected stroke, or sunstroke.

Additional pressure can be applied with the fingers or a padded object to a supplying artery. To slow bleeding, vessels may be squeezed at specific body points where they pass near the surface over bony parts. Such arteries are called pressure points.

If none of these methods are effective in controlling bleeding, a tourniquet should be used. A tourniquet is a constricting band that is used to cut off the supply of blood to an injured limb. It cannot be used to control bleeding from the head, neck, or body, since it would obviously

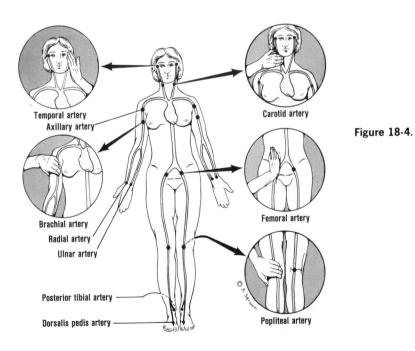

Figure 18-4.

621

result in greater injury or death. A tourniquet should be used *only* if the control of hemorrhage by other means proves to be difficult or impossible.

Internal Bleeding

Internal bleeding is an extremely serious condition. Pressure from internal bleeding on nerves can cause great pain or paralysis. Extensive swelling can cut off blood circulation to a limb and cause gangrene. Hidden bleeding is hard to diagnose and can rapidly prove fatal. When the mechanisms of injury indicate the possibility of internal damage, and the signs of shock are present but there is no obvious injury, internal bleeding should be expected.

If you suspect internal bleeding, take the following steps: (1) Lay the victim on a flat, level surface, and treat him for shock; (2) Apply cold cloths or ice to the area where you think there is internal bleeding; (3) If the bleeding is in an extremity, apply pressure to the injury site with a pressure dressing; (4) Keep the victim warm until medical help arrives. Cover him with blankets, a coat, or towels. If he is lying on a cold or damp surface, place a blanket or coat under him; (5) Do not give the victim a stimulant of any kind, including coffee or tea. Anticipate that the victim may vomit — give him nothing by mouth; (6) Summon medical help immediately.

POISONS ━━━━━━━━━━━━━━━━━━━━━━━

A poison is any substance — solid, liquid, or gas — that impairs health or causes death when introduced into the body or onto the skin surface. Almost any sign of bodily distress or disturbance may indicate poisoning. Acute symptoms may be delayed for hours. Signs and symptoms vary according to the poison and the length of time that it has been in the system. The following signs and symptoms may indicate poisoning:

1. Severe nausea, vomiting, or diarrhea.
2. Muscular twitching, convulsions, collapse, paralysis.
3. Delirium, drowsiness, unconsciousness.
4. Signs of burns about the mouth or on the skin.

5. Corrosion, swelling, bleaching of the skin.
6. Pain, tenderness, cramps — especially sudden pain with no apparent cause.
7. Characteristic odor on the breath.
8. Unusual urine color (red, green, bright yellow, black).
9. Slow or labored breathing.
10. Presence of an empty bottle or other signs that would indicate possible poisoning.

First Aid for Ingested Poisons

Waste no time. Call a doctor, poison control center, or rescue squad promptly. Follow their advice if it differs from these instructions.

If so directed by a poison control center or physician, make the victim vomit. To accomplish this, give a full tablespoon of syrup of ipecac to anyone over one year of age, plus at least one glass of water (several more if possible). If no vomiting occurs in twenty minutes, this dose may be repeated once only. As a last resort, try gagging the victim to induce vomiting. Do not, however, waste time waiting for vomiting. Transport the victim promptly to medical facilities.

Do not induce vomiting if the victim is unconscious or having convulsions; if the swallowed poison is known to be caustic or corrosive (lye, strong acid, drain cleaner, etc.) or has caused burns of the lips or throat; if the swallowed poison contained kerosene, gasoline, or other petroleum distillate; or if the victim has a heart condition that may be aggravated by the strain of vomiting.

If so directed, give activated charcoal mixed in a glass of water. This is contraindicated if the victim is unconscious or is having convulsions. It is also not advised until after ipecac has not induced vomiting.

Always take the package, container, enclosure, any vomited material, food, pills, and any remaining poison with you to the medical facility to provide additional information. Give artificial respiration if necessary.

First Aid for Inhaled Poisons

Get the victim to fresh air immediately. If this is impossible, call the fire department or a rescue squad. If the victim is in a closed room, garage, or other small space, take a deep breath and hold it before entering. Loosen the victim's tight-fitting clothing. If the victim is not breathing, start artificial respiration promptly, and do not stop until the patient is breathing well or help arrives. Send someone else for help. Do not interrupt artificial respiration for anything.

Transport the victim to a medical facility promptly.

First Aid for Absorbed Poisons

Poisons, chemicals, and poisonous plants that come in contact with the skin may cause burning, allergy, and other severe body reactions. Absorbed poisons are rapidly taken into the body, and quick first aid measures are necessary.

Remove contaminated clothing, and flush the affected skin immediately with large quantities of water or other available liquid as you remove the clothing. No medication should be used on the skin unless ordered by a physician. Do not leave the victim alone. Treat for shock, and give artificial respiration if necessary.

Give the victim ample quantities of water or other liquids to drink unless he is having convulsions or is unconscious. Protect yourself by using rubber gloves if immediately available; wash any area of skin that made contact with the victim.

BURN INJURIES ▬▬▬▬▬▬▬▬▬▬▬▬▬▬

Burns are classified in severity according to the degree (depth) and extent of body surface injured. The deeper the burn and the more total body surface burned, the more severe the injury. It is difficult to determine the extent of a burn upon initial examination, so it is wise to consider what caused it. Often the degree will vary in different parts of the same affected area. See Table 18-1 for a description and first aid for the three degrees of burns.

FRACTURES ▬▬▬▬▬▬▬▬▬▬▬▬▬▬▬▬

A fracture is a broken or cracked bone. Generally speaking, only a

Table 18-1

	Burn	Treatment	Consequence
1	First degree is red, sore, not blistered.	Cool the burn with tap water or cool compresses.	Heals without scarring about six days.
2	Second degree is blistered and painful. It may ooze fluid.	Apply cool water. Remove clothing that is not stuck to the wound; remove jewelry. Lay victim flat. Use cool compresses on the way to the hospital. Do not	Heals in two weeks with slight scarring.
3	Third degree is white, brown, or charred; it may be painless at first.	cool a large portion of the body — shock may occur. If the burn area is large, cover the person loosely with a clean sheet. If he has chills, cover him with a blanket too. Second and third degree burns require emergency care, maybe hospitalization.	Can take months, even years to treat. Grafting operations reduce scarring and deformity, but scars are inevitable.

physician using an x-ray examination can accurately diagnose a fracture. But a fracture should be suspected when any of the following signs or symptoms are present:

1. Pain in the region of the fracture.
2. Loss of function (an inability to move the affected limb).
3. Deformity or irregularity of the affected part of the body, such as crookedness, limb rotation, angulation, open wounds over a bone, or differences in shape and length of corresponding bones.
4. Moderate or severe swelling and discoloration of the surrounding skin due to hemorrhage.
5. The victim may:
   a. Feel broken bones grating against each other.
   b. Have felt or heard a bone snap.
   c. Remember how the accident occurred and recall how he fell, whether he hit, etc.

The main objectives in first aid care for fractures are to immobilize the injured area and treat for shock. When an accident occurs, however, the vital life signs should be checked first before attempting to treat fractures. If you render first aid at an accident site, do not move the victim unless some life-threatening situation (such as fire, gas poisoning, explosion, or drowning) is present or if an ambulance or rescue squad will not reach the accident scene within a short period of time. Check to see if the victim is breathing. If he is not, clear an airway, and give artificial respiration.

In open fractures, control severe bleeding. Cut away the victim's clothing around the wound. Apply a large, sterile pressure dressing to control hemorrhage. Do not wash, probe, or put your fingers in the wound. If a bone fragment is protruding, cover the entire wound with a large, sterile pad. Do not attempt to replace the bone in its normal position.

Whether the fracture is simple or compound, treat for shock. Protect the victim from further injury.

If an ambulance is not available or if there is delay in transportation, apply splints to the suspected fracture area. Do not try to straighten a joint that is out of alignment.

Self-Evaluation

FIRST AID: READY OR NOT!

Directions: Rendering first aid seems to be an on-going process required of most people. Evaluate your readiness to render first aid by using the below assessment. If improvement is needed, by all means obtain the necessary knowledge and skills to save lives and alleviate pain and suffering.

Can you . . .?	Yes	Maybe, but a review would help	No
Open an airway?	10	5	0
Perform the Heimlich maneuver for all situations (pregnant woman, obese, unconscious, etc.)	10	5	0
Give mouth-to-mouth resuscitation	10	5	0
Administer CPR	10	5	0
Treat for shock	10	5	0
Care for a heart attach victim (no cardiac arrest involved)	10	5	0
Control external bleeding	10	5	0
Apply properly necessary dressings and bandages	10	5	0
Give syrup of ipecac	10	5	0
Treat first, second, and third degree burns	10	5	0
Identify the signs of a fracture	10	5	0
Splint a fracture (on various parts of the body)	10	5	0

Scoring:

108-up	Very good!
96-107	Good work on the weaknesses
84-95	There's definitely room for improvement
72-83	A good first aid course is highly recommended
0-71	You had better let the victim treat himself

APPENDIX:
Methods of
Birth Control

THE PILL
Prescription required

"The pill" refers to any of the oral contraceptives. The most widely used contains two female hormones, estrogen and progestin, and is taken 21 days each month. Another (sometimes called the "mini-pill") contains progestin only and is taken continuously. A woman should be sure to receive from the druggist, doctor, or person who gives her the pills an FDA-required brochure that explains the use, benefits, and risks of the product in greater detail.

Effectiveness	Advantages-Disadvantages	Side Effects	Health Factors to Consider	Long-term Effect on Ability to Have Children
Effectiveness depends on how correctly the method is used. Of 100 women who use the combination estrogen and progestin pill for one year, less than one will become pregnant. Of 100 women who use the progestin-only pill (mini-pill) for one year, 2 or 3 will become pregnant.	Advantages: The combination pill is the most effective of the popular methods for preventing pregnancy. No inconvenient devices to bother with at the time of intercourse. Decreased menstrual flow, less cramping, decreased pre-menstrual discomfort. Disadvantages: Must be taken regularly and exactly as instructed by the prescribing physician.	Side effects may include tender breasts, nausea or vomiting, gain or loss of weight, unexpected vaginal bleeding, higher levels of sugar and fat in the blood, darkening of the facial skin, depression, increased tendency for abnormal blood clotting, increased risk of heart attack or stroke, small increase of liver or gall bladder disease, fatigue, high blood pressure, vision changes, rash, swelling and water retention, secretion from the	Women who smoke should not use the Pill because smoking increases the risk of heart attack or stroke. Other women who should not take the Pill are those who have had a heart attack, stroke, angina pectoris, blood clots, cancer of the breast or uterus, scanty or irregular periods. Also don't plan on oral contraceptives use if you have had any of the following: active liver disease, any eye disorder, chronic illness leading to immobility, a family his-	There is no evidence that using the Pill will prevent a woman from becoming pregnant after she stops taking it, although there may be a delay before she is able to become pregnant. Women should wait a short time after stopping the Pill before becoming pregnant. During this time another method of contraception should be used. After childbirth, the woman should consult her doctor before resuming use

nipples, jaundice, intolerance to contact lenses, changes in appetite, loss of scalp hair, impaired kidney function, complexion problems, mood changes, more severe epilepsy, changes in libido, nervousness.

tory of breast cancer, a family history of vascular diseases, depressive reactions, or varicose veins.

of the Pill. This is especially true for nursing mothers because the drugs in the Pill appear in the mild and the long-range effect on the infant is not known.

Pill users have a greater risk than non-users of having gall bladder disease requiring surgery.

A woman who believes she may be pregnant should not take the Pill because it increases the risk of defect in the fetus.

Some Pill users tend to develop high blood pressure, but it is usually mild and may be reversed by discontinuing use.

Health problems such as migraine headaches, mental depression, fibroids of the uterus, heart or kidney disease, asthma, high blood pressure, diabetes, or epilepsy may be made worse by use of the Pill.

There is no evidence that taking the Pill increases the risk of cancer. Benign liver tumors occur very rarely in women on the Pill. Sometimes they rupture and cause

Risks associated with the Pill increase with age, and as a woman enters her late 30's it is generally advisable to seek another method of contraception.

THE PILL (continued)

Advantages-Disadvantages	Side Effects	Health Factors to Consider	Long-term Effect on Ability to Have Children
	fatal hemorrhage.	Young women who have not reached full growth should not take the Pill.	
	The ACHES that indicate possible serious side effects of the pill:		
	Five Signals **Possible Problem**		
	Abdominal pain Gall bladder disease or liver tumor		
	Chest pain (severe) or shortness of breath Blood clot in the lungs or myocardial infarction		
	Headaches (severe) Stroke or high blood pressure		
	Eye problems: blurred vision, flashing lights, or blindness Stroke or high blood pressure		
	Severe leg pain (calf or thigh) Blood clot in the legs		

(From: Robert Landesman. "Basic Facts About Contraception," *Drug Therapy*, July 1978, p. 123)

THE HUMAN SYSTEMS

The Skeletal System 2
The Respiratory System 5
The Muscular System 3
The Digestive System 6
The Circulatory System 4
The Urinary and Endocrine System 7
The Nervous System 8

INDEX

Achilles tendons, 3
Adrenal gland, 4, 7
Alveoli, 5
Aorta, 4
Appendix, 6
Arterial blood, 4
Artery (cross section), 4
Autonomic nerves, 8
Basilic vein, 4
Biceps brachii, 3
Biceps femoris, 3
Brachial artery, 4
Brachial nerves, 8
Brachialis, 3
Bronchi, 5
Bronchioles, 5
Capillaries, 5
Carpals, 2
Carotid artery, 4
Cephalic vein, 4
Cerebellum, 8
Cerebrum, 8
Cervical vertebrae, 2
Clavicle, 2
Colon, ascending, 6
Colon, descending, 6
Colon, transverse, 6
Common hepatic duct, 6
Convolutions, 8
Coccyx, 2
Corpus Callosum, 8
Cranium, 2, 8
Deep flexors, 3
Deltoid, 3
Diaphragm, 5
Dorsalis pedis artery, 4
Duodenum, 6, 7
Endocrine glands, 7
Endothelium, 4
Epiglottis, 5
Esophagus, 5, 6
Excretory system, 7
Extensions of forearm, 3
External elastic membrane, 4
External oblique, 3
Facial artery, 4
Femoral nerve, 8
Femoral vein, 4
Femur, 2
Fibula, 2
Frontalis, 3
Gall bladder, 6
Ganglia, 8

Gastrocnemius, 3
Gluteus maximus, 3
Gullet, 6
Heart, 4, 8
Humerus, 2
Hypothalamus, 8
Intercostals, 3
Internal elastic membrane, 4
Internal oblique, 3
Intestines, 8
Jugular veins, 4
Kidney, 4, 7, 8
Large intestine, 4, 7
Larynx, 5
Latissimus dorsi, 3
Left ventricle, 4
Liver, 4, 6, 7
Iliac artery, 4
Lumbar vertebrae, 2
Lung, 4, 7, 8
Main pancreatic duct, 6
Mandible, 2
Masseter, 3
Maxilla, 2
Medulla, 8
Meninges, 8
Metacarpals, 2
Metatarsals, 2
Nasal passage, 5
Nostril, 5
Orbicularis oculi, 3
Obicularis oris, 3
Pancreas, 6, 7
Parathyroid glands, 7
Patella, 2
Pectoralis major, 3
Pectoralis minor, 3
Pelvis, 2
Phalanges, 2
Pharynx, 5
Pineal body, 7, 8
Pituitary, 8
Pituitary body, 7
Pons, 8
Popliteal artery, 4, 5
Portal vein, 4
Pulmonary arteries, 4
Radial artery, 4
Radius, 2
Rectum, 6
Rectus abdominus, 3
Rectus femoris, 3
Renal artery, 4

Respiratory bronchiole, 5
Rib cartilages, 2
Right atrium, 4
Right ventricle, 4
Sartorius, 3
Sciatic nerves, 8
Serratus, 3
Serratus posterior inferior, 3
Semitendonosus, 3
Sinuses, 4
Small intestine, 6
Sacrum, 2
Soleus, 3
Spinal cord, 2, 8
Spinal nerves, 8
Spleen, 4, 8
Splenius capitus, 3
Sternomastoid, 3
Sterno-cleido-mastoid, 3
Sternum, 2
Stomach, 6, 8
Superficial flexors, 3
Superior vena cava, 3
Suture lines, 2
Tarsals, 2
Temporalis, 3
Tendons, 3
Thoracic vertebrae, 2
Throat muscles, 3
Thymus glands, 7
Thyroid glands, 7
Tibia, 2
Tibialis anterior, 3
Tongue, 4
Trachea, 4
Trapezius, 3
Triceps, 3
Tunica adventitia, 4
Tunica intima, 4
Tunica media, 4
Turbinates, 5
Ulna, 2
Ureter, 7
Urethra, 7
Urinary bladder, 7
Vagus, 8
Vastus Lateralis, 3
Vastus medialis, 3
Vein (cross section), 4
Venous blood, 4
Vertebra, 8
Vocal cords, 5

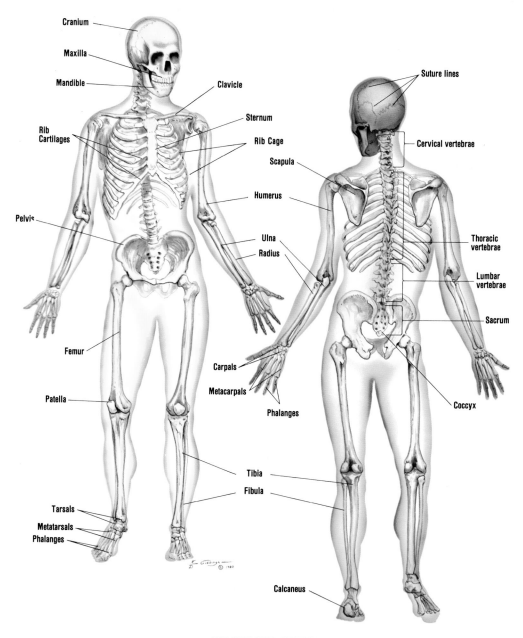

Cranium

Maxilla

Mandible

Clavicle

Sternum

Rib Cartilages

Rib Cage

Scapula

Humerus

Pelvis

Ulna

Radius

Femur

Carpals

Metacarpals

Phalanges

Patella

Tibia

Fibula

Tarsals

Metatarsals

Phalanges

Calcaneus

Suture lines

Cervical vertebrae

Thoracic vertebrae

Lumbar vertebrae

Sacrum

Coccyx

THE SKELETAL SYSTEM

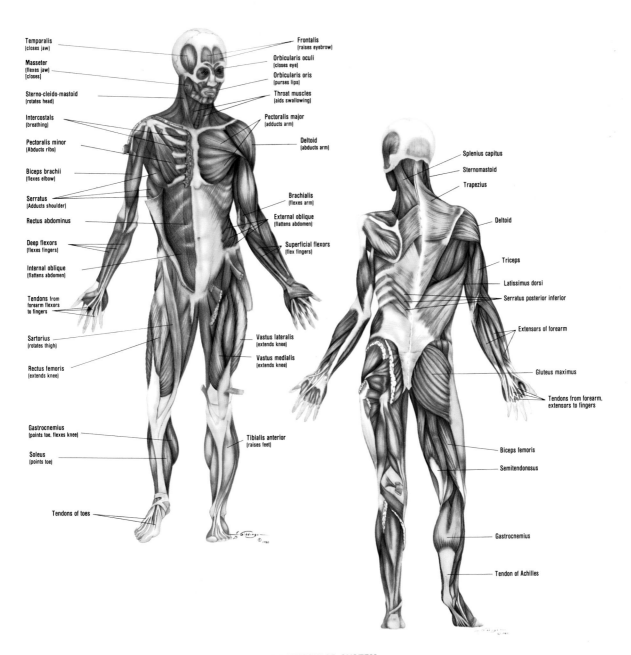

Temporalis
(closes jaw)

Masseter
(flexes jaw)
(closes)

Sterno-cleido-mastoid
(rotates head)

Intercostals
(breathing)

Pectoralis minor
(Abducts ribs)

Biceps brachii
(flexes elbow)

Serratus
(Adducts shoulder)

Rectus abdominus

Deep flexors
(flexes fingers)

Internal oblique
(flattens abdomen)

Tendons from
forearm flexors
to fingers

Sartorius
(rotates thigh)

Rectus femoris
(extends knee)

Gastrocnemius
(points toe, flexes knee)

Soleus
(points toe)

Tendons of toes

Frontalis
(raises eyebrow)

Orbicularis oculi
(closes eye)

Orbicularis oris
(purses lips)

Throat muscles
(aids swallowing)

Pectoralis major
(adducts arm)

Deltoid
(abducts arm)

Brachialis
(flexes arm)

External oblique
(flattens abdomen)

Superficial flexors
(flex fingers)

Vastus lateralis
(extends knee)

Vastus medialis
(extends knee)

Tibialis anterior
(raises feet)

Splenius capitus

Sternomastoid

Trapezius

Deltoid

Triceps

Latissimus dorsi

Serratus posterior inferior

Extensors of forearm

Gluteus maximus

Tendons from forearm,
extensors to fingers

Biceps femoris

Semitendonosus

Gastrocnemius

Tendon of Achilles

THE MUSCULAR SYSTEM

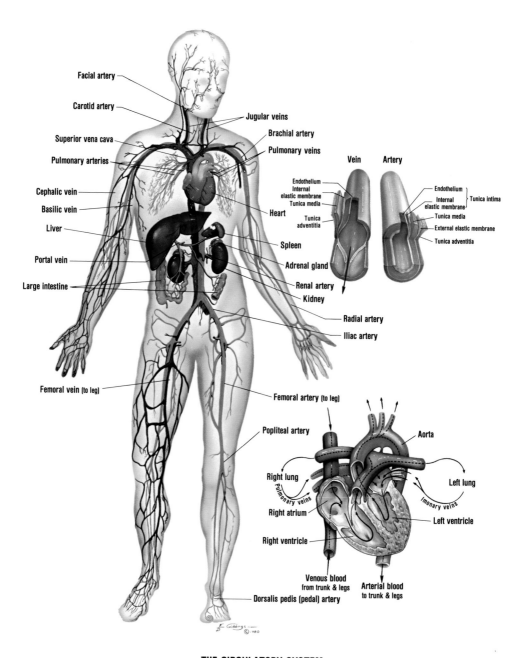

Facial artery

Carotid artery

Jugular veins

Superior vena cava

Brachial artery

Pulmonary arteries

Pulmonary veins

Cephalic vein

Vein

Artery

Basilic vein

Heart

Endothelium
Internal
elastic membrane
Tunica media

Endothelium

Liver

Spleen

Internal
elastic membrane

Tunica intima

Tunica
adventitia

Tunica media

Portal vein

Adrenal gland

External elastic membrane

Large intestine

Renal artery

Tunica adventitia

Kidney

Radial artery

Iliac artery

Femoral vein (to leg)

Femoral artery (to leg)

Popliteal artery

Aorta

Right lung

Left lung

Pulmonary veins

Imonary veins

Right atrium

Left ventricle

Right ventricle

Venous blood
from trunk & legs

Arterial blood
to trunk & legs

Dorsalis pedis (pedal) artery

THE CIRCULATORY SYSTEM

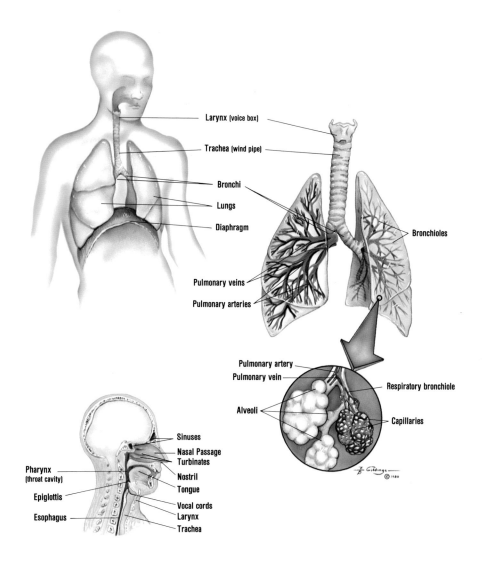

Larynx (voice box)

Trachea (wind pipe)

Bronchi

Lungs

Diaphragm

Pulmonary veins

Pulmonary arteries

Bronchioles

Pulmonary artery

Pulmonary vein

Alveoli

Respiratory bronchiole

Capillaries

Sinuses

Nasal Passage
Turbinates

Pharynx
(throat cavity)

Nostril

Epiglottis

Tongue

Vocal cords

Esophagus

Larynx

Trachea

THE RESPIRATORY SYSTEM

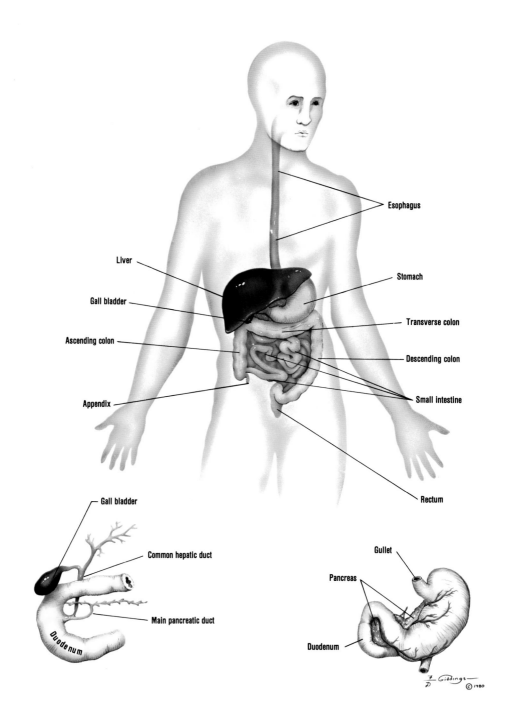

Esophagus

Liver

Stomach

Gall bladder

Transverse colon

Ascending colon

Descending colon

Appendix

Small intestine

Rectum

Gall bladder

Common hepatic duct

Main pancreatic duct

Duodenum

Gullet

Pancreas

Duodenum

THE DIGESTIVE SYSTEM

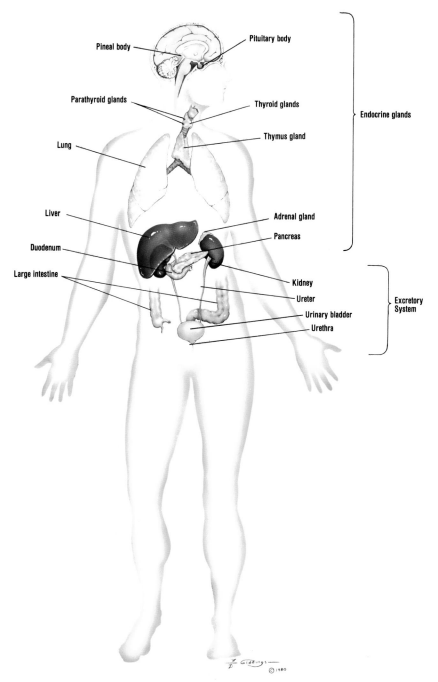

Pineal body

Pituitary body

Parathyroid glands

Thyroid glands

Thymus gland

Lung

Liver

Adrenal gland

Pancreas

Duodenum

Large intestine

Kidney

Ureter

Urinary bladder

Urethra

Endocrine glands

Excretory System

THE URINARY AND ENDOCRINE SYSTEM

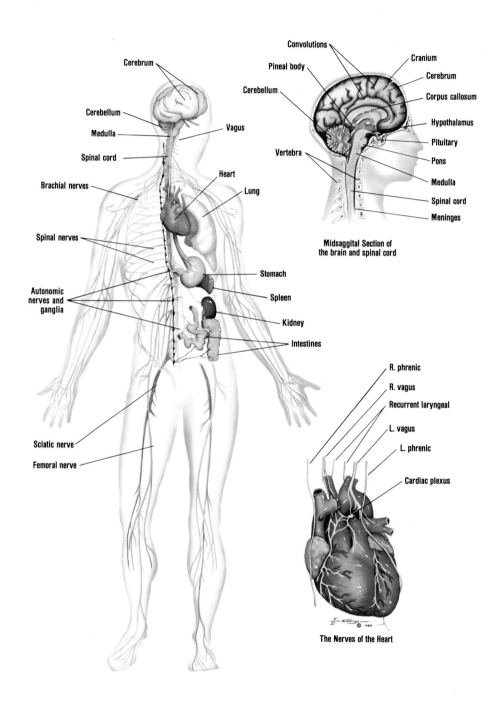

Cerebrum

Cerebellum

Medulla

Spinal cord

Brachial nerves

Spinal nerves

Autonomic
nerves and
ganglia

Sciatic nerve

Femoral nerve

Vagus

Heart

Lung

Stomach

Spleen

Kidney

Intestines

Convolutions

Pineal body

Cerebellum

Vertebra

Cranium

Cerebrum

Corpus callosum

Hypothalamus

Pituitary

Pons

Medulla

Spinal cord

Meninges

**Midsaggital Section of
the brain and spinal cord**

R. phrenic

R. vagus

Recurrent laryngeal

L. vagus

L. phrenic

Cardiac plexus

The Nerves of the Heart

THE NERVOUS SYSTEM

INTRAUTERINE DEVICE (IUD)
Prescription required

The IUD is a small plastic or metal device that is placed in the uterus (womb) through the cervical canal (opening into the uterus). As long as the IUD stays in place pregnancy is prevented. How the IUD prevents pregnancy is not completely understood. IUD's seem to interfere in some manner with implantation of the fertilized egg in the wall of the uterus. There are 5 kinds of IUD's currently available — Copper-7, Copper-T, Progestasert, Lippes Loop, and Saf-T-Coil. IUD's containing copper (Copper-7 and Copper-T) should be replaced every three years; those containing progesterone (Progestasert) should be replaced every year.

Effectiveness	Advantages-Disadvantages	Side Effects	Health Factors to Consider	Long-term Effect on Ability to Have Children
Effectiveness depends on proper insertion by the physician and whether the IUD remains in place. Of 100 women who use an IUD for one year, 1 to 6 will become pregnant.	Advantages: Insertion by a physician, then no further care needed, except to see that the IUD remains in place (the user can check it herself but should be checked once a year by her doctor). Disadvantages: May cause pain or discomfort when inserted; afterward may cause cramps and a heavier menstrual flow. Some women will experience adverse	Major complications, which are infrequent, include anemia, pregnancy outside the uterus, pelvic infection, perforation of the uterus or cervix, and septic abortion, irregular period A woman with heavy or irregular bleeding while using an IUD should consult her physician. Removal of the IUD may be neces-	Before having an IUD inserted, a woman should tell her doctor if she has had any of the following: cancer or other abnormalities of the uterus or cervix; bleeding between periods or heavy menstrual flow; infection of the uterus, cervix, or pelvis (pus in fallopian tubes); prior IUD use; recent pregnancy, abortion, or miscarriage; uterine surgery; venereal disease; severe	Pelvic infection in some IUD users may result in their future inability to have children.

THE PILL (continued)

Effectiveness	Advantages-Disadvantages	Side Effects	Health Factors to Consider	Long-term Effect on Ability to Have Children
	effects that require removal of the IUD. The IUD can be expelled, sometimes without the woman being aware of it, leaving her unprotected.	sary to prevent anemia. Women susceptible to pelvic infection are more prone to infection when using an IUD. Serious complications can occur if a woman becomes pregnant while using an IUD. Though rare, cases of blood poisoning, miscarriage, and even death have been reported. An IUD user who believes she may be pregnant should consult her doctor immediately. If pregnancy is confirmed, the IUD should be removed. Although it rarely happens, the IUD	menstrual cramps; allergy to copper; anemia; fainting attacks; unexplained genital bleeding or vaginal discharge; suspicious or abnormal "Pap" smear.	

can pierce the wall of the uterus when it is being inserted. Surgery is required to remove it.

DIAPHRAGM (With Cream, Jelly, or Foam)
Prescription required

A diaphragm is a shallow cup of thin rubber stretched over a flexible ring. A sperm-killing cream, jelly, or foam is put on both sides of the diaphragm, which is then placed by the woman inside the vagina before intercourse. The device covers the opening of the uterus, thus preventing the sperm from entering the uterus.

Effectiveness	Advantages-Disadvantages	Side Effects	Health Factors to Consider	Long-term Effect on Ability to Have Children
Effectiveness depends on how correctly the method is used. Of 100 women who use the diaphragm with a spermicidal product for one year, 2 to 20 will become pregnant.	Advantages: No routine schedule to be kept as with the Pill (can use only when needed). The diaphragm with a spermicidal product is inserted by the user (or possibly the partner). Can be inserted up to two hours before intercourse. No discomfort or cramping as with the IUD. No effect	No serious side effects. Possible allergic reaction to the rubber or the spermicidal jelly. Condition easily corrected.	None	None

635

DIAPHRAGM (continued)

Effectiveness	Advantages-Disadvantages	Side Effects	Health Factors to Consider	Long-term Effect on Ability to Have Children
	on the chemical or physical processes of the body, as with the Pill or the IUD. Thus, there is no medical risk. No need to interrupt intercourse because the diaphragm is inserted before intercourse begins. Once in place, usually neither you nor your partner can feel the presence of the diaphragm. Disadvantages: Must be inserted before each intercourse and stay in place at least six hours afterward. May become dislodged when woman on top during intercourse. Must add more			

cream, foam, or jelly to diaphragm with additional acts of intercourse. This may be messy.

Size and fit require yearly checkup, and should be checked if woman gains or loses more than 10 pounds. Should be refitted after childbirth or abortion.

Requires instruction on insertion techniques. Some women find it difficult to insert and inconvenient to use.

Some women in whom the vagina is greatly relaxed, or in whom the uterus has "fallen," cannot use a diaphragm successfully.

Foam, Cream, or Jelly Alone
No Prescription Required

Several brands of vaginal foam, cream, or jelly can be used without a diaphragm. They form a chemical barrier at the opening of the uterus that prevents sperm from reaching an egg in the uterus; they also destroy sperm.

Effectiveness	Advantages-Disadvantages	Side Effects	Health Factors to Consider	Long-term Effect on Ability to Have Children
Effectiveness depends on how correctly the method is used. Of 100 women who use aerosol foams alone for one year, 2 to 29 will become pregnant. Of 100 women who use jellies and creams alone for one year, 4 to 36 will become pregnant.	Advantages: Easy to obtain and use. Can use only when needed. Disadvantages: Must be used one hour or less before intercourse. Enough must be used to insure contraception (must cover the cervix) If douching is desired, must wait 6 to 8 hours after intercourse.	No serious side effects. Burning or irritation of the vagina or penis may occur. Allergic reaction may be corrected by changing brands.	None.	None.

Vaginal Suppositories
No Prescription Required

Vaginal suppositories are small waxy "tablets" that are placed at the opening of the uterus just before intercourse. Note: Very few vaginal suppositories are intended for birth control. Ask before you buy.

Effectiveness	Advantages-Disadvantages	Side Effects	Health Factors to Consider	Long-term Effect on Ability to Have Children
No figures available, considered fair to poor.	Advantages: No devices needed. Can use only when needed. Easy to use and carry. Disadvantages: Must be inserted 15 minutes before intercourse. If placed earlier, they may become ineffective. If placed later (too close to intercourse) the suppository will not have time to melt and will be ineffective. Rare instances of sensitivity reactions.	No adverse side effects.	None.	None.

Condom (Rubber)
No Prescription Required

The condom is a thin sheath of rubber or processed lamb cecum that fits over the penis.

Effectiveness	Advantages-Disadvantages	Side Effects	Health Factors to Consider	Long-term Effect on Ability to Have Children
Effectiveness depends on how correctly the method is used. Of 100 women whose partner uses a condom for one year, 3 to 36 women will become pregnant.	Advantages: In addition to contraception, may afford some protection against venereal disease. Easily available. Requires no "long-term" planning before intercourse. Can use only when needed. Easily carried; inexpensive. Disadvantages: Some people feel the condom reduces pleasure in the sex act. The male must interrupt foreplay and fit the condom in place before sexual entry into	No serious side effects. Occasionally an individual will be allergic to the rubber, causing burning, irritation, itching, rash, or swelling, but this can easily be treated. Switching to the natural skin condom may be a solution.	None.	None.

the woman.

The condom can slip or tear during use or spill during removal from the vagina.

FEMALE STERILIZATION

The primary method of sterilization for women is tubal sterilization, commonly referred to as "tying the tubes." A surgeon cuts, ties, or seals the fallopian tubes to prevent passage of eggs between ovaries and the uterus. Several techniques are available which are listed below:

Operation	Description	Complication Rate	Failure Rate	Recovery Time	Cost	Unsuitability for Some Women
Mini-laparotomy	Surgeon closes off the tubes through a 1" incision above the pubic hairline.	2.9 per 100 operations	Generally accepted figure is 4 per 1,000 for all methods. (A sterilization is termed a "failure" when a patient becomes pregnant after the operation).	Several hours to 2 days	$350 and up in clinic; $750-$1000 in hospital	Not for women who are very obese, pregnant, or have an abnormal uterus.
Laparoscopy	Using special instrument inserted through an abdominal incision, a surgeon can look at tubes and seal them.	3.5 per 100 operations		2 days	Same as for mini-lup.	Not for women who have heart or lung problems or pelvic infection.
Laparotomy	Surgeon closes the tubes through a 2-3"	Cannot be determined since it is		One week or more.	$350 and up	Generally suitable for most women.

FEMALE STERILIZATION (continued)

Operation	Description	Complication Rate	Failure Rate	Recovery Time	Cost	Unsuitability for Some Women
	abdominal incision. Usually done in connection with childbirth or surgery.	done in association with other surgery.				
Culdoscopy	Using special instrument inserted through an incision in the back of the vagina, surgeon can look at the tubes and seal them.	3.9 per 100 operations		Several days	$1000	Same as for luparoscopy plus vaginal or cervical infections, last trimester of pregnancy or just after childbirth.
Colpotomy	Surgeon closes off tubes through an incision in back of the vagina.	4.3 per 100 operations		Several days	$1000	Same as for culdoscopy.

Hysterectomy, a surgical procedure involving removal of all or part of the uterus, also prevents pregnancy, but is performed for other medical reasons and is not considered primarily as a method of sterilization.

From: Midge Lasky Schildkraut. "Sterilization: Now It's Simpler, Safer. Reversible? Maybe? *The Better Way,* January 1978, p. 2.

FEMALE STERILIZATION (continued)

Effectiveness	Advantages-Disadvantages	Side Effects	Health Factors to Consider	Long-term Effect on Ability to Have Children
Virtually 100 percent.	Advantages: A one-time procedure — never any more bother with devices or preparations of any kind. Surgery and recovery time are minimal. Disadvantages: Surgery is required. Although in some cases a sterilization procedure has been reversed through surgery, the procedure should be considered permanent.	As with any surgery, occasionally there are complications such as severe bleeding, infection, or injury to other organs which may require additional surgery to correct.	There is some risk associated with any surgical procedure, which varies with the general health of the patient.	Procedure should be considered non-reversible. Once the surgery is performed successfully, the woman cannot become pregnant. There have been exceptions, but they are very uncommon.

MALE STERILIZATION

Sterilization of men involves severing the tubes through which the sperm travel to become part of the semen. The man continues to produce sperm, but they are absorbed by the body rather than being released into the

MALE STERILIZATION (continued)

semen. This operation, called a vasectomy, takes about half an hour, and may be performed in a doctor's office under local anesthetic. A vasectomy does not affect a man's physical ability to have intercourse.

Effectiveness	Advantages-Disadvantages	Side Effects	Health Factors to Consider	Long-term Effect on Ability to Have Children
Virtually 100 percent	Advantages: A one-time procedure that does not require hospitalization and permits the man to resume normal activity almost immediately. Simpler, quicker, and safer than female sterilization. Virtually free of adverse side effects. Disadvantages: Although in some cases a vasectomy may be reversed, it should be considered permanent. The man is not sterile immediately after the operation; usually it takes a	Complications occur in 2-4% of the cases, including infection, hematoma (trapped mass of clotted blood), granuloma (an inflammatory reaction to sperm that is absorbed by the body), and swelling and tenderness near the testes. Most such complications are minor and are treatable without surgery. Studies by the National Institute of Health show that vasectomy does not affect a man's sexual desire or ability.	None.	Procedure is considered non-reversible. Once surgery is performed successfully, the man cannot father children. There have been exceptions, but they are very uncommon.

644

few months. Other
means of
contraception must
be used during that
time.

RHYTHM METHOD

The woman must refrain from sexual intercourse on days surrounding the predicted time of monthly ovulation or, for a higher degree of effectiveness, until a few days after the predicted time of ovulation. Ways to determine the approximate time of ovulation include a calendar method, a method based on body temperature, and a mucous method.

Calendar Method: Using the calendar method requires careful recordkeeping of the time of the menstrual period, and calculation of the time in the month when the woman is fertile and must not have intercourse. Before you practice the rhythm method according to the calendar, you must learn the duration of your longest and shortest menstrual cycle. To do this, keep a record of how often you have a menstrual period. Keep this record for six months to one year. Next, write down the number of days in your longest and shortest cycle. Subtract 18 from the number of days in your shortest cycle, and subtract 11 from the number of days in your longest cycle. The two numbers you obtain are the days in your cycle when you might become pregnant, and you should not have intercourse on these days.

Temperature Method: To use the temperature method, the woman must use a special type of thermometer and keep an accurate daily record of her body temperature. You should take a rectal or vaginal temperature at the same time each morning before getting up or eating anything. After the menstrual period, the body temperature is generally between 97°F and 98.6°F. The day ovulation occurs, the body temperature drops to between 96.8° and 97.7°F. Then, it climbs to between 98.6° and 99.5°F and stays there until the menstrual period begins. It is difficult to detect the temperature drop because it lasts only a few hours. So, you look for the temperature rise because it is more noticeable, and it remains constant. One to two days after the temperature rise, the safe period begins.

Mucous Method: To use the mucous method, the woman must keep an accurate daily record of the type of vaginal secretions present. The cervical mucous changes from a thick, sticky, opaque fluid to a thin, watery, stretchy, clear fluid around the time of ovulation.

645

RHYTHM METHOD (continued)

The temperature method or the mucous method used alone or concurrently with the calendar method are more effective than the calendar method alone.

Effectiveness	Advantages-Disadvantages	Side Effects	Health Factors to Consider	Long-term Effect on Ability to Have Children
Effectiveness depends on how correctly the method is used.	Advantages: No drugs or devices needed.	No physical effects, but because the couple must refrain from having intercourse except on certain days of the month, using this method can create pressures on the couple's relationship.	None.	None.
Of 100 women who use the calendar method for one year, 14 to 35 will become pregnant.	Disadvantages: Requires careful recordkeeping and estimation of the time each month when there can be no intercourse.			
Of 100 women who use the temperature method for one year, 6 to 10 will become pregnant.	To use any of the three methods properly a physician's guidance may be needed, at least at the outset.			
Of 100 women who use the mucous method for one year, 10 to 25 will become pregnant.	If menstrual cycles are irregular, it is especially difficult to use this method effectively.			
Of 100 women who use for one year the temperature or mucous method with intercourse	Dissatisfaction because of extended			

only after ovulation, time each month less than 1 to 7 will when sexual become pregnant. intercourse must be avoided.

Instructions may be poor

WITHDRAWAL (Coitus Interruptus)

This method of contraception requires withdrawal of the male organ (penis) from the vagina before the man ejaculates so the male sperm are not deposited at or near the birth canal. The failure rate with this method is high and it should not be considered effective for preventing pregnancy.

DOUCHING

Use of a vaginal douche immediately after sexual intercourse to wash out or inactivate sperm is completely ineffective for preventing pregnancy.

ABORTION

Abortion refers to the interruption of pregnancy sometime within the first twenty weeks before the fetus can survive outside the womb.

There are several kinds of abortion:

Spontaneous. Also called miscarriage, spontaneous abortion is usually due to some condition in the mother that would have prevented normal fetal growth. About one in ten-fifteen pregnancies end in miscarriage, and about 75 percent of all miscarriages occur during the first three months of pregnancy. Common causes of miscarriage include disease in the mother, abnormalities in the placenta, or abnormalities in the developing fetus.

Psychogenic. Psychogenic abortions are miscarriages that are emotionally produced.

Self-Induced. Probably the most commonly attempted form, self-induced abortion refers to "home remedy" methods used by the mother to terminate the pregnancy. Unfortunately, most such crude methods are insufficient to end the pregnancy, and most result in serious damage to the mother instead.

TYPES OF THERAPEUTIC ABORTIONS

Type	Methodology	When Performed	Associated Hazards
Endometrial Aspiration	Suction removal of all of the uterine contents.	A few days after the last missed period (9-16 days after). Before 13th week of gestation.	Generally safe and effective if done under controlled conditions. Uterine perforation and hemorrhage are risks.
D & C (Dilation and Curettage)	Cervix is dilated and a small, spoon-shaped instrument is used to scrape uterine walls.	1st trimester.	Perforation and hemorrhage.
Saline Injection	Amniotic fluid is withdrawn through a long needle, replaced with concentrated saline solution. Fetus dies within hours followed in 12-48 hours by labor.	21-24 weeks is safest period.	Simplest and safest method of late abortion. Frequently disturbing to mother because it resembles normal childbirth. Clotting disorders, hemorrhage and adverse central nervous system effects. Risk three times greater than endometrial aspiration.
Hysterotomy; Hysterectomy	A miniature Cesarean Section — removal of uterine contents through abdominal wall; removal of uterus and contents.	1st and 2nd trimester.	High incidence of complications. Should be avoided if at all possible.

Index

A

abortion, 393-395
accidents, 4, 10, 527-531
Achilles tendon, 349
acne, 593-597
acrophobia, 100
addiction, *see* drugs
additives, *see* food additives
adipocytes, 288, 289
adjustment, 9, 25-26, 55-62
    resistance, 68
adolescence,
    sexuality, 117-118
adrenal glands, 68
age, 11, 226-238
aging process, 226-231
alcohol, 11-12, 85, 145-151
    and pregnancy, 403
    old age, 237
alcoholism, 150-151

allergies, 476-481
American Cancer Society, 449
amino acids, 247
amphetamines, 168-170
amyl nitrite, 170
aneurysm, 10
ankle, 348
anoretic,
    appetite suppressant, 168
anorexia nervosa, 303-304
antibody, 501
antigen, 501
antioxidants, 263
anxiety, 87
    amphetamine-induced, 169
arteriosclerosis, 5, 430
arthritis, 350, 471-473
    obesity, 292-293
assault,
    sexual, 128-132

649

asthma, 479-480
atheroma, 430
atherosclerosis, 294, 422, 430
attitudes, 8

B
bacteria, 498
Bartholins glands, 359
behavior,
    diet, 308-309
    gender-related, 115-116
    sexual, 119-128
biopsy, 450
biotin, 276
birth, 63
    defects, 397-400
    home, 389
    see also childbirth
birth control, *see* Appendix
birthing room, 388-389
bladder,
    and smoking, 155
    urinary, 359
blisters, 347
blood pressure, 10, 416-422
    and exercise, 329
    and obesity, 293-294
    and stress, 73
    taking, 574-575
body image, 28
bone, *see* fractures
botulism, 263
Bradley method, 387
breast,
    cancer, 451-453
    feeding, 390, 401
bubonic plague, 507
Burkitt, Dr. Denis P., 266
burns, 530, 624

C
caffeine, 256
    during pregnancy, 391, 404-405
calcium, 256, 277
calories,
    common snacks, 296-297
    exercise burn off, 305-307
    fast foods, 260, 261, 285-287
    representative foods, 310-311
    substitution foods, 315-318
cancer, 3, 10, 443-468
    and fiber, 266
    and heavy drinking, 146-147
    causes of, 445-449
    diagnosing, 449-451
    major types of, 451-459
    treatment of, 459-460
carbohydrates, 249, 259
cardiac arrest, 617
cardiovascular disease, 415-440
    and fiber, 266
    and obesity, 294
    and smoking, 155
catheterization,
    cardiac, 434
cerebrovascular disease,
    and smoking, 155
cervix, 360, 383, 397
cesarian section, 387
chemotherapy, 460
Chiari's syndrome, 10
child abuse, 193-202, 205
    and alcohol, 150
    causes of, 198-199
    emotional, 195-198, 200-201
    physical, 194-195
    sexual, 198
childbirth, 383-389
    kinds of, 385-389
    stages of, 383-384

childhood,
   depression, 82-83
   self-esteem, 31-33
   sexual identity, 113-118
chiropractic physician, 557-558
choking, 618-620
cholesterol, 12, 252, 424, 430
   and fiber, 266-267
cigarettes, 151-156, 292
   see also smoking
cirrhosis,
   of liver, 5
claustrophobia, 100
clitoris, 358-359
cocaine, 172-173
cognitive self, 28
cold, 576-578
compression,
   as tumor, 427
   cardiac, 434
constipation, 583-585
contagious disease, 495
contractions,
   uterine, 63, 383
coronary bypass, 435
cough, 578-579
Cowper's glands, 369
crises, 55-62, 193-241

D

death and dying, 210-220
   and obesity, 292
decision making, 40-44
dentist, 556-557
depressant,
   alcohol, 145
   barbiturate, 166-168

depression, 57, 79-87
   causes of, 81-82
   drug withdrawal, 170
   kinds of, 80-81
   postnatal, 82
diabetes, 5, 12, 424, 473-475
   and birth defects, 399
   and fiber, 266
   and obesity, 294
   and stress, 73
diarrhea, 582-583
Dick-Read method, 387
diet, 256, 301-302, 420
   drugs, 299-301
   fads, 295, 298
   guidelines, 264-265
disease,
   cancer, 443-468
   cardiovascular, 415-440
   chronic, 471-493
   defenses against, 501-503
   infectious, 495-524
   risk factors, 9-13
   stages of, 498-501
   stress, 73-75
distress, 66
divorce, 202-210
douching, 364-365
Downey cells, 581
DPT, 506
drugs, 85, 141-182, 449, 477-478,
   560-564
   abuse, 141-182
   addiction, 174-178
   alcohol, 145
   alternatives to, 181-182
   amphetamines, 168-170
   and pregnancy, 400-405
   barbiturates, 166-168

drugs (continued)
  cigarettes, 151-156
  cocaine, 172-174
  diet, 299-301
  heroin, 157-159
  high-risk populations, 142-143
  inhalants, 170-172
  marijuana, 159-164
  of public concern, 143-145
  over-the-counter, 560-561
  PCP, 164-165
  prescription, 561-562

E
ears, 588-590
  earache, 589-590
eating habits, 311-314
echocardiography, 434
education, 8
ejaculation, 369
  premature, 370-371
elderly,
  and drugs, 143
  health status, 234-236
  see also old age
electrocardiogram, 434
embolism, 10
emergency care, 607-628
emotions, 7, 73
  stress, 418, 420
empathy, 86
employment, 8
endocrine glands, 289-290
environment, 7, 8, 527-543
  and diseases, 496
  and pregnancy, 399-400
Environmental Protection
  Agency, 446
epididymis, 369, 458

epilepsy, 481-484
Epstein-Barr (EB) virus, 581
erythroblastosis fetalis, 392
esophageal sphincter (LES), 484
esophagus, 484
eustress, 66
euthanasia, 215-220
exam, see physical checkup
exercise, 7, 60, 85, 325-355,
  421-422, 475
  benefits of, 333-335
  calories used, 305-307
  injuries, 346-349
  old age, 237
  program, 336-346
  warning signs, 350-351
exhaustion, see fatigue
eyes, 585-588

F
fallopian tubes, 360, 373, 380
falls, 530
family planning, 393
fats, 249-252, 259
  brown fat theory, 290
fatigue, 351, 475
  exhaustion, 68
feelings, 36
  see also specific topic, i.e.,
    depression, love, etc.
female,
  hygiene, 363-365
  reproductive system, 358-363
  see also women
fertilization, 373-374
fetus, 114
  and problems with smoking, 155
  Fetal Alcohol Syndrome
    (FAS), 148

fever, 580
fiber, 261, 266-267
fibrillation, 422
first aid, 607-609
    see also emergency care
fitness, *see* exercise
fluoroscopy, 434
fluorine, 278
folic acid, 275
follicle, 594
food additives, 262-265
Food and Drug Administration,
    255, 262, 446
foods, 257-279, 448-449
    fast foods, 259-262
    organic and natural, 272-274
    see also calories
fractures, 624-626
frigidity, 371
fungi, 498

G
gall bladder, 295
gender (physical), 114
genetics, 290
genital herpes, 514-516
genitalia,
    female, 358-360
German measles, 431
goals, 35, 44-49
gonorrhea, 511-513
grief, 220-226
    awareness, 223-224
    denial, 220-223
    idealization, 225-226
    resolution, 224-225
    restitution, 224
guilt,
    depression, 81
    masturbation, 120
    Type A personality, 70-71

H
halothane, 170
happiness, 38-40, 72
hay fever, 478-479
headache, 600-601
health, 2, 7-9
    clubs, 351-352
    consumer, 547-567
heart,
    and exercise, 330, 341-343
    and smoking, 154-155
    and stress, 73
    attack, 422-426, 617-618
    congenital defects, 431-433
    congestive failure, 426-427
    disease, 3, 10, 415-430
heartburn, 484
Heimlich maneuver, 619
hemorrhage,
    artery, 427
    first aid, 620-622
    pregnancy, 381
hemorrhoids,
    and fiber, 266
hepatitis, 502, 507
heredity, 9, 290, 397-400
    cancer, 447
    hypertension, 418
hermaphrodite, 116
hernia, 295
heroin, 157-159
Hodgkin's disease, 453
home,
    influences on gender identity,
        114-116
homosexuality, 122-126
    female, 124-125
    male, 122-124
hormones, 446

hostility,
    Type A personality, 70-71
humus, 273
hymen, 359
hyperplasia, 287
hypertension, 416
    and obesity, 293
    see also blood pressure
hypertrophy, 287
hypochondria, 75, 81
hysterectomy, 366-367

I
identity, 113-118
illness, 56
    mental, 96-104
    psychosomatic, 75
    signs of, 570
    stress-related, 64
immunity, 502
impotence, 370
inactivity, 288-289, 335-336
incubation, 499
individualism, 26-28
infancy,
    diseases of, 5-6
    see also childhood
infertility, 395-397
    female factors, 396-397
    male factors, 396
influenza, 5, 507-509, 580-581
insulin, 473-475
insurance,
    medical, 554-556
intelligence, 8
    I.Q., 30-31
iodine, 277
iron, 256, 277
isometrics, 329-330
isotonics, 330

J
joint, 472-473

K
kidneys, 10, 68, 254, 420
knee, 348
Kurzman-Seppala, Teresa, 180

L
labia, 358
labor, *see* childbirth
lactic acid, 359
laetrile, 460-461
Lamaze method, 386
laughter, 66
LeBoyer method, 385-386
leukemia, 453-454
life-style, 7
    personality, 78
linoleic acid, 249
lipoproteins, 252
liver, 5, 10
loneliness, 60-61
loss, 82
love, 132-136
lung cancer, 454
    smoking, 153

M
male,
    prostate cancer, 456-457
    reproductive system, 367-369
    testicular cancer, 458
manic depression, 99
March of Dimes, 397
marijuana, 159-164
marriage,
    mature love, 134-136
mastectomy, 453
masturbation, 120-121, 371

meals, 257-262
measles, 504
medication,
    self-, 60, 560-561
    see also drugs
menopause, 365-366
menstruation, 360-363
    and acne, 595
    cramps, 599-600
mental illness, 96-104
    prevention of, 100-104
midwife, 388
minerals, 252, 259-260, 275-278
miscarriage, 377, 378
mononucleosis, 502, 581-582
moral judgments,
    criteria for, 118
mumps, 505-506
muscles, 329-333
    endurance, 331-332
    flexibility, 332-333
    strength, 329-330
myocardial infarction, 422

N

narcolepsy, 168
National Dairy Council, 255-256
neuroses, 99-100
niacin, 255, 256, 276
nicotine, 151
    see also cigarettes
    see also smoking
nitrate, 274
nitrite, 263, 274
nitrous oxide, 170
nongonococcal urethritis, 516
nutrition, 8, 245-282
    see also foods

O

obesity, 10, 285-323, 420
    brown fat theory, 290
old age, 226-238
    emotional changes, 228
    health status, 234-236
    mental changes, 229-231
    myths, 231-233
    problems, 233-234
    process, 226-231
    physical change, 226-228
    reducing effects of, 236-238
    social changes, 228-229
oral cancer, 454-455
oral contraceptive, 256
organic psychoses, 99
orgasmic difficulty, 371
os, 360
ovaries, 360, 397
oviducts, 360
ovum, 360, 372-374, 397

P

pacemaker, 434
pancreas,
    and smoking, 155
pantothenic acid, 276
pap smear, 451
papule, 594
paranoia, 98
    inhalant-induced, 171
Parkinson's disease, 10
pathogen, 496, 498, 501
PCP (phencyclidine), 164-166
Peale, Dr. Norman Vincent, 84
penis, 367-368
pepsin, 485
personality, 69-79
    determining, 106-107
    heart attack, 426

personality (continued)
  Type A, 69-71, 76
  Type B, 71-73, 78
phosphorus, 277
physical checkup, 62, 549-552
  old age, 237
physical fitness, *see* exercise
physician, 547-549
placenta, 383
pneumonia, 5, 10
poisoning, 530-531
  first aid, 622-624
polio, 504
pollution, 531-538
  air, 531-534
  noise, 535-536
  pesticides, 537
  radiation, 537-538
  solid, 535
  water, 531-534
pornography, 126-128
  negative aspects of, 127
potassium, 277
pregnancy, 256, 372-383
  complications, 380-381
  due date, 381
  ectopic, 380
  symptoms of, 376-377
prevention,
  of cancer, 461-462
  of disease, 2, 14-16
  of drug abuse, 180-182
prodromal period, 499-500
prostate,
  cancer, 456-457
  gland, 369
protein, 247-249, 259-260
protozoa, 498

psychiatric,
  nurse, 103
  social worker, 103
psychiatrist, 103
psychoanalyst, 103
psychologist, 103
psychology, 8
psychoses, 97-99
  inhalant-induced, 171
  organic, 99
pulse rate, 326-328, 573-574
pustule, 594

Q
quackery,
  cancer, 460-461
  medical, 559-560
  psycho-, 101

R
rabies, 509
race (ethnicity), 11
  blood pressure, 418
  drugs, 142-143
radiation, 448
rape, 128-132
  alcohol and, 149
  prevention of, 129-132
reaction,
  anxiety, 99
  conversion, 99
  depressive, 99
  dissociative, 99-100
  obsessive compulsive, 100
  phobic, 100
Recommended Dietary Allowances (RDA), 246-247, 267
recovery, 500-501
rectum, 359
  cancer, 453

relationships,
    companionate, 134-136
    marriage, 134-136
relaxation, 76
reproduction, 357-410
respiration,
    measuring, 574
    obesity, 292
resuscitation,
    cardiopulmonary, 617
    mouth-to-mouth, 616
    mouth-to-nose, 616-617
    pulmonary, 613
retirement, 233-234
Rh incompatibility, 391-392
rheumatic fever, 431
Rhogam, 392
riboflavin, 255, 256
rickettsia, 498

S
salt, 262, 263, 278
Schifferes, Justus J., 98
schizophrenia, 97-98
scrotum, 368, 458
seizure,
    focal, 484
    grand mal, 482
    petit mal, 482
    psychomotor, 484
self-actualizing, 36-38
self-care, 569-605
self concept, 28-33
self-esteem, 26, 28-36
    low, 33-34
self-evaluation, 17-20, 51-53, 106-
    111, 138-139, 184-190, 240-241,
    280-282, 320-323, 354-355,
    407-410, 438-440, 465-468,
    488-492, 522-524, 539-543,
    565-567, 602-605, 627-628

Selye, Dr. Hans, 68
seminal vesicles, 369
seminiferous tabules, 369
sex,
    diseases, 510-516
    disorders, 369-371
    during pregnancy, 390-391
    see also reproduction
sexuality, 113-119
    cross-identification, 116
    normal and abnormal, 121-122
shin splints, 349
shock,
    anaphylactic, 480-481
    crisis, 56
    first aid for, 612-613
    signs of, 609-611
sinus,
    headache, 601
skin cancer, 457-458
sleep, 597-599
smallpox, 506
smoking, 10-11, 151-156
    and pregnancy, 401-403
    blood pressure, 420
    old age, 237, 256
social self, 28
sodium, see salt
sonogram, 383
sore throat, 579-580
spasm, 351, 427-428
sperm, 367-369, 372-374, 396
sphygmomanometer, 574-575
stillbirth, 399
strep throat, 431
stress, 11, 62-79
    alarm, 68, 418, 420
    and disease, 73-75, 496
    drugs, 178-180

657

stroke, 3, 10, 427-430
sugar, 261, 263, 267-271
suicide, 6, 10, 88-96
   prevention of, 94-96
   victim characteristics, 91-92
   warning signs, 92-94
Surgeon General, 14
surgery, 459, 553-554
syphilis, 513-514

T
teeth, 590-593
temperature, 571-573
   oral, 571
   rectal, 572-573
tension,
   headache, 601
testicles, 368-369
testosterone,
   alcohol effects on, 148
thiamin, 255, 256
throat,
   sore, 579-580
   strep, 431
thrombosis, 427
thyroid gland, 290, 399, 420
thyroxine, 290
tomboy, 114
toxemia, 380-381, 420
tuberculosis, 10
tumor, 443, 446, 460
typhoid fever, 506-507

U
ulcer,
   gastric, 485
   peptic, 485-487
   smoking, 155
ultrasound, 382-383
urethra, 359

uterine cancer, 459
uterus, 359-360, 373

V
vaccination, 503
vagina, 359
vaginismus, 371
value systems, 39-40, 59
vas deferens, 369
vectorcardiography, 434
vegetarianism, 271-272
virus, 497-498
vital signs, 570-575
vitamins, 252-254, 275-278
   A, 249, 256, 275
   additives, 263
   B, 256, 275
   C, 66, 253-254, 256, 258, 276
   D, 249, 251, 256, 275, 366
   E, 249, 256, 275
   fast foods, 261
   K, 249, 256, 276
voyeurism, 271-272

W
water, 254
weight, 285-323
   diet, 251
   old age, 237
women,
   and drug abuse, 142
   cancer, 454, 459
   diabetes, 475
   see also female

X
xenophobia, 100
x-ray, 550-552, 625

Y
yellow fever, 507
youth,
   and drugs, 142

Notes

Notes

Notes

Notes

Notes

Notes